The Second Sickness

The Second Sickness

Contradictions of Capitalist Health Care

Revised and Updated Edition

HOWARD WAITZKIN

ROWMAN & LITTLEFIELD PUBLISHERS, INC.
Lanham • Boulder • New York • Oxford

ROWMAN & LITTLEFIELD PUBLISHERS, INC.

Published in the United States of America
by Rowman & Littlefield Publishers, Inc.
4720 Boston Way, Lanham, Maryland 20706
http://www.rowmanlittlefield.com

12 Hid's Copse Road
Cumnor Hill, Oxford OX2 9JJ, England

British Library Cataloging in Publications Information Available

Library of Congress Cataloging-in-Publication Data

Waitzkin, Howard.
    The second sickness : contradictions of capitalist health care / Howard Waitzkin. —
revised and updated ed.
        p. cm.
    Includes bibliographical references and index.
    ISBN 0-8476-9886-6 (cloth: alk. paper) — ISBN 0-8476-9887-4 (pbk.: alk. paper)
    1. Social medicine. 2. Medical care—United States. I. Title.

RA418 .W349 2000
362.1′042—dc21

                                                                    99-046590

Printed in the United States of America

♾ ™The paper used in this publication meets the minimum requirements of American
National Standard for Information Sciences—Permanence of Paper for Printed Library
Materials, ANSI/NISO Z39.48-1992.

To Abe Waitzkin—
housepainter, trade unionist,
poker player, cancer victim, socialist

And as a doctor I suffered from two very difficult diseases. I was only beginning to make my way as a surgeon when I came down with a bad case of tuberculosis. . . . My second "sickness" . . . well, that wasn't so simple. I caught it from no one— and I caught it from everything. I got it as a boy, as a man, as a doctor. It was much worse than tuberculosis. It wasn't like curing an infection. I couldn't get rid of it by drugs. And many of the things I saw as a doctor only made it worse. . . . But there came a time when I no longer gave in to it. That was after I came to understand that tuberculosis was not merely a disease of the body but a social crime. . . . I have learned what must be done to cure this second sickness.

—Norman Bethune, M.D., surgeon to the liberation forces of China, 1939

Contents

List of Figures and Tables   ix
Preface to the Second Edition   xi
Preface to the First Edition and Acknowledgments   xv

PART ONE: Medicine, Social Structure, and Social Pathology

Chapter 1. Health Care, Social Contradictions, and the Dilemmas
       of Reform   3

Chapter 2. Social Structures of Medical Oppression   37

Chapter 3. The Social Origins of Illness: A Neglected History   55

PART TWO: Problems in Contemporary Health Care

Chapter 4. Technology, Health Costs, and the Structure of Private Profit   77

Chapter 5. Social Medicine and the Community   97

Chapter 6. The Micropolitics of the Doctor-Patient Relationship   119

PART THREE: Policy, Practice, and Social Change

Chapter 7. Medicine and Social Change: Lessons from Chile and Cuba   165

Chapter 8. Conclusion: Health Praxis, Reform, and Political Struggle   189

Notes   209
Selected Bibliography   227
Index   233
About the Author   238

Figures and Tables

FIGURES

1.1   Mortality Trends during the Last Century, England and Wales,
       with More Recent Expenditure Trends   25
1.2   National Health Expenditures, United States, 1960–1995   30
1.3   Income of Selected Health-Care Personnel in the United States,
       1950–1995   32
4.1   Overview of the Development, Promotion, and Proliferation of
       Coronary Care Units and Similar Medical Advances   94
7.1   Structure of Popular Participation in Health Care under the Unidad
       Popular Government in Chile   177
7.2   Structure of Popular Participation in Health Care in Cuba   183

TABLES

1.1   Physicians per Population, by State, 1995   17
1.2   Physicians per Population, New Mexico, by County, 1990   18
1.3   Median Annual Net Income by Profession, 1994   31
4.1   Growth of Coronary Care in the United States, by Region,
       1967–1974   81
4.2   Studies Comparing Coronary Care Unit and Ward Treatment
       for Myocardial Infarction   82
4.3   Studies Comparing Hospital and Home Care for Myocardial
       Infarction   82
5.1   Medical Expansion in the 20 Largest Cities in the United States,
       Late 1970s   100
5.2   Participating Clinics in the Alameda Health Consortium,
       Alameda County, California, 1997   112
5.3   Funding Sources, La Clínica de la Raza, Oakland,
       California, 1998–1999   114

Preface to the Second Edition

Since the first edition of *The Second Sickness* appeared in 1983, momentous events, so to speak, shook the world (1).

In the late 1980s, after Mikhail Gorbachev introduced *Perestroika* as a strategy of reform in the Soviet Union, that country's socialist system crumbled, as did those of other Eastern European countries. Gorbachev saw market-oriented reform as a return to the vital economic policies of Lenin, and as a route toward a strengthened socialism rather than toward capitalism (2). Nevertheless, a combination of economic and political crises ensued, partly choreographed by the United States through its influence on the policies of international lending agencies and through the effects of the Central Intelligence Agency in Soviet political processes (3). The "triumph of capitalism" in the former Soviet Union and in Eastern Europe coincided with the emergence of extreme poverty alongside enormous wealth, the dismantling of public health and welfare systems, and an overall deterioration of health outcomes. This deterioration included a decline in male life expectancy in Russia from 63.8 years in 1990 to 59.0 years in 1993—apparently the most rapid and serious decline in health indicators under peacetime conditions in the history of civilization (4). As the Cold War and nuclear competition between the United States and Soviet Union declined, nuclear weapons proliferated among other Third World countries. Global economic crises have rendered such countries more unstable politically.

Along with the failure of some existing socialist systems, the global capitalist economy has expanded at an unprecedented rate. In the United States, the Clinton Administration advanced beyond the Reagan and Bush Administrations to enhance the ability of finance capital to move swiftly throughout the world, with few constraints of national borders or government regulation. Both within the United States and other capitalist countries, the gap between rich and poor increased; the luxuries of great wealth became more resplendent, even as the suffering of the poor has become more entrenched. Influenced by the policies of the Clinton Administration, international lending agencies led by the World Bank and International Monetary Fund have insisted on the dismantling or privatization of public health and welfare systems. These "structural adjustment" policies, imposed as requirements for new loans, have reduced the capacity of Third World countries to provide a safety net for their citizens, while opening up their economies to free-market principles that have benefited international investors. The same policies have been associated with extreme financial crises that have emerged throughout the Third World, including many Asian countries, the former Soviet Union, and Latin America.

Within the United States, corporate dominance of the economy has coincided with an unprecedented penetration of corporations within the health-care system. Especially under the rubric of managed care, for-profit corporations have taken over an ever increasing proportion of hospitals, clinics, home care agencies, and physicians' practices. Since 1989, all newly initiated managed care organizations have operated as for-profit corporations, often under the control of private insurance companies. A majority of the U.S. population is covered by managed care organizations. With the burgeoning power of managed care organizations, physicians' work satisfaction has declined along with their professional dominance. Although physicians' income generally has remained high, their control over the conditions of professional work has deteriorated, as corporate administrators have initiated micromanagement of clinical decisions including both diagnostic studies and treatments. With reference to the fate of professionalism in medicine, Marx and Engels' observations of more than 150 years ago remain prescient: "The bourgeoisie has stripped of its halo every occupation hitherto honored and looked up to with reverent awe. It has converted the physician, the lawyer, the priest, the poet, the man of science, into its paid wage-laborers" (5).

Meanwhile, barriers to health-care access become more pervasive in the United States, even as expenditures continue to climb. As of 1999, more than 43 million people in the United States did not hold any form of public or private health insurance, while health-care expenditures totaled more than one trillion dollars annually, equivalent to about 14 percent of the gross domestic product. Many people with insurance coverage still experienced major barriers to access, due to copayments or other deductible provisions. Most strikingly, every proposal for a national health program in the United States, intended to address the problems of inadequate access and high costs, failed. As the United States enters the new millennium, it remains the only economically developed country without a national health program that ensures universal access to care.

Given such changes outside and inside the health-care system, a book like this one predictably would require extensive revision, but drastic modifications—surprisingly enough—have not proven necessary. Although I have updated material throughout the book, including references, the overall analytic approach remains the same. Despite the crisis associated with the fall of state socialism in the Soviet Union and Eastern Europe, a Marxist-oriented analysis of the contradictions in society that form the basis of problems in the health-care system remains a trenchant way to understand these problems. The structures of oppression and the social origins of illness, as discussed in part one, have emerged as even greater problems as corporate penetration of health care has increased. Similarly, the issues of technology and profit, community medicine, and the micropolitics of the doctor-patient relationship, analyzed in part two, have remained crucial for an adequate understanding of contemporary health care. Most important, although changing political conditions have required some modifications in part three, the overall directions of desirable praxis and nonreformist reform in health care remain close to those spelled out originally.

In view of the purported triumph of capitalism and failure of state socialism in the Soviet Union and Asia, how can one justify the stability of the analysis presented here? At many points, the original edition alluded to the ideological processes by which very injurious structures under capitalism are legitimated and accepted as the only reasonable alternative. That capitalism could be thought to have triumphed in the face of such widespread misery becomes another manifestation of ideology's remarkable impact. In addition, the original edition also referred frequently to the failures of state socialism in the Soviet Union and Eastern Europe, including such difficulties as the reemergence of class structure and the destruction of the environment in the name of societal productivity rather than private profit. The remarkable changes that have occurred since the book's first edition have confirmed many of the critical perspectives on health care under capitalism and state socialism that a Marxist-oriented analysis originally suggested.

As the downsides of capitalism's purported triumph have become more obvious, so has the need for further critique and praxis aimed at progressive change in medicine and in medicine's societal context. This work will continue to address the profound social contradictions that affect health and health care. Events of the past twenty years have done nothing to diminish the importance of criticism and struggle to change the societal origins of illness and suffering. The "second sickness" remains very much with us.

Preface to the First Edition and Acknowledgments

This book began with some simple ideas that provide the history of social medicine—that much illness and suffering have origins in society, that the organization of medical practice ultimately is inseparable from broader social organization, and that meaningful solutions of health problems often demand fundamental social change. My motivation for studying what Bethune called "the second sickness" also grew from my personal experience. I want to clarify the circumstances that helped shape the book's content.

First of all, the book emerged from troubling events in my family and from various inadequacies I perceived in my schooling. My grandfather was a housepainter and union organizer in Ohio. He died from a form of liver cancer undoubtedly caused by toxic solvents used in paint thinning; his union unsuccessfully had requested government monitoring of these chemicals. The doctors who cared for him before his death maintained a circle of lies and distortions that left him confused and dispirited. My parents are clerical workers who still suffer the emotional effects of my father's being laid off, at age 55, from a job he had held for twenty-five years. They believe that this outcome was their responsibility, since my father had not been able to attend college during the Depression and since it was a college graduate who replaced him. As a student of sociology in college and graduate school, I found little to explain such social origins of illness and suffering. Later, in medical school, my clinical instructors taught me that shaping the truth was often a necessary and desirable skill, since patients' morale determined whether they would maintain a productive life at work, in the family, and so forth. As an intern and resident in medicine, I saw the enormous profits that drug companies and medical equipment manufacturers were making for innovations that had dubious effectiveness in patient care. While working for the health programs of the Black Panther Party in Boston, the United Farm Workers Union in rural California, and La Clínica de la Raza in Oakland, California, I also witnessed the cruel irrationalities of a system that does not provide even the most rudimentary services for the poor and minority groups.

It was my political rather than my academic experience that helped explain these observations. The civil rights movement, which in Ohio focused on segregated housing, exposed racial injustices and the hypocrisy of equality. The Indochina War and the military coup in Chile revealed the inhuman excesses fostered by capitalism and imperialism. Conflict between my neighborhood and my medical school, while I was living in Boston, showed the pernicious effects of purportedly benign institutions. Political action in each of these areas motivated me to study other histories, other theories, and other strategies than those I had learned in school. To the chagrin of some of my mentors, these experiences also convinced me that I no longer could separate my intellectual work from political activism.

Intertwined with personal experience, this book contains large elements of advocacy, whose political orientation is obvious. There is purportedly a fine line between committed scholarship and polemic. Personally, I have not found this distinction helpful. Although one may try to hide one's value commitments behind various literary devices, the effort to put values aside is, in my view, dishonest, misleading, and ultimately unsuccessful for both writer and reader. The problems this book describes are complex, and the solutions not at all straightforward. Partly for this reason, I have tried to avoid sermonizing and dogmatism, while making my own commitments clear. Arguments and evidence, in any case, are here for appraisal. My guess is that the book's style and tone will be most troublesome for those least distressed by our current predicament.

Some notes on the book's organization may be useful. Part one, which offers a general framework, grew from an attempt to find explanations for illness and suffering in social structure, as well as social solutions to health problems. In chapter 1, I analyze the social contradictions from which many problems in medicine arise, the exploitation of illness for profit, and the deficiencies of health-care systems that do not adequately serve the urban and rural poor, racial minorities, and other disadvantaged groups. Chapter 2 concerns social structures of oppression in medicine that both mirror and reproduce oppressive features of the wider society. This chapter also gives an overview of Marxist studies in social medicine that examine structures of oppression which the social organization of health care fosters. In chapter 3, I consider the social origins of illness—the conditions of society that generate disease and early death—in the context of previous work in social medicine that has been largely overlooked.

Part two presents several concrete studies linking medicine and society. The coverage of these studies is intentionally broad. One purpose of these chapters, which developed partly from specific problems and experiences in my own sociomedical practice, is to convey the wide scope that is necessary for social medicine. In chapter 4, pursuing a concern from clinical observations, I focus on the technologic imperative that increases both costs and profits, while having little impact on death or disease. Chapter 5 analyzes medicine at the level of the community, especially the plight of public hospitals, community-worker control of primary health services, and the often detrimental impact of private medical expansion in urban areas; my interest in these issues came from community organizing and practice in New England and California. In chapter 6, I consider the micropolitics of the doctor-patient relationship, including distortions of communication like those I witnessed in my family and as a medical student. The studies in part two deal with different levels of analysis: the impact of technology, the local community, and the interpersonal relationship between doctor and patient. Although the issues are diverse, underlying contradictions of society are major determinants of problems at each level. Taken together, these studies try to present a practically grounded approach to the range of problems with which social medicine currently must contend.

What to do about these problems is, of course, a key question. Part three considers policy issues and directions of needed change. The main thrust of this discussion is that basic improvements in the health-care system depend on fundamental change in society as a whole. Chapter 7 explores this troubling proposition by analyzing social change and health policy in comparative international perspective; I emphasize Cuba and Chile, two countries whose very different social realities determined the outcomes of ambitious new health-care programs. Extending this analysis to health-care reform in the United States, chapter 8 criticizes justifications for cutbacks in services, reviews the strengths and weaknesses of current reform proposals, and suggests possibilities for sociomedical activism. This chapter reaches pessimistic conclusions concerning health policy that is unattached to broader social change. On the other hand, activism that explicitly links health care and political struggle permits an optimism that confronts present realities with more than wishful thinking.

I want to thank Roberto Belmar, Stephany Borges, Rick Brown, Claire Douglas, Dan Doyle, Ray Elling, June Fisher, David Himmelstein, Hal Holman, Charles Houston, Annie Johnston, Alice Jones, Elliot Mishler, Hilary Modell, Vicente Navarro, Byron Randall, Lillian Rubin, Frank Sampson, Steven Schear, Herb Schreier, Jim Scott, Victor Sidel, Larry Sirott, John Stoeckle, Paul Sweezy, Assefa Taye, Barbara Waterman, and Stephanie Woolhandler. At crucial times and in unique ways, they gave me the encouragement, criticism, love, and feeling of *compañerismo* I needed. Several organizations—Roxbury Tenants of Harvard, *Movimiento de Izquierda Revolucionaria* (MIR) and allied groups throughout Latin America, the student-faculty-worker movement of the University of Oaxaca Medical School in Mexico, the United Farm Workers Union, La Clínica de la Raza, Science for the People, and the *Medicina en la Comunidad* programs of the Cuban Ministry of Health—provided inspiration and practical models of progressive political work in health care. David Himmelstein, Richard Lichtman, Joyce Seltzer, Gladys Topkis, Marlie Wasserman, and Barbara Waterman gave me valuable editorial advice. My grandfather, Abe Waitzkin, taught me that the struggle toward a better life involves the humor, timing, and strategic sense of playing a poker hand well.

Part One

Medicine, Social Structure, and Social Pathology

1

Health Care, Social Contradictions, and the Dilemmas of Reform

As a 30-year-old worker in the pesticide division of a chemical company in Lathrop, California, T. B. and his co-workers in this division began to wonder why they and their wives were not having children. After several years, they contacted a local medical clinic, where sperm examinations revealed sterility or decreased fertility. Later studies showed similar findings among pesticide workers in other states. Eventually the problem was traced to DBCP, a soil fumigant used to kill worms that feed on crop roots. Laboratory experiments showed that DBCP caused testicular damage in rats; reports of testicular cancer in DBCP workers began to appear. The California Department of Health found hazardous DBCP levels in more than forty municipal water wells; the chemical had leached down to groundwater after surface applications. Health officials estimated that about 200,000 people had been drinking water contaminated by DBCP. Although the Department of Health issued a ban on DBCP, chemical and agricultural corporations resisted the ban by legal actions and tried to use similar compounds instead.

R. L. was a 32-year-old Spanish-speaking mother of five, who moved from rural Mexico to Oakland, California, where she began to work as a part-time housekeeper. She knew no English, held no legal documents regarding residency in the United States, and had no insurance. She became pregnant again in 1979. During the last month of her pregnancy, she came to the emergency rooms of two private hospitals because she felt that labor might have begun. Emergency room staff refused to see her because she did not have insurance and, as an undocumented alien, was not eligible for public support through MediCal. She then went three times within one week to the emergency room of the county hospital; the interns who examined her found high blood pressure but did not test for fetal distress and did not refer her to a prenatal program. Twelve hours after her last visit, she delivered a stillborn infant at home. Three months later, the county hospital threatened to send her bill to a collection agency for nonpayment.

G. M. was a 74-year-old Italian American man who was admitted to a medical center in Boston because of rectal bleeding. As part of his evaluation on admission, an electrocardiogram showed that he was having a heart attack, although he had no chest pain or other symptoms. He was taken to the intensive care unit; studies of cardiac enzymes confirmed that a heart attack in fact had occurred. The doctor who had followed him at a neighborhood health center reported that several months earlier the patient had presented to him with chest pain and a pattern of electrocardiogram changes consistent with a heart attack. On this previous occasion, the doctor had chosen not to admit the patient to a hospital but instead had followed him at home, where he recuperated uneventfully. During the current admission, he had no further symptoms or cardiac instability. He was transferred from the intensive care unit to the ward after four days and discharged after eight days. A plan was made to evaluate the source of his rectal bleeding about six weeks after discharge.

The health systems of the United States and other advanced capitalist countries reveal many troubling deficiencies; these case summaries illustrate only a few. Occupational and environmental hazards threaten survival in ways that are difficult to predict. Needed services remain inaccessible to the poor and to minority groups. Technologically oriented medicine increases the cost of care. Solutions remain elusive, despite attempted improvements.

Why do such problems persist in wealthy and powerful nations? These difficulties have received wide attention in research and policy. Generally, each separate problem is the object of analysis, debate, and limited reform. Superficially, the issues appear diverse, and proposals to deal with them reflect this diversity. The more general social conditions that are responsible for a variety of health problems and that impede solutions escape serious study. The cases of a man suffering infertility from pesticide exposure, a woman whose infant dies needlessly, and a man who endures expensive, technologic medicine seem isolated from one another. But the social conditions that their case histories reflect are not isolated problems; it is important to seek the underlying realities that provide a more unified explanation and a more coherent strategy for change.

Major problems in medicine are also problems of society; the health system is so intimately tied to the broader society that attempts to study one without the other are misleading. Difficulties in health and medical care emerge from social contradictions and rarely can be separated from those contradictions. These interconnections are not only important for clearer understanding; they also suggest directions of change. From this view, health reforms that do not address the relationships between the health system and broader social structure are doomed to failure.

One strength of the Marxist explanation is an analysis of the linkages between the health system and the broader political, economic, and social systems of the society. Without attention to these connections, the health system falsely takes on the appearance of an autonomous, free-floating entity, whose defects purportedly can be corrected by limited reforms in the medical sphere. To explain problems like those the case histories raise, a consistent theoretical orientation is helpful. The theoretical basis of the analysis that follows derives from dialectic and historical materialism. This approach, which is the principal analytic tool of Marxism, is complex. Others have discussed the nuances, strengths, and limitations of materialist theory (1); a thorough exposition is not my purpose here. However, several key features are worth noting.

First, social reality contains structural contradictions. Contradictions are antagonistic or opposing characteristics that arise among social groups, within organizations and institutions, across nations, and in the realm of ideas. Contradictory tendencies in a social system are more than simply problems or difficulties; they are destructive tendencies that emerge from and are intertwined with a system's creative capacities. If a specific feature in necessary for a system's accomplishments, a contradictory feature is one that undermines those accomplishments. Both sides of the contradiction are integrally related to each other. A central purpose of the dialectic approach is to clarify the "unity of opposites" — the social contradictions that are at once creative and destructive.

Certain social contradictions, which have received extensive analysis in Marxist theory and are major focuses of this book, illustrate this theoretical approach. A primary structural contradiction in capitalist societies is that of social class. Ownership and control of the means of economic production create a fundamental contradiction between the capitalist class and the working class; accumulation of wealth by the capitalist class depends on the productive activity of workers. In historical periods of higher wages, fringe benefits, and easier working conditions, the contradiction of class may become less obvious. Yet the potentially antagonistic relationship between classes is inherent in a system that aims toward the amassing of wealth by some, largely through the work of others.

Additional contradictions lie behind paradoxical features of both capitalist and socialist societies. Under capitalism, the private accumulation of capital tends to occur more in some specific geographic areas than in others; wealthy regions contrast with areas of stark poverty. Natural resources tend to flow from the countryside to cities and from poor nations to wealthy ones. Social policies to redistribute wealth on a geographic basis are weak or lacking. This contradiction, between development and underdevelopment, manifests itself in regional inequalities within nations and international disparities among nations. Moreover, in capitalist societies, the state assumes contradictory roles. Inconsistent public policies provide limited social welfare to citizens but also protect the ability of private enterprise to accumulate great wealth. In the realm of ideas, contradictory ideologies justify and legitimate contradictions of social structure. For instance, the notion of equality masks the continuing inequities of class structure. Structural contradictions do not disappear in socialist societies. An example is the tendency toward reemergence of class structure based on expertise and bureaucratic authority rather than on ownership of economic production.

The complexities of such contradictions deserve exploration later. For now, it is enough to point out the analytic approach that links puzzling and seemingly diverse health-care problems to underlying structural contradictions. A man's childlessness from pesticide exposure, for example, emerges in large part from a contradiction between profit and safety. The drive to maximize profits in industry and agriculture interferes with the costly testing and precautions that would be necessary to protect workers' health fully. Illegal immigration is one outcome of the contradiction of development and underdevelopment, where regions of wealth exist in close geographic proximity to regions of poverty. Preventable infant mortality also results partly from contradictory social policies that foster a strong private sector in health care, while public services that are profoundly needed remain unavailable. The inappropriate use of expensive technology reflects contradictions in medical science. On the one hand, medical science encourages technically complex treatments but, on the other hand, tends not to demand a rigorous scientific appraisal of the treatments' effectiveness in reducing morbidity and mortality. The promotion of high technology also reinforces economic contradictions. Sustained corporate profit generally requires expansion, diversification into different product lines, and creation of new markets. Medical technology provides a lucrative direction for numerous industries, as rates of profit in other areas become sluggish. Meanwhile, as expensive technology proliferates, cheap and mundane medical practices receive little attention, even though they may be more appropriate. Such linkages between medical problems and social contradictions will receive more attention in this and subsequent chapters. The purpose here is to illustrate the theoretical analysis that traces many issues of health care to contradictions in society.

A second and related theme in materialist theory is that social problems occur in the context of whole societies, rather than simply in parts of societies. The Marxist perspective assumes that, although limitations of focus are necessary, the interconnections among social structures are of utmost importance. Particular difficulties, like those in the case histories, may arise in such areas as occupational and environmental health, maternal and infant care, and high technology. However, it is a mistake to analyze such problems in isolation from the social structures of the entire society. Too narrow an analysis not only overlooks the dynamics that create and reinforce specific problems but also obscures directions of meaningful reform.

A third thrust of dialectic and historical materialism is its emphasis on conflict. Structural contradictions imply conflict between social groups; conflict also can occur at different levels. Class conflict, for instance, can arise in workplaces and other organizations, within regions, throughout one nation, and across nations. The contradiction of international development and underdevelopment is a seed of struggles against imperialism and for national liberation. In socialist societies, contradictions deriving from professional expertise and bureaucratization also lead to conflict, but of a much different type from that under capitalism. In short, the contradictory nature of social reality implies a process of dialectic change, by which old contradictions reach resolution through conflict and by which new contradictions emerge. To return to the case histories, the contradictions that foster occupational illness, infant mortality, and inappropriate technology can be major points of conflict. Struggles in the medical arena can succeed most fully if they go beyond medical problems to attack the social contradictions that are responsible at a deeper level.

Another theme in materialist analysis concerns exploitation. Under capitalism, illness is exploited for a variety of purposes by a number of groups, including profit-making corporations, health-care professionals, and medical centers. The contradictions of the health system are linked to these patterns of exploitation. One cautionary remark, however, is necessary. Exploitation is a structural problem. The Marxist framework is not a conspiratorial model. The individuals who own or control corporations and individual clinicians associated with medical centers do consciously consider their financial resources, power, and prestige in policy decisions. These advantages to individuals, however, are not the point. The nature of capitalism reinforces current deficiencies of health care; from the standpoint of private profit, there is no reason that corporations should view medicine differently from other goods and services. The commercialization of health care and its associated technology is a necessary feature of the capitalist politicaleconomic system. It is the structure of the system, rather than decision making by individual entrepreneurs and clinicians, that is the appropriate level of analysis. This distinction makes all the difference for policy and social action.

The materialist approach also requires historical specificity. Marxist analysis tries to explain social problems with historical concreteness and with reference to specific material reality. Although general analytic principles may be appropriate to the study of different problems, each problem has its own context which demands concrete explanation. The irony here, of course, is that Marxism has suffered from a dogmatic application of the theories developed by its founders to later historical issues. Classic Marxist theories have been unable to predict the course of social revolution in precapitalist societies, the precise nature of class conflict in advanced capitalist societies like the United States, and events in postrevolutionary societies. These failures do not detract from Marx's critique of early capitalism, nor from later nondogmatic Marxist attempts to grapple with current realities that the classics of Marxism did not anticipate.

The next sections of this chapter deal with several major problems in the health systems of advanced capitalist countries. Although the emphasis is on North America (including illustrative examples from my own clinical work in California and New England), comparisons with other capitalist and noncapitalist countries appear at various points. The description of these problems is not particularly new or surprising. What is surprising, however, is that most discussions of these problems accept them mainly as problems in medicine—that is, problems of health and health care—rather than as problems of society. With the analytic approach outlined above, I try to show that problems in medicine emerge from and reflect broader structural contradictions in the society at large.

PROFIT AND SAFETY

Ecological threats to the survival of humanity and other life forms have reached grotesque proportions. During the past decade, consciousness about the potentially devastating effects of nuclear power, toxic wastes, occupational and environmental carcinogens, and related problems has heightened. Whether this concern can overtake the scope of present and future devastation remains unclear. Perhaps more than in any other area, the analysis of illness, work, and the environment must consider the connections between these issues and the contradictions of capitalism.

The basic contradiction which accounts for many problems in this area is that between profit and safety. Safety in the workplace, in almost all instances, means increased cost of production and, as a result, decreased profits. The technical improvements necessary to protect workers from dust, fumes, radioactivity, accidents, and stress entail inevitable expenses and seldom lead to increased productivity. On the contrary, a safe workplace often means a slower pace of work as well as a more cautious appraisal of substances and technologies needed for the manufacture of new products. Corporations cannot simply raise prices to absorb these higher costs without adversely affecting the demand for goods. The constraint of private profit is a structural basis for resistance to changes in production that would ensure occupational health and safety.

The contradiction between profit and safety also extends beyond the workplace to the general environment. Considerations of profit not only limit the feasibility of safe working conditions; they also encourage the dumping of waste products of the production process into the wider community. Industrial production generally requires the emission of wastes into air, water, or land supplies. In some situations, technology can reduce the amount or toxicity of such emissions, although such interventions always involve costs that in one way or another infringe on profit. In other instances, particularly that of nuclear power, truly adequate waste disposal may be both costly and technically impossible with current knowledge.

When considering these issues, one must distinguish between capitalism and industrialization. There is no question that industrialization itself is associated with increases in some illnesses, especially occupational illnesses, that are linked to the nature of industrial work. In socialist societies, where private profit per se is not an impediment to a safe workplace and environment, illness-generating conditions still arise. As analysts have openly recognized in several socialist countries, a new contradiction emerges that resembles, in certain respects, that between profit and safety; this new contradiction involves productivity and safety. Even when the means of production are socially owned, socialist societies need to adopt stringent goals of high productivity in industry, agriculture, or both. These goals are especially important where conditions of prior underdevelopment have undermined the population's health and welfare. Yet the drive to raise productivity discourages attempts to reduce occupational risks in the workplace and to control the emission of toxic wastes. Such improvements to protect workers and the environment necessarily consume already scarce time and social resources. The drive toward productivity in some socialist nations like the former Soviet Union has created complex and unanticipated health problems, and programs to deal with these problems have been only partially successful.

Because most socialist countries have emphasized public health, however, there have been numerous attempts to deal with these issues. In several instances, rapid improvements in occupational and environmental health problems have been possible. For example, Cuban trade unions and the national institute of occupational health blocked or delayed production in several key industries until hazards to workers were corrected. Nationally organized occupational safety and health programs also have received high priority in several Eastern European and newly independent African countries with socialist systems. Therefore, the contradiction between productivity and safety does not seem an inherent and insurmountable feature of socialism.

While it is important to acknowledge that problems of illness, work, and the environment do not disappear under socialism, the connections between these problems and the constraints of private profit under capitalism are quite profound. To analyze occupational and environmental health problems without reference to the contradiction between profit and safety is misleading. It is also foolish to believe that meaningful improvements in these problems are possible without basic change in the structure of private profit. The examples that follow are brief accounts of four occupational or environmental health problems. Rather than giving a detailed analysis of these or many similar problems, the purpose here is to explore the linkages between these problems and the structural contradiction of profit versus safety.

Plastic Workers' Liver Cancer

Plastic is everywhere in modern society. It wraps food, upholsters furniture, transports water in pipes, amuses children as toys, entertains as phonograph records, and attracts attention as signs. During the past three decades, plastic production and consumption have increased rapidly.

A basic component of plastic is polyvinyl chloride. Through chemical reactions polyvinyl chloride (a solid) is manufactured from vinyl chloride (a gas). Beginning in 1938, a series of reports showed toxic damage of the liver and other organs in animals exposed to vinyl chloride in laboratory experiments. Studies conducted under several different conditions verified these findings. Although many scientists and officials in the plastic industry knew about these results, they did not change the utilization of vinyl chloride in the manufacturing process.

In 1974 three workers in a plastic factory in Louisville, Kentucky, developed angiosarcoma of the liver, previously a very rare cancer. During the next two years investigators found that more than twenty-six other cases of angiosarcoma were linked to occupational exposure to vinyl chloride; these people with cancer attracted worldwide attention. New studies showed an association between vinyl chloride exposure and cancer in organs besides the liver; they also found increasing rates of many types of cancer among people exposed to the chemical. Some researchers believed that an epidemic of cancer related to vinyl chloride had begun.

Despite unambiguous evidence that vinyl chloride causes cancer of the liver and other organs, the plastic industry has resisted attempts to reduce occupational exposure. The production process itself has several steps. During one step, the cleaning stage when workers crawl into the reactors where polyvinyl chloride is formed, the concentration of vinyl chloride may exceed 1,000 parts per million (ppm). In experiments with rodents, investigators have found liver damage at exposures of 50 ppm. Although the minimum toxic level for humans is unknown, occupational health officials recommended engineering changes that would ensure exposure levels of 1 ppm or less; the plastic industry's response was that a reduction to 1 ppm would raise the cost of production by 50 percent. As a compromise, the U.S. Occupational Safety and Health Administration set a standard that allowed exposure levels up to 25 ppm. The plastic industry challenged even this intermediate level by court appeals, which delayed implementation of the new regulations.

Although the impact of increased production costs on profit is industry's main concern, a related issue has affected the activism of organized labor. Since implementation of safer standards is costly and time-consuming, it is likely that many plants producing polyvinyl chloride would close, either permanently or temporarily. If plants were closed until completely safe production procedures or substitutes for polyvinyl chloride were developed, many workers would lose their jobs for extended periods of time.

This is labor's classic dilemma in occupational diseases. Workers frequently face a choice between job safety and continued employment. Workmen's compensation laws provide financial benefits only after a worker has suffered injury or disability from the work process; there are no adequate provisions for financial assistance during changes in the production process that would prevent the development of occupational diseases. Workers' desire for a safe workplace thus is an ambivalent desire; the threat of unemployment is present in any struggle to reduce occupational hazards. Historically, organized labor has favored safety legislation and tighter regulations, but when workers confront job loss, they often have accepted compromises that they recognize are inadequate.

As the dangers of vinyl chloride have become clear, plastic workers' unions have supported the recommendation of 1 ppm, but political and economic realities have restrained the unions' activism. In general, unions have not opposed the compromise regulation of 25 ppm. Since society gives no assurance of alternative employment during industry's transition to safer standards, the unions have little choice. Profitability imposes a structural impediment on industry's willingness to modify production in order to ensure a safe workplace. To keep their jobs, workers frequently must accept a risk of cancer.

Asbestos Workers' Lung Disease and Cancer

Asbestos is one of several compounds that cause occupational lung disease. Industries that expose workers to asbestos include manufacturers of insulation (pipes, heatproof screens, and so on), construction, shipyards, and textile makers. The disease asbestosis occurs in the following way. Industrial dusts containing asbestos settle in the small airways of the lungs, from dust deposits, and cause inflammation. The inflammation leads to scarring (fibrosis) in the cell layers between airways and small blood vessels. As a result of fibrosis, it becomes more and more difficult for oxygen to move from the lungs into the bloodstream. Workers in many industries develop similar chronic lung disease from exposure to other types of dust: aluminosis ("bauxite lung") from aluminum in smelting, explosives, paints, and fireworks manufacturing; baritosis from barium sulfate in mining; beryllium disease from beryllium in aircraft manufacturing, metallurgy, and rocket fuels; byssinosis ("brown lung") from cotton, flax, and hemp dust in textile manufacturing; coal workers' pneumoconiosis ("black lung") from coal dust in mining, coal trimming, and the graphite industry; kaolinosis from hydrated aluminum silicates in china making; platinum asthma from platinum salts in electronics and chemical industries; siderosis from iron oxides in welding and iron ore mining; silicosis from silica in mining, pottery, sandblasting, foundries, quarries, and masonry; stannosis from tin oxide in smelting; and talcosis from hydrated magnesium silicates in the rubber industry.

Although many of these diseases produce chronic disability and early death from lung pathology alone, asbestos has the added danger of cancer. Since 1935 the medical literature has contained reports of lung cancer associated with asbestosis. The industry's response followed a pattern of denial and suppression of information; for many years major asbestos companies in the United States and Canada publicly claimed that the evidence that asbestos caused cancer was not convincing enough to reduce exposure levels. Several companies also gave financial support to researchers whose published studies showed no relation between asbestos and cancer. Retrospectively all these studies used inadequate methods. For example, industry-sponsored research studied young people who had worked in asbestos production for short periods of time; this research generally ignored the latent period between exposure and development of disease.

During the 1960s several investigators not receiving industry support, for the first time, were able to study workers who had longer periods of exposure. These definitive studies showed a clear-cut association between asbestos exposure and cancer (including mesothelioma, an otherwise rare cancer growing from the lining of the chest or abdominal cavity). Fifty years after the initial reports of asbestosis, and forty years after the observed association between asbestos and cancer, only during the past two decades have there been serious attempts to reduce workers' exposure to safe levels.

As in other occupational health problems, industry's profits stand in the way of change. The prospect of unemployment also inhibits unions of asbestos workers from taking a strong stand on working conditions. Many asbestos workers have lost their jobs during production cutbacks resulting from environmental protection regulations. The threat of job loss and the changes that can occur when workers take control of their factories are clear from an example, that of the Vermont Asbestos Company (VAC).

For many years the GAF Corporation of New York (a multinational corporation controlling numerous industrial subsidiaries) had owned and operated an asbestos mine in northern Vermont. The mine served as the main employer for two towns. In 1974, the U.S. Environmental Protection Agency and the Vermont Occupational Safety and Health Administration asked the mine to install dust-control devices and procedures to lower asbestos exposure to acceptable levels. The estimated cost of these changes was about $1 million. Rather than spend the money, GAF decided to close the mine.

Facing massive unemployment, workers at the mine began to consider an alternative—owning and running the mine themselves. At first the price, $5 million, seemed impossible. With outside technical support, however, workers obtained the necessary loans, bought the mine, and began operating it themselves. Workers and their families purchased shares in the company. Productivity increased rapidly; within a year, VAC repaid all outstanding loans. In one and one-half years it was making a profit, which the board (composed jointly of manual and managerial workers, all of whom held shares in the company) decided to invest in a new plant that would make construction material from asbestos waste products and would be located in an area of high unemployment. VAC also quickly corrected the hazardous asbestos exposure levels. Within one year of assuming ownership, workers installed dust-control devices that brought asbestos levels within recommended standards.

The contradiction between profit and safety largely disappears when "profit" returns to workers. Since VAC's revenues no longer went to an external corporation that owned the means of production, they were hardly profits in the traditional sense. Monetary rewards mean little if workers face disability, cancer, and early death. The importance of safety in the workplace becomes a high priority when workers own the workplace. The successes of VAC and similar cooperative ventures in worker ownership, of course, do not imply that such a strategy will solve occupational health problems under capitalism. Worker ownership within the overall framework of capitalism faces basic structural limitations. However, such experiments clarify the contradiction of profit versus safety, as well as the improvements that become possible when profit is no longer an impediment to change in the production process.

Farmworkers' Back

The contradiction between profit and safety arises not only in industry but also in agriculture. Chronic back injury, for example, is one of the commonest occupational diseases that farmworkers have endured in the United States. This disease has had essentially nothing to do with industrialization; it has occurred in agricultural work that historically has had little mechanization and that has depended almost entirely on manual labor.

Although contradictions like that between profit and safety manifest themselves mainly at the level of social structures, they also have direct effects on the lives of individuals. Therefore it is again useful to consider these effects more concretely. The following case history concerns a patient followed at a clinic of the United Farm Workers Union in California.

> J. C. was a 32-year-old Chicano father of five. He began working as a farm laborer at age 14. He generally worked eight to ten hours a day, in stoop labor with an arched back, on such crops as lettuce. For about ten years he used the "short hoe" required of many farmworkers in the Western states. At age 28, while bending at work, he suddenly felt a sharp pain in his back with radiation down his left leg.
>
> Physical exam at that time showed tenderness over the L4–L5 intervertebral space of the back, decreased reflexes and sensation of the left leg, and positive straight-leg-raising test (a test for slipped disk). X-rays showed advanced degenerative arthritis of the entire lower spine and a slipped disk at the L4–L5 level.
>
> Severe pain on bending persisted after back surgery. The patient knew no English, could not find a job outside farm labor, and was applying for permanent disability benefits.

The short hoe has a short wooden handle—about one foot in length. To use the short hoe, a person must work in a stooped posture, bent forward at the waist, so that the hoe can reach the ground. The short hoe has no intrinsic advantage over the long-handled hoe, which a farmworker can use in an erect posture. The only reason for the short hoe is supervision. If the foreman sees that all workers in a crew are bent over, he can be more sure that everybody is working. With long-handled hoes, people can stand with straight backs and supervision becomes somewhat more difficult. It is harder for a small number of supervisors to be sure that a large number of workers are really working.

Farmworkers' back is a preventable disease. It occurs in an unindustrialized, agricultural sector of the economy which is highly oriented toward profit. The short hoe's human toll is crippling back disease for thousands of farmworkers; the main injuries are slipped disks and degenerative arthritis of the spine. These problems occur in young workers who do stoop labor, and their physical effects are irreversible. Since migrant workers most often lack educational opportunities and frequently know little English, farmworkers' back usually means permanent economic disability.

There is nothing new about this disease. Medical specialists have testified about the short hoe's devastating effects for several decades. Yet for many years farm owners, especially the agribusiness corporations that have gained control of many agricultural enterprises, refused to stop the short hoe's use. Farm owners usually gave no reason for this policy, except that long-handled hoes would require higher costs of supervision. (A few companies also argued that the wood for longer handles increased costs. When analyzed, the costs of longer handles were minimal.) The profit motive and the nature of agricultural production led directly to this illness-generating labor practice.

Until the mid-1960s, farmworkers were largely unorganized. A reserve army of migrant workers were available to replace individuals who were crippled by farmworkers' back or who objected to the conditions of work. Powerlessness resulted from lack of organizations; individual farmworkers had no alternative to the crippling effects of the short hoe, because resistance meant loss of work.

The UFW has organized farmworkers through the West, Southwest, and Southeast. Like other unions, the UFW has fought for basic improvements in wages and benefits. Beyond these economic goals, however, the union has focused on the conditions of work. The UFW has launched organizing and publicity campaigns concerning the short hoe, dangerous insecticides and chemicals, and other occupational health issues.

In response to this pressure, the California legislature ultimately passed a law banning the short hoe. Agribusiness corporations then obtained a series of court injunctions against the new law; these rulings accepted the companies' claims that conversion to the long-handled hoe would lead to excessive costs. Other courts later reversed these injunctions. But even after legislation, California farmworkers—as well as workers in other states without such laws—continued to use and to suffer from the short hoe. Meanwhile, activists have hardly scratched the surface of such occupational health problems as pesticides, herbicides, and toxic chemicals. The contradiction between profit and safety persists in agriculture as it does in industry.

Brain Disease from Mercury Poisoning

It is also important to understand how this contradiction extends beyond the workplace to affect entire communities and larger populations. In 1907 a chemical company built a factory in Minamata, Japan. Minamata is a small seacoast community whose economy for centuries had been based on fishing. Over the years, the factory grew and became part of a large petrochemical conglomerate, the Chisso Corporation. Because the factory dumped its waste products into Minamata Bay, fish began to die or to avoid the area. In 1925 Chisso started to give payments to local fishermen who complained. In 1932 Chisso began to produce acetaldehyde, a chemical used in the manufacture of drugs, perfumes, plastics, and many other products. Organic mercury is a catalyst in acetaldehyde production.

Beginning in 1952, cats in Minamata began to die after developing convulsions, bizarre behavior, and paralysis. Between 1956 and 1957, 52 children and adults started to show similar neurologic disorders; 21 people died. Outside investigators reported that the cause of the disease probably was heavy-metal poisoning carried to humans and cats who ate the fish from Minamata Bay.

In 1959, a scientist working for Chisso fed material from an acetaldehyde waste pipe to a cat in his laboratory. Soon the cat showed the typical signs of Minamata Disease. The scientist reported this finding to the Chisso management. The management suppressed the finding and ordered the scientist not to conduct more experiments concerning Minamata Disease. The scientist remained silent; the results of his experiment came to light during trials that took place in the late 1960s. The company publicly announced that there was no scientific proof that Minamata Disease was related to Chisso manufacturing processes. The company installed a purification device in 1959. Nevertheless, Chisso continued to dump waste products containing mercury into Minamata Bay until 1968, when it switched to catalysts that were technically more efficient than mercury.

During the late 1960s and early 1970s, over three thousand patients brought legal suit against Chisso for financial compensation and medical expenses. Residents also held demonstrations, sit-ins, and other protests at the Minamata plant. Company guards, together with unionized workers at the plant, physically attacked the protesters several times; there were many injuries, some serious. In 1973 the Central Pollution Board decided that Chisso would pay medically "verified" patients $68,000 for "heavy" cases and $60,000 for "lighter" cases. By the mid-1970s, 798 patients had been verified, and approximately 2,800 other applicants were waiting for decisions. Many of these patients were children with congenital Minamata Disease, whose mothers had eaten mercury-containing fish during pregnancy. Meanwhile the provincial government announced that fish outside Minamata Bay, marked by buoys, were safe to eat. This decision ignored the fact that fish throughout the Shiranui Sea, of which Minamata Bay is a part, can swim past buoys. Researchers in Japan estimated that as many as 10,000 people, previously eating fish from the Shiranui Sea, eventually fell ill with Minamata Disease (2).

The structure of capitalist production is responsible for such tragedies of environmental poisoning. For more than a decade, Chisso management suppressed evidence of the company's responsibility for Minamata Disease; management recognized the financial burden it would face if it accepted responsibility. Indemnity payments would drastically affect profits. There were no mechanisms by which Japanese society as a whole would compensate the victims or pay their medical expenses. Moreover, in this situation, workers at Chisso had structural interests that overlapped with management's. By reducing profitability, major payments to Minamata victims or a less efficient production process without mercury catalysts would ultimately threaten workers' jobs. During the protests and suits, these economic realities led unionized workers at Chisso to side with managers and against their injured neighbors. If profit were not the guiding motivation of industry, and if the society guaranteed people's material subsistence, prevention and protection from industrial poisoning would not encounter such fundamental resistance.

The implications of Minamata Disease go far beyond Japan and mercury. During the 1960s a paper company in northern Ontario, Canada, dumped mercury-containing wastes into the English-Wabagoon River (3). This region of Canada is fairly isolated; the people who live there are mainly Native Americans and the operators of popular tourist camps. Several citizens, concerned about the mercury problem, obtained tests that showed toxic levels in the river fish. Government officials investigated the situation. The paper company reduced but did not eliminate the mercury in its waste discharges. Although it is estimated that river fish will contain toxic mercury levels for about seventy years, the government did not stop the company's mercury dumps, nor did the government ban fishing—apparently responding to pressures from the tourist industry that caters to visiting sports fishermen. Inaction persisted despite the fact that several people living in the region developed classic symptoms of Minamata Disease and showed high mercury levels in tests of blood and hair.

Outbreaks of mercury and other heavy-metal poisoning occur periodically in many parts of the United States and in other countries. In the early phases of the Minamata epidemic, investigators found that Chisso was pouring into the sea more than fifty chemicals that can cause disease in humans. Later research showed that thallium, manganese, and selenium—all present in high concentration in Chisso's effluents—were not the cause and that mercury was. Other industries have discharged these elements and related compounds, including lead, hydrocarbons, asbestos, and radioactive spills. Environmental poisons have caused temporary epidemics of acute illness; their chronic effects, especially in the development of cancer, are only recently receiving more attention. The social, economic, and political issues involved in many geographic areas, and related to many specific poisons, resemble those of Minamata. While the structure of capitalist production remains what it is, one can expect more of the same devastation that the people of Minamata have faced. The contradiction between profit and safety is a major source of illness, suffering, and death.

PLENTIFUL RESOURCES AND MEDICAL MALDISTRIBUTION

A second widely recognized problem of health systems in capitalist societies is maldistribution. Strong social policies to improve maldistribution have accompanied the advent of socialism in some countries. Historically, social barriers limiting recruitment into medicine have created numerical shortages of doctors and other health workers. To highlight the problem of maldistribution, some data are revealing. These patterns apply not only to the United States, but also to countries like Canada and Sweden, where reforms creating national or provincial health insurance programs have not fully corrected distributional inequities.

One form of maldistribution relates to geography. Rural areas like Appalachia and the Great Plains states, as well as urban districts with largely black or Hispanic populations, experience extreme shortages of health workers. On the other hand, more affluent parts of cities and suburbs, especially on the East Coast and West Coast, have large concentrations of medical personnel. Table 1.1 gives a state-by-state breakdown in the distribution of active physicians. (Doctor-to-population ratios provide a rather insensitive measure of maldistribution.) The variation is enormous. For instance, there is a heavy concentration of doctors in such places as Washington, D.C., New York, and Massachusetts; other states like Mississippi, Alabama, and South Dakota have a startling lack of health workers.

Even states with seemingly adequate doctor-population ratios contain severe internal maldistribution. For example, the state of New Mexico appears to have an adequate number of health workers when compared to other states. Data from

Table 1.1   Physicians per Population, by State, 1995

State	Total	Rate*	State	Total	Rate*
Alabama	7,814	184	Montana	1,569	181
Alaska	890	153	Nebraska	3,236	199
Arizona	8,315	198	Nevada	2,391	157
Arkansas	4,256	171	New Hampshire	2,451	214
California	75,496	241	New Jersey	21,895	276
Colorado	8,425	227	New Mexico	3,320	199
Connecticut	10,919	334	New York	65,299	361
Delaware	1,546	217	North Carolina	15,159	214
D.C.	3,623	662	North Dakota	1,291	204
Florida	31,053	220	Ohio	24,402	219
Georgia	13,984	198	Oklahoma	5,203	160
Hawaii	2,814	248	Oregon	6,648	212
Idaho	1,583	137	Pennsylvania	32,919	273
Illinois	28,765	244	Rhode Island	2,942	298
Indiana	10,426	180	South Carolina	6,904	190
Iowa	4,703	166	South Dakota	1,206	166
Kansas	4,961	198	Tennessee	11,846	226
Kentucky	7,416	193	Texas	35,100	189
Louisiana	9,604	222	Utah	3,766	194
Maine	2,449	198	Vermont	1,577	270
Maryland	17,463	349	Virginia	14,676	227
Massachusetts	23,471	387	Washington	12,032	224
Michigan	20,061	210	West Virginia	3,582	196
Minnesota	11,007	239	Wisconsin	10,903	213
Mississippi	3,703	138	Wyoming	716	150
Missouri	11,594	218			

Source: U.S. Bureau of the Census, *Statistical Abstract of the United States: 1997* (Washington, D.C.: U.S. Bureau of the Census, 1997), p. 124, No. 179.
*Per 100,000 residents

1995 showed a ratio of 199 doctors per 100,000 population; this figure was somewhat below the national ratio of 236 per 100,000. However, when the statewide figure is broken down by counties, one finds large discrepancies (Table 1.2). Most doctors are concentrated in a single county (Bernalillo), where the state medical school and the largest city (Albuquerque) are located. In more rural counties there are severe shortages of health workers, and the statewide figures mask these short-

Table 1.2   Physicians per Population, New Mexico, by County, 1990

County	Active Physicians	Resident Population	Rate*
Bernalillo	1,585	499,262	330
Catron	3	2,533	117
Chaves	67	58,582	116
Cibola	15	23,819	63
Colfax	18	12,996	139
Curry	41	45,559	97
DeBaca	3	2,254	133
Doña Ana	171	146,619	126
Eddy	54	51,111	111
Grant	40	28,621	145
Guadalupe	2	4,097	48
Harding	—	995	—
Hidalgo	2	5,995	34
Lea	40	56,659	72
Lincoln	15	13,116	123
Los Alamos	42	18,179	232
Luna	10	19,713	55
McKinley	93	65,179	153
Mora	3	4,261	70
Otero	48	51,868	92
Quay	37	10,457	351
Rio Arriba	26	34,891	76
Roosevelt	9	17,463	54
Sandoval	51	68,779	81
San Juan	93	95,112	102
San Miguel	27	26,468	105
Sante Fe	235	105,178	238
Sierra	8	9,845	81
Socorro	8	14,983	54
Taos	24	24,228	104
Torrance	3	10,701	29
Union	4	4,042	97
Valencia	21	48,305	46

Source: U.S. Department of Commerce, *County and City Data Book,* 12th ed. (Washington, D.C.: Department of Commerce, 1994), pp. 368, 371, 382, 385.
*Per 100,000 residents

ages. Several counties have extremely poor doctor-population ratios, some worse than the state average of Mississippi.

Besides geography, there is maldistribution based on income. Low-income patients cannot buy health care and medications as easily as can higher-income patients. In addition, poor people often have to use emergency rooms and outpatient departments of public hospitals for their care. Here they frequently face bureaucracy, impersonality, and lack of continuity because of rotating interns and residents who can follow their patients only for brief periods of time. The effects of past and present racism reinforce those of poverty; blacks, Hispanics, Asians, Native Americans, and other racial minorities face inaccessibility and communication barriers to obtaining services. To some extent, this situation has improved since the passage of Medicaid and Medicare legislation in 1965. But private practitioners often refuse to accept Medicaid or Medicare patients because of paperwork and delays in payment. In general, it is still more difficult for poor and lower middle-income people to gain access to adequate health care than it is for the wealthy.

Before examining the social contradictions that account for maldistribution, one should realize that this is not simply a theoretical problem; maldistribution has effects that are often devastating. General health statistics for a nation or region tend to mask the impact of maldistribution in smaller geographical areas or at different income levels. Many people in the United States and other capitalist countries do not have consistent access to even the simplest form of care. Because of maldistribution, there are still individuals who suffer permanent disability every year. The case presentations that follow involve patients who have used the clinics of the United Farm Workers (UFW) Union in California. It is important to note that the Union set up this system of clinics because of maldistribution and farmworkers' inadequate access to health services.

A Girl with Acute Glomerulonephritis

O. O. was an 11-year-old girl. Her family, migrant workers, were living temporarily in a shanty camp without running water. The patient and her family were Spanish-speaking and knew very little English. About a week before she came to the clinic, she scraped both feet on a rock in a fall. She and her parents washed the wounds with water from a well and bandaged them with a makeshift bandage. Four days later, both her feet became painful, hot, red, and swollen. Two days after that, her ankles, fingers, and eyelids became puffy, and she began to feel very sleepy. Her family brought her to a union organizer, who drove then 75 miles to the clinic in Salinas—the closest medical facility the family could afford.

At the clinic, physical exam showed a sleepy girl in no acute distress, with a slight fever and elevated blood pressure. There was no heart murmur. Infected lesions were present on both feet. Her ankles, fingers, and eyelids contained edema fluid. Abnormal lab work confirmed a diagnosis of acute glomerulonephritis (kidney inflammation) that was a complication from a streptococcal skin infection.

The patient's wounds were cleaned and dressed with an antibiotic ointment. A course of penicillin, rest, and a nutritive diet was started. After two weeks, the patient felt better. After three weeks, she could resume her usual activities. At six months, her tests of kidney function were still about 60 percent of normal.

In a criticism/self criticism session at the clinic, it was felt there was little the Union could have done to prevent the complication of the skin infection, mainly because of the family's physical isolation and unavailability of health workers in the local area.

A Boy with Congenital Heart Disease

B. C. was a 5-year-old boy whose grandmother brought him to a UFW clinic because of poor appetite. The child had been delivered at home and had not been seen by a doctor previously. No one in the family spoke English.

Physical exam revealed a very small boy, with height and weight below the third percentile. The child's fingernail beds and lips were slightly blue; the fingernails showed clubbing. Examination of the heart showed a harsh murmur. Electrocardiogram showed right ventricular hypertrophy (thickened muscle of the right side of the heart).

The tentative diagnosis was pulmonic stenosis (narrowing of the pulmonic valve of the heart) with septal defect (hole in the muscle separating the chambers of the heart) and possible pulmonary hypertension (high pressure in the lung vessels because of the heart abnormality).

The child was referred to a university medical center. Catheterization study of pressures inside the heart confirmed the above diagnoses at a severe level. He underwent surgery to correct the pulmonic stenosis and septal defect. Most expenses were paid by the Crippled Children's Service. The surgeons believed that residual pulmonary hypertension would remain postoperatively.

This child faced the probability of a permanent functional deficit from heart and lung disease. If he had had access to a health worker by age three, the defect probably could have been corrected without permanent deficit.

These young people are victims of society. The girl with glomerulonephritis probably would not have suffered permanent kidney impairment if services that the family could afford were available close to home. The boy with congenital heart disease could have lived a normal life if he had been examined by age three — usually a routine for wealthier families in the United States.

The root of medical maldistribution is the structural contradiction of development and underdevelopment. Uneven development is most obvious on an international scale, where the economic disparities between underdeveloped and advanced capitalist nations are evident. National underdevelopment is an important determinant of ill health and early death in Third World countries. However, uneven development also occurs within nations, including those whose aggregated measures of economic and physical well-being indicate highly desirable levels of wealth and health. Even in countries like the United States, the distribution of health workers and facilities is closely correlated to the distribution of economic resources. Although these correlations are not perfect, regions of the country with higher levels of personal income, more concentrated economic enter-prises (particularly industrial corporations), and more plentiful nonmedical ser-vices (including universities, housing, and cultural facilities) generally command larger numbers of both generalist and specialist physicians, as well as hospitals and other health facilities. Rural-urban differences show these relationships most clearly, but the same pattern emerges even within cities, where maldistribution of health services coincides with income differentials and other measures of eco-nomic development for small units like census tracts.

The dynamics of uneven development in the health-care system are complex. Regarding health institutions, finance capital has become more and more concen-trated in a smaller number of medical centers and corporations. As discussed in a later chapter, the concentration of capital in the health sector has paralleled the emergence of monopoly capital in other sectors of the economy. The growth of medical centers has required a large capital base, especially to support advanced diagnostic and therapeutic technologies. This trend has led to some bizarre con-trasts. In many North American cities, one sees densely concentrated hospitals in specific geographic areas. These hospitals often contain the world's most advanced medical technology, with duplicated and overlapping equipment located in a perimeter of several city blocks. On the other hand, nearby urban and rural areas frequently lack clinics and hospitals altogether, and patients—usually poor and often from minority backgrounds—must travel miles for primary services.

For health workers, the nature of professional education reinforces the contra-diction of uneven development. Doctors, nurses, and other health workers receive their training in medical schools and teaching hospitals that emphasize advanced technology and specialization. This training encourages people to use diagnostic tests and treatments that require extensive laboratory and X-ray facilities, drugs, complex therapies, and other advanced techniques. Specialists become accus-tomed to technologic facilities and to patients who present challenging diagnostic and therapeutic problems. Upon completion of training, professionals often feel dissatisfied by the range of relatively commonplace ailments they find in commu-nity settings. As a result, they tend to remain closely associated with large med-ical centers and slowly advance along academic medical hierarchies in medicine, nursing, or allied fields. Likewise, they hesitate to practice in rural or urban areas where their training might remain largely unutilized and where advanced techno-logic facilities are unavailable.

Practitioners frequently justify the decision to practice close to medical centers on intellectual grounds. On the other hand, specialization itself leads to a relative inability to manage even simple problems outside the sphere of one's specific competence. Thus, the surplus of personnel and facilities near medical centers attracts a further surplus. Practicing in a setting more detached from medical cen-ters becomes a fear-evoking experience. Inside academic teaching hospitals, physicians often deride the relatively unsophisticated management of patients with complex problems, who are referred for specialized treatment. Specialists associated with referral hospitals often view the "local medical doctor" as a technically inferior physician. The true gravity of the situation, however, is that many doctors grow so dependent on large medical centers that they themselves feel inhibited from practicing in areas of great medical need. In this sense, practitioners' education leads to a trained incapacity, involving a dependency on technology that itself is highly concentrated.

Although such institutional and personal dynamics reinforce medical maldistribution, this problem is only one manifestation of uneven development. The incredible contrast of technically advanced medicine and inaccessible services emerges organically from an uncoordinated socioeconomic system, in which planning does not comprehensively address the health and welfare needs of the population. Uneven development under capitalism means, for example, that workers in specific sectors of the economy face cyclical patterns of unemployment and inadequate income. Such problems typically arise when profit considerations lead companies to reduce their workforces (as in the auto industry) or to relocate the site of production (as in the runaway shop seeking a lower-cost labor force). In these situations, corporate decisions seek to maintain or to increase the rate of profit. Because of the system's structure, the well-being of individual workers and local communities is a subordinate consideration in corporate decision making.

Economically underdeveloped areas, in general, are also medically underdeveloped, and similar forces determine both forms of underdevelopment. Those geographic regions of the United States that face shortages of health workers and facilities tend to be the same regions that are most depressed economically. This association applies in particular to Appalachia, parts of the South, and the Great Plains states. Within regions, as in the case of New Mexico, medical resources are inversely related to general economic impoverishment.

Under capitalism there is no consistent and forceful planning that prevents either the economic or medical disadvantages of uneven development. Major decisions regarding the allocation of social resources follow mainly the short-term needs of corporations. State intervention—in the forms of health and welfare benefits, regional health planning, and hospital construction in underdeveloped areas—remains uncoordinated and largely symbolic. Major examples of such governmental activity are the Hill-Burton Programs for hospital construction and the Regional Medical Programs. Both highly touted efforts, though explicitly recognizing the problem of medical maldistribution, proved largely unsuccessful in improving accessibility of medical care in underserved areas. A primary but seldom recognized reason for these failures is the lack of coordinated central planning that links health-care services to general socioeconomic development. Limited reforms to improve medical maldistribution convey the symbolic trappings of concern for the public health. However, the expectation that redistributional policies in medicine can succeed in the context of general socioeconomic impoverishment remains profoundly misguided.

Uneven development also rests on certain ideologic contradictions in capitalist society. One such contradiction is that between freedom and equality. This contradiction mystifies the problem of medical maldistribution. For health professionals, the ideology of freedom holds that practitioners should be free to select the conditions of their practice. For clients, a similar ideology teaches that patients should be free to select their own doctors and sites of care. Such principles resonate with a more general ethos of individualism and voluntarism. One motivation of entering professional life is the opportunity of private practice, including the presumed ability to be one's own boss. Many professionals do not want to be told where to practice, how much to charge, how to improve what they are doing, or how to respond to organized consumer groups. Similarly, it is argued that clients should have freedom of choice.

Yet freedom of choice is heavily class-linked. As Marx and Engels noted, in a simple observation yet to be refuted, freedom is greatest for those who control property and wealth (4). This conclusion applies no less to health care than to other goods and services. Poor people have not had as much freedom as have the wealthy to choose their sources of health care. More often than not, the poor have relied on the fragmented and depersonalized services of public hospitals and outpatient departments. As noted earlier, many public facilities have closed largely because of financial cutbacks deriving from general economic trends. Freedom of choice is an important ideologic structure, but the reality of freedom is that some groups have enjoyed its fruits more than have others.

Equality also is an ideologic goal in the United States. This is not the place to discuss many of the nuances of inequality, except to reiterate that maldistribution and uneven development are two of its manifestations. There is also a growing concern, in the United States and many other countries, that citizens should have equal access to health care—in short, that health care is a fundamental right, analogous to the right of public education. Major reorganizational changes in the health system must occur, however, if equality is to become more than a rhetorical goal.

One such change necessarily would limit the freedom that health professionals historically have enjoyed. Professionals would be less free to practice where, how, and when they choose. Other countries have used several mechanisms to reduce financial and distributional impediments to equality. (Although these policy issues are a major focus of the last chapter of this book, they are pertinent to the underlying ideologic contradictions of maldistribution.) In some countries health workers receive payments directly from an arm of government for services to low-income patients, or alternatively the government reimburses patients for payments they make to health workers; the financial structure is a system of national health insurance. In countries with socialist or mixed capitalist-socialist economic systems, health workers generally are employees of a national health service; they obtain a salary from government revenues and receive either no or nominal fees from individual patients. These financial arrangements reduce health workers' freedom to set an independent price for their services, and health care ceases to be a commodity paid for like other goods and services. The model of a national health service recognizes that a "free market" structure does not provide equal access to health care.

Other measures also are necessary to reduce maldistribution. If health workers are entirely free to work where they choose, maldistribution will continue. Some countries have used financial incentives, through higher salaries, to motivate health workers to serve in rural areas and urban districts with shortages. This technique remains essentially voluntary. Despite financial incentives, since health workers may choose to practice in areas of surplus, there is no way to ensure redistribution according to need. As a result, maldistribution tends to persist to a greater or lesser degree.

Another method to overcome inequality of access involves compulsory measures, which require workers to serve, for at least a specific period of time, in needy areas of a country. Some nations combine compulsory policies with training a corps of paraprofessional health workers. These workers perform most duties of doctors but refer people with difficult problems to urban centers. Compulsory assignment of health workers to needy areas has been the only technique that consistently has relieved maldistributional problems. The implementation of such policies always depends on basic social changes that include a strong emphasis on collective goals—even if these goals imply, for periods of time, the subordination of individual preferences.

None of this implies that these solutions are simple and unproblematic. In postrevolutionary socialist societies, as already discussed, new inequalities emerge, including those based on professional expertise. Likewise, the inefficiencies and inflexibilities of socialist bureaucracies in dealing with distributional inequalities are well known (the concluding chapter also addresses these issues). Yet, to correct medical maldistribution, a society must address the ideologic contradiction of freedom and equality as well as the material contradiction of uneven development.

RISING COSTS AND DIMINISHING RETURNS

Since World War II, the cost of health care has risen rapidly in all capitalist nations. The problem of cost plagues the health systems of not only the United States but also nations like Great Britain, in which some industries have been nationalized. Higher costs, however, have not coincided with improved health. Instead, evidence has accumulated to show decreasing returns in the face of escalating costs. Figure 1.1, from the work of Powles, summarizes this problem (5). This figure shows the gradual declines in infant mortality and increases in life expectancy that have occurred during the last century. There has been little apparent relationship between these trends and the specific advances of modern medicine. In the meantime, health-care expenditures have risen dramatically.

Figure 1.1   Mortality Trends during the Last Century, England and Wales, with Recent Expenditure Trends

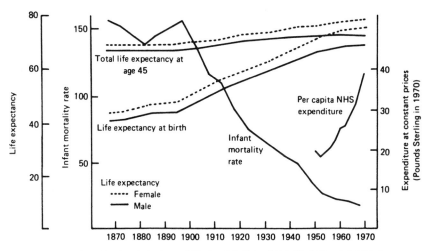

Source: J. Powles, "On the Limitations of Modern Medicine," *Sci. Med. Man* 1 (1973): 2.

Modern medicine's effectiveness in improving health is very difficult to prove for large populations. To place high costs in perspective, one must examine the effectiveness of that for which money is spent. A convergence in public health research has shown that, with a few exceptions, the technical advances of modern medicine have not led to major improvements in measures of health, illness, life expectancy, or death. Instead, the health status of large populations seems more closely related to broad changes in society, including socioeconomic development, better sanitation, environmental conditions, and nutrition.

Critical epidemiologists have questioned medicine's effectiveness by examining trends in general mortality and life expectancy as well as mortality from specific diseases (6). Major historical improvements in both general and specific mortality patterns antedated rather than followed medicine's technical advances. Despite the undeniable usefulness of certain diagnostic and therapeutic techniques with individual patients, such techniques have exerted little historical impact on the health of large populations.

Although these conclusions apply to a wide variety of diseases, they are most startling in the field of infection. When one considers problems that respond to medical treatment, infectious diseases seem most obvious. It has been shown that antibiotics have reduced deaths from a few infections—for example, pneumonia and meningitis. But the major improvements in reduction of deaths and illness that have occurred for most other infections were not clearly related to the development of antibiotics or similar technical advances.

In a paper written as president of the Infectious Diseases Society of America, Kass searched for evidence that modern medicine had been effective in reducing the impact of infection. He traced death rates back over a century for several diseases thought responsive to antibiotics (tuberculosis, diphtheria, and scarlet fever) or immunization (whooping cough and measles). For each disease studied, Kass found that the major declines in mortality preceded the diagnostic tests and specific treatments developed by modern medicine. This observation held true for diseases caused by bacteria, for which antibiotics had been discovered, and by viruses, for which immunization had been introduced. Kass concluded that, contrary to popular belief, improvements in the incidence of infectious diseases generally did not result from advances of modern medicine but rather from broad social changes that were difficult to pinpoint:

> This decline in the rate of certain disorders, correlated roughly with improving socioeconomic circumstances, is merely the most important happening in the history of man, yet we have only the vaguest and most general notions about how it happened and by what mechanisms socioeconomic improvement and decreased rates of certain diseases run in parallel (7).

All this is not to say that antibiotics or other modern treatment is inappropriate for individual patients with specific infections. The point is that the most impressive improvements in these diseases have not occurred because of modern medicine.

Such conclusions may seem inconsistent with one thrust of the last section of this chapter, which argued for well-distributed medical services. If the effectiveness of modern medicine cannot be demonstrated, why are accessible services needed? In fact, one possibly unintended consequence of research on medical effectiveness has been a trend toward nihilist social policy. From this view, since more health services do not necessarily create better health, such goals as correcting maldistribution decline in urgency.

It is important to acknowledge medicine's limited impact on the health status of large populations. This understanding leads one to search for the underlying structural contradictions that permit ever-increasing costs for health care, in the face of medicine's dubious overall effectiveness. While more accessible medical care may have a profound impact on deprived groups in cities or rural areas, these improvements are difficult to document with traditional methods.

Great improvements in health outcomes predictably would follow more fundamental socioeconomic change. Using British data, for instance, McKeown documented a strikingly higher infant mortality rate in the poorest social classes than in the wealthiest. Despite the impact that more accessible obstetrical care might have on these class differences, McKeown argued: "There is little doubt that the difference in health experience is attributable mainly to the direct or indirect effects of poverty, and would be largely eliminated if it were possible to raise the lower standards of living and medical care to the level of the highest" (8). The key point here is that general standards of living and medical care are intertwined. Deprived living conditions and inaccessible services have effects that are theoretically separable but realistically related to one another. This analysis leads to an argument for better medical care and broad social change as complementary facets of political strategy.

Thus far, several conclusions are evident about the problem of diminishing returns. For large populations, the effectiveness of modern medical techniques is difficult to prove. For smaller, previously deprived subpopulations, the redistribution of fairly simple services can achieve undeniable improvements in health, especially in infant mortality. On the other hand, broad socioeconomic changes that lead to higher standards of living (including better nutrition, housing, and occupational and environmental conditions) have a more profound impact on morbidity and mortality than do improved medical services alone.

The problem of rising costs and diminishing returns has many nuances. Underlying this problem, however, are several social contradictions. One is the contradiction of uneven development, which was discussed earlier. Differential morbidity and mortality rates in small geographical areas and between social classes, as well as improvements that follow redistribution of services to deprived subpopulations, reflect the general unevenness of socioeconomic development. Other contradictions, often overlooked, also are roots of decreasing returns and escalating costs.

A major contradiction is at an ideologic level; it involves the ideology of medical science and the scientization of social problems. An obvious feature of health systems in advanced capitalist countries since World War II has been the proliferation of complex and extremely expensive medical technology. Examples include radiologic techniques (ranging from the frequent use of chest X-rays, to arteriography, to mammography for breast cancer, to computerized tomographic scanning), radiation therapy, coronary artery bypass surgery, fetal monitoring, and the widespread adoption of intensive care units. These technologic innovations depend on scientific discoveries in medicine and convey a symbolic impression of technical effectiveness. The irony here is that the scientific evaluation of these technologies' actual effectiveness in improving morbidity or mortality has been quite superficial.

Detailed studies evaluating these technologies in clinical practice have begun mainly since the 1970s, when concern about their costliness started to increase. For many of the new technologies, controlled clinical trials have not demonstrated improvements in measurable outcomes. One such example is the coronary care unit (CCU), which uses an extremely expensive collection of technologies to treat patients who suffer heart attacks. As discussed in chapter 4, CCUs proliferated throughout the United States and other countries, without consistent evidence that they were effective in achieving their goal of improving survival. Yet CCUs have gained such widespread acceptance that their dismantling, or even restrictions on their further proliferation, are unthinkable—for the medical profession, regulatory agencies, and the general public.

In short, the ideologic symbolism of science, rather than the strict scientific evaluation of new techniques, has justified the spread of costly medical technology. On the ideologic level, there is a contradiction between what one might call the complex and the mundane. Technologic medicine, grounded in the complexities of scientific technique, carries symbolic trappings of effectiveness. Because of complexity, laypersons and many professionals have difficulty in skeptically appraising high technology. Although methods of evaluating technologic innovation (especially the random controlled trial) are fairly simple, such evaluation often does not occur before the wide adoption of technical innovations.

On the other hand, mundane and simply understood practices—like the reduction of occupational stress and prenatal care for indigent pregnant women—do not convey a symbolic aura of technical effectiveness. The latter mundane practices may exert much more profound impacts on cardiac and perinatal diseases than will CCUs, fetal monitoring, and similar technologies. Yet the conceptual simplicity of such practices, which have little basis in scientific technique, has much to do with their de-emphasis in health-care policy.

Despite their technical simplicity from the standpoint of medical science, mundane practices to improve the public health may be quite complex from the standpoint of the capitalist social system. For instance, although occupational stress may be a primary risk factor in heart disease, its reduction may call for basic changes in the organization of economic production. Likewise, while accessible prenatal care is a major determinant of perinatal survival, the provision of services to indigent and geographically isolated women challenges basic assumptions of private-sector medicine and implies an extension of public-sector financing.

Theorists writing from a Marxist perspective have analyzed the scientization of social problems and the wide social impact of scientific ideology. As Habermas points out, by defining an ever-increasing range of problems as amenable to scientific solutions, scientific ideology tends to remove these issues from critical scrutiny and to depoliticize them:

> Science involves not rationality as such but rather, in the name of rationality, a specific form of acknowledged political domination. Because this sort of rationality extends to the correct choice among strategies, the appropriate application of technologies, and the efficient establishment of systems . . . it removes the total social framework of interests in which strategies are chosen, technologies applied, and systems established, from the scope of reflection and rational reconstruction (9).

The technologic complexity of scientific medicine tends to mystify and depoliticize the social origins of disease and early death. The same technologic orientation diverts attention from simple solutions that would challenge current patterns of social organization, both inside and outside medicine.

Complex and costly technology conveys the aura of effectiveness, restricts critical scrutiny, and is consistent with broader socioeconomic structures of capitalist society. Mundane medical practice, though technically simpler and potentially more effective in many circumstances, may require a direct, political appraisal of the underlying social roots of health problems. All this is not to argue against technologic approaches to certain limited diseases; instead, the purpose is to clarify the forces that encourage expensive technology and discourage inexpensive practice—no matter how ineffective the former and effective the latter may be.

The problem of diminishing returns and escalating costs also rests in part on contradictions in the capitalist economy. Historically, capitalist enterprises face a declining rate of profit from the successful production and sale of a particular type of product. The specific historic details of this contradiction vary by industry, but the overall structure is broadly similar. As the market for a given product becomes saturated, the rate of profit falls. Corporations then seek additional sources of profit by diversifying into new product lines, by expanding into international markets, and by entering entirely different fields. A nonmedical example is the steel industry, which has faced a declining rate of profit from domestic steel production, has closed older steel plants, has opened new plants in foreign countries, and has moved into entirely different areas like petrochemicals where the rate of profit is higher (10).

In the health-care sector, this general economic contradiction motivates corporations to acquire or to start subsidiaries that produce medical goods or provide medical services. Since World War II, a corporate invasion of health care has occurred; the most obvious example is the development and promotion of expensive medical technology. While the effectiveness of this technology in improving morbidity and mortality often remains dubious, its proliferation has provided an expanding source of profit for corporations. Regarding pharmaceuticals, petrochemical companies like American Cyanamid and Dow, as well as previously nonmedical firms like Greyhound, have purchased major drug houses. Ramada Inns and other hotel chains have organized subsidiaries that control networks of proprietary hospitals and nursing homes. Perhaps most important, large corporations have diversified into the provision of direct primary care health services, particularly in the development of health maintenance organizations. Since the mid-1970s, the following corporations involved themselves in planning health maintenance organizations, both for their own employees and as quasi-independent profit-making entities: North American Rockwell, Zenith, DuPont, Texas Instruments, Goodyear, General Electric, Westinghouse, IBM, General Foods, General Mills, Inland Steel, U.S. Steel, Mobil Oil, and Standard Oil of Indiana. The commercialization of health care follows organically from the needs of capital. Structurally, the exploitation of illness for corporate profit is no different from the exploitation of other human frailties, like the needs for food, housing, and transportation.

Corporations are not the only source of escalating health-care costs. The structure of the capitalist state also has contributed to costs, especially through the private-public contradiction. This contradiction, which later chapters discuss in

Figure 1.2   National Health Expenditures, United States, 1960–1995

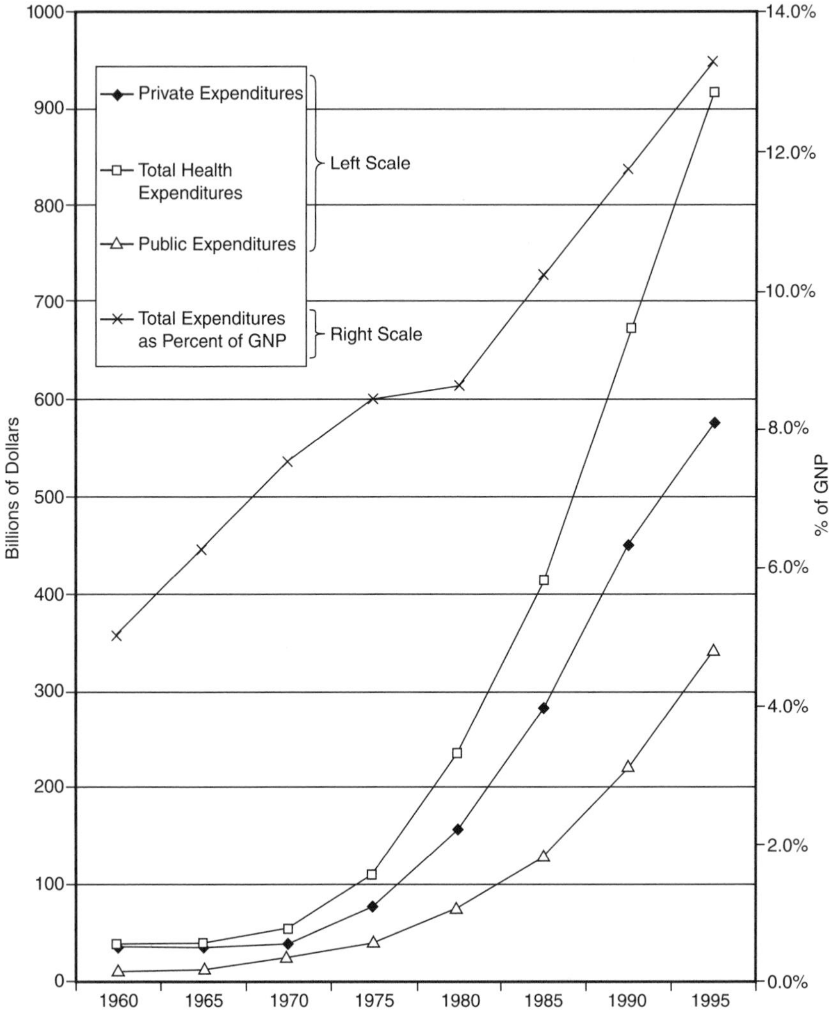

Source: U.S. Bureau of the Census, *Statistical Abstract of the United States* (Washington, D.C.: The Bureau, 1980, 1990, 1991, 1997), pp. 103 (101st ed., 1980), 426 (110th ed., 1990), 431 (111th ed., 1991), 113 and 452 (117th ed., 1997).

greater depth, encourages the public subsidization of private practice and health-care facilities. This subsidization occurs in many ways. For example, in the United States federal grants have supported private hospital construction, frequently resulting in excess bed capacity. Funding for private construction has come not only from the national Hill-Burton program, but also from government agencies offering special-purpose support for specific diseases like cancer and heart disease.

This paradox of increasing public subsidization of the private sector, together with a decline of institutions that are formally part of the public sector, is an inherent feature of the private-public contradiction. Figure 1.2 shows one facet of this contradiction's impact on health-care costs. Both public and total health expenditures began to rise rapidly in 1965, the year that Medicare and Medicaid legislation was enacted. Much of this increase in public expenditures ultimately has gone to private practitioners, hospitals, corporations, and other private facilities.

The corporate invasion of medicine and the private-public contradiction are structural sources of escalating costs that are relatively subtle and seldom discussed—in comparison to the fees of private physicians. This more obvious component of costly medicine is appropriate to emphasize last. The health-care labor force is a caricature of the contradictions of class structure more generally. The enormous discrepancy in income among health workers is analyzed in the next chapter. Here it is important to observe the changes in these income differentials over time and the relation to overall costs for health care. Doctors consistently have maintained the highest level of income among the professions (Table 1.3). Physicians' incomes have risen much more rapidly than those of nonprofessional health workers (Figure 1.3). Several factors have contributed to these excess earnings. Because professional associations historically have limited access to the practice of medicine, the price of services generally has risen without major constraints of competition. Also, doctors directly affect the demand for services through requests for return visits, referrals, consultations, and similar clinical decisions. This "derived demand," created by the producers of services, tends to drive costs upward.

While physicians' earnings are important, it is an error to overrate them. Professional fees have their impact within a nexus of social contradictions that encourage costly practices, inappropriate technology, uncritical acceptance of innovations, corporate exploitation of illness, and the public subsidization of private medicine. Attempting to control health-care costs as a single-sector effort, without reference to these underlying contradictions, is a foolhardly endeavor.

Table 1.3   Median Annual Net Income by Profession, 1994

Professions	*Income ($)*
Physicians	160,000
Attorneys	71,328
Professors (full)	64,860
Engineers	56,191
Accountants	39,815
Teachers	35,764

Source: Bureau of Labor Statistics, March 1998 (http://stats.bls.gov/oco/ocos074.htm. earnings).

Figure 1.3   Income of Selected Health-Care Personnel in the United States, 1950–1995

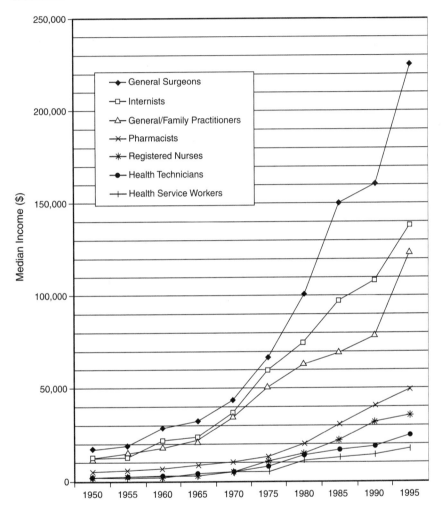

Sources: V. Navarro, *Medicine under Capitalism* (New York: Prodist, 1976); U.S. Bureau of Labor Statistics, *Occupational Outlook Handbook* and on-line data, 1984–1998 (http://stats.bls.gov/oco/ocos074.htm.#earnings).

TECHNOLOGIC PROGRESS AND HUMANISTIC DECLINE

The problem of humanism in medicine is clear from even the most cursory glance at modern health systems. Despite their frequently unproven effectiveness, technologic approaches to health care have become the norm. During the twentieth century, as many have complained, the dominant goals of medicine shifted on balance from caring to curing. The emphasis moved away from nurturant support for a person under physical and emotional stress. Instead, the curing of specific physical abnormalities, through technical means if possible, became a primary goal. Although the curing-caring dichotomy perhaps is too simplistic, it does convey the concern that technical components of modern medicine have tended to overwhelm its humanistic goals.

Some of the most sophisticated critics of medicine's technical effectiveness, like McKeown, have argued that medicine still has an important role to play. In brief, this role is medicine's pastoral function (11). Even if their effectiveness is difficult to prove for large populations, medical professionals can offer nurturance, counseling, and emotional support for clients when they are ill or troubled. This service is analogous to what religious practitioners provided in less secularized societies.

One of the cruel paradoxes of maldistribution, of course, is that even simple technology is inaccessible where needed and underutilized where highly concentrated. The goals of compassion and humanism are beyond reproach; an overemphasis on technologic medicine has tended to impede these goals. The purpose here is to link the problem of humanism to more general social contradictions and to point out some ambiguities of humanism.

In the first place, the historic decline of the caring function in medicine has followed broader changes and contradictions in capitalist societies. Although unrealistic nostalgia about the past is unwarranted, prior medical traditions acknowledged the close emotional relationship between health-care professionals and clients. This emphasis was primary in homeopathy, folk healing, midwifery, and other medical traditions that flourished in the United States and other countries. During the early decades of this century, laboratory-based scientific medicine grew and other traditions became disenfranchised.

These changes inside medicine reflected similar forces that were transforming other facets of society. Engineering approaches that fostered health-care technology also shaped the course of modern industry and the organization of social services. The growth of technologically oriented medicine paralleled the historical consolidation of monopoly capitalism, and these historical trends affected one another. Laboratory-based medicine received financing from capitalist corporations and philanthropy. On the other hand, corporations found in modern medicine a source of profits on an international scale (12). In short, the cure-oriented, engineering approach was an outcome of a long-term historical process that both reflected and reinforced more general developments in capitalism.

A contradiction underlying the problem of humanism involves alienation and the distribution of technical knowledge. Structural sources of alienation in the industrial workplace and in medical care have been quite similar. As Marx pointed out in his early analyses, workers under capitalism lose control over the means of production and must surrender their products to the capitalist. Workers' alienation results when the pride of fashioning a completed product is lost, since capitalists own the facilities needed for manufacture and extract surplus value from the sale of products. Braverman and other analysts have noted the "deskilling" of labor during the twentieth century. As engineering principles have rationalized the work process, the conception of tasks has become separated from their execution. That is, supervisory personnel, usually with more advanced technical training, decide which workers are to carry out what tasks according to predetermined methods. Workers' loss of autonomous decision making, discretion, and creativity within the work process has been a pervasive source of alienation (13). Deskilling and alienation are the contradictory underside of rationalized, managerial control over the work process.

The deskilling of labor has occurred in service work as well as economically "productive" work in industry. In medicine, this process has affected workers in many of the so-called health professions. For nurses and "allied" health workers (laboratory technicians, X-ray technicians, respiratory and occupational therapists, and so forth), formal professionalization has coincided with increasing specialization, fragmentation, and preprogramming of the work process. Caring concern for the totality of patients' social, psychological, and physical problems is not a simple matter when many specialized workers must attend to limited and fragmented tasks. The diversity of these tasks and the variety of health-care workers who carry them out lead to a frequently unintegrated and dissatisfying situation for patients and workers alike. Technologically advanced hospitals are alienating places in which to work, for many of the same structural reasons as are technically advanced factories. This of course does not mean that humanism is impossible in such settings. However, a contradictory work process, one which is alienating while highly rationalized, makes the caring function more difficult.

The importance of caring in medicine is undeniable, and contradictions which impede it are unfortunate. Nevertheless, caring itself has certain ambiguities. Attention to the totality of patients' experience seems a laudable goal of holistic health care. Caring for problems outside the realm of technical medicine, however, tends to "medicalize" a wide range of psychological, social, economic, and political problems. Medicalization is a subtle process, whose negative effects can arise despite health workers' best intentions. Historically, numerous areas of life gradually have fallen under medical control. Examples include issues of sexuality and family life, work dissatisfaction, problems of life cycle (including birth, adolescence, aging, dying, and death), difficulties in the educational system (learning disabilities, maladjustment, and students' psychological distress), environmental pollution, and many other fields.

By participating in these areas, practitioners may believe that they are extending the caring function of the medical role. On the other hand, medicalization has been the subject of a critique that focuses on health workers' expanding role in social control (14). As medical professionals assume responsibility for managing problems beyond the illnesses of individuals, attention shifts away from the underlying structural conditions that often are sources of individual distress. By defining social problems as medical, medicine becomes an institution of social control. Through medicalization, the structural roots of personal distress become mystified and depoliticized. That is, by caring for the nontechnical realm of patients' life experiences, medical practitioners tend to remove these problems as potential objects of organized political action.

Thus, for instance, occupational stress is translated into a doctor's note stating that a patient needs to rest for a week because of muscular tension. Or a worker with black lung receives medical certification of permanent disability. Or a woman's emotional upset about the demands of child care and the boredom of housework leads to a prescription for a minor tranquilizer. Or a young woman on welfare who cannot support her family financially hears a physician's recommendation that she be sterilized after her next delivery. The health professional may feel a positive motivation to care for the patient, in the totality of the patient's experience. In each instance, however, a problem at the level of social structure — stressful work demands, unsafe working conditions, sexism, and poverty — is transformed into an individual problem under medical control.

The medicalization of social problems is not limited to capitalism. One troubling feature of medical practice in the former Soviet Union, during quite different historical periods, has involved similar issues. During the Stalinist period, a physician's certification of illness was the only mechanism by which a worker could be excused from responsibilities in production. Beyond the predictable strains in the doctor-patient relationship, this policy medicalized and diverted attention from a wide range of problems in government, industry, and family life. During more recent years, psychiatric diagnosis and hospitalization became a major technique to defuse political opposition to the Soviet regime (15). Medicalization clearly can occur in the context of socialism, but it is important to recognize the growing impact of this process in advanced capitalist societies. While the engineering approach and structural sources of alienation among health workers have impeded the caring function of modern medicine, the medicalization of social problems has revealed the ambiguities of medical humanism.

CONTRADICTIONS OF REFORM

Linking problems of health care to underlying social contradictions raises the question of political strategy. If health-care reforms do not address the social roots of medical problems, solutions will remain limited and ultimately unsatisfactory. A comprehensive political strategy pointing to revolutionary social change, needless to say, is beyond the scope of this book — however profoundly it is desired. Because of the complexities of advanced capitalist countries, realistic political strategizing aimed at fundamental social change is quite difficult to accomplish, despite many (sometimes dogmatic) attempts to do so.

It is important to acknowledge the contradictions of reform. The quest for progressive change, in the context of capitalism, is often quite difficult because reform can slide into reformism. That is, improved material circumstances may seem beneficial but ultimately may reinforce the status quo by reducing the potential for social conflict. This contradictory quality of reform needs careful attention. When oppressive conditions exist, improvements seem reasonable. However, the history of health and welfare reform in capitalist countries has shown that reforms most often follow social protest, make incremental improvements that do not change overall patterns of oppression, and face cutbacks when protest recedes (16).

A distinction developed many years ago by Gorz clarifies this problem (17). "Reformist reforms" provide small material improvements while leaving intact current political and economic structures. These reforms may reduce discontent for periods of time, while helping to preserve the system in its present form: "A reformist reform is one which subordinates objectives to the criteria of rationality and practicability of a given system and policy. . . . [It] rejects those objectives and demands—however deep the need for them—which are incompatible with the preservation of the system."

"Nonreformist reforms" achieve true and lasting changes in the present system's structures of power and finance. They do not simply modify material conditions; instead, they provide the potential for mass political action. Rather than obscuring sources of exploitation by small incremental improvements, nonreformist reforms expose and highlight structural inequities. Such reforms ultimately increase frustration and political tension in a society; they do not seek to reduce these sources of political energy. As Gorz puts it: "Although we should not reject intermediary reforms (those that do not immediately carry their anti-capitalist logic to its conclusion) it is with the strict proviso that they are to be regarded as a means and not an end, as dynamic phases in a progressive struggle, not as stopping places." From this viewpoint, in health care as in other fields, one must try to discern which reform proposals are reformist and which are nonreformist. One also must take an advocacy role, supporting the latter and opposing the former.

The distinction between reformist and nonreformist reforms is seldom easy. For each problem area discussed in this chapter—profit and safety, maldistribution, diminishing returns and escalating costs, and humanism in medicine—a variety of piecemeal solutions have received consideration. Few of these proposals, as I argue later, address the underlying social contradictions which are root causes of medical problems. It is essential to understand and to criticize piecemeal reformism. It is also necessary to examine carefully the much smaller number of health reforms and progressive directions of health activism that truly challenge broad social contradictions and that heighten the potential for basic social change. Without these links between medicine and social structure, both problems and solutions will continue to float in a haze of confusion and mystification.

2

Social Structures of Medical Oppression

Modern medicine combines liberating potentialities with oppressive realities. Health care aims to free humanity from needless suffering and death, yet contradictions of society create obstacles to this goal. The social organization of medicine also fosters patterns of oppression that are antithetical to medicine's more humane purposes. These patterns within medicine mirror and reproduce oppressive features of the wider society as well.

Structures of oppression that link medicine and society are a major focus of Marxist scholarship in social medicine. The focus is not a new one; similar perspectives date back more than a century. Interruptions of many years have separated major advances in the field. These interruptions have stemmed in part from circumstances discouraging Marxist scholarship and in part from the political priorities of early contributors. Some historical highlights give a background for current work on the social organization of medicine.

HISTORICAL DEVELOPMENT OF THE FIELD

The first major Marxist study of health care was Engels' *The Condition of the Working Class in England* (1), originally published in 1845, three years before Engels coauthored with Marx *The Communist Manifesto* (2). This book described the dangerous working and housing conditions that created ill health. In particular, Engels traced such diseases as tuberculosis, typhoid, and typhus to malnutrition, inadequate housing, contaminated water supplies, and overcrowding. Engels' analysis of health care was part of a broader study of working-class conditions under capitalist industrialization, but his treatment of health problems was to have a profound effect on the emergence of social medicine in Western Europe, particularly on the work of Rudolf Virchow.

37

Virchow's pioneering studies in infectious disease, epidemiology, and social medicine (a term Virchow popularized in Western Europe) appeared with great rapidity after the publication of Engels' book on the English working class. Virchow himself acknowledged Engels' influence on his thought (3). In 1847, based on an investigation of a severe typhus epidemic in rural East Prussia, Virchow recommended a series of profound changes that included increased employment, better wages, local autonomy in government, agricultural cooperatives, and a more progressive taxation structure. Virchow advocated no strictly medical solutions, such as more clinics or hospitals; he saw the origins of ill health in societal problems. The most reasonable approach to epidemics, then, was to change the conditions that permitted them to occur (4). In 1848 he joined the first major working-class revolt in Berlin. During the same year he strongly supported the short-lived spring uprising in Paris (5). In his scientific investigations and in his political practice, Virchow expressed two overriding themes. First, the origin of disease is multifactorial; among the most important factors in causation are the material conditions of people's everyday lives. Second, an effective health-care system cannot limit itself to treating the pathophysiologic disturbances of individual patients. Instead, to be successful, improvements in the health-care system must coincide with fundamental economic, political, and social changes.

After the revolutionary struggles of the late 1840s suffered defeat, Western European governments heightened their conservative and often repressive social policies. Marxist analysis of health care entered a long period of eclipse. With the onset of political reaction, Virchow and his colleagues turned to relatively uncontroversial research in laboratories and to private practice.

During the late nineteenth century, with the work of Ehrlich, Koch, Pasteur, and other prominent bacteriologists, germ theory gained ascendancy and created a profound change in medicine's diagnostic and therapeutic assumptions. A unifactorial model of disease emerged. Medical scientists searched for organisms that caused infections and single lesions in noninfectious disorders. The discoveries of this period undeniably improved medical practice. Still, as numerous investigators have shown, the historical importance of these discoveries has been overrated. For example, the major declines in mortality and morbidity from most infectious diseases preceded rather than followed the isolation of specific etiologic agents and the use of antimicrobial therapy. In Western Europe and the United States, improved outcomes in infections occurred after the introduction of better sanitation, regular sources of nutrition, and other broad environmental changes. In most cases, as discussed in the last chapter, improvements in disease patterns antedated the advances of modern bacteriology (6).

Why did the unifactorial perspective of germ theory achieve such prominence? And why have investigational techniques that assume specific etiology and therapy retained a nearly mythic character in medical science and practice to the present day? A serious historical reexamination of early-twentieth-century medical science, which attempts to answer these questions, has begun only in the past few years. Some preliminary explanations have emerged; they focus on events that led to and followed publication of *The Flexner Report* (7).

During most of this century, *The Flexner Report* held high esteem as the document that helped change modern medicine from quackery to responsible practice. One underlying assumption of the report was that laboratory-based scientific medicine, oriented especially to the concepts and methods of European bacteriology, produced a higher quality and more effective medical practice. Although the comparative effectiveness of various medical traditions (including homeopathy, traditional folk healing, chiropractic, and so forth) had never been subjected to systematic test, the report argued that medical schools not oriented to scientific medicine fostered mistreatment of the public. The report called for the closure or restructuring of schools that were not equipped to teach laboratory-based medicine. The report's repercussions were swift and dramatic. Scientific, laboratory-based medicine became the norm for medical education, practice, research, and analysis.

Historical studies cast doubt on the assumptions in *The Flexner Report* that have comprised the widely accepted dogma of the past half century. They also document the uncritical support that the report's recommendations received from parts of the medical profession and the large private philanthropies (8). At least partly because of these events, the Marxist orientation in medical care stayed in eclipse.

Although some of Virchow's works gained recognition as classics, the multifactorial and politically oriented model that guided his efforts has remained largely buried. Without doubt, Marxist perspectives had important impacts on health care outside western Europe and the United States. For example, Lenin applied these perspectives to the early construction of the Soviet health system. Salvador Allende's treatise on the political economy of health care, written while Allende was working as a public health physician, exerted a major influence on health programs in Latin America. The Canadian surgeon Norman Bethune contributed analyses of tuberculosis and other diseases, as well as direct political involvement, that affected the course of postrevolutionary Chinese medicine. Che Guevara's analysis of the relations among politics, economics, and health care—emerging partially from his experience as a physician—helped shape the Cuban medical system (9).

Partly reflecting political ferment and widespread dissatisfaction with various aspects of modern health systems, serious Marxist scholarship of health care began in Western Europe and spread to the United States. The following sections of this chapter give an overview of the social structures of medical oppression which contemporary Marxist research has examined; later chapters develop these themes in greater detail.

CLASS STRUCTURE

The Marxist definition of social class emphasizes the relations of capitalist economic production. Although a brief summary perhaps oversimplifies, Marxist analysis notes that one group of people, the capitalist class, own or control the means of production: the machines, factories, land, and raw materials necessary to make products for the market. The working class, who do not own or control the means of production, must sell their labor for a wage. But the value of the product that workers produce is always greater than their wage. Workers must give up their product to the capitalist; by losing control of their own productive process, workers become alienated from their labor. Surplus value, the difference between the wage paid to workers and the value of the product they create, is the objective basis of the capitalist's profit. Surplus value also is a structural source of exploitation; it motivates the capitalist to keep wages low, to change the work process (by automation and new technologies, close supervision, lengthened work day or overtime, speedups, and dangerous working conditions), and to resist workers' organized attempts to gain higher wages or more control in the workplace (10). The contradiction between profit and safety, as noted earlier, emerges in large part from the economic relations of class structure.

Although they acknowledge the historical changes that have occurred since Marx's time, contemporary Marxist studies have reaffirmed the presence of highly stratified class structures in advanced capitalist societies and Third World nations. Another topic of great interest is the persistence or reappearance of class structure, usually based on expertise and professionalism, in countries where socialist revolutions have taken place. These theoretical and empirical analyses show that relations of economic production remain a primary basis of class structure.

The health system mirrors the class structure of the broader society (11). The "corporate class" includes the major owners and controllers of wealth. They comprise 1 percent of the population and own 80 percent of all corporate stocks and state and local government bonds; their estimated median annual income in 1997 was $714,000. The "working class," at the opposite end of the scale, makes up about 49 percent of the population. It is composed of manual laborers, service workers, and farm workers, who earn a median income of about $16,500. Between these polar classes are the "upper middle class" (professionals like doctors, lawyers, and so forth, comprising approximately 14 percent of the population and earning about $100,000; and middle-level business executives, 6 percent of the population and earning about $45,000) and the "lower middle class" (shopkeepers, self-employed people, craftsmen, artisans, comprising 7 percent of the population, earning about $22,000; and clerical and sales workers, 23 percent of the population, earning about $19,300 per year). Although these definitions provide summary descriptions of a very complex social reality, they are useful in analyzing manifestations of class structure in the health system.

Control over Health Institutions

Navarro has documented the pervasive control that members of the corporate and upper middle classes exert within the policy-making bodies of North American health institutions (12). These classes predominate on the governing boards of private foundations concerned with health care, private and state medical teaching institutions, and local voluntary hospitals. Only on the boards of state teaching institutions and voluntary hospitals do members of the lower middle class or working class gain any appreciable representation; even there, the participation from these classes falls far below their proportion in the general population. Community-based research has documented corporate dominance of health institutions in many parts of the United States. Navarro has argued, based partly on these observations, that control over health institutions reflects the same patterns of class dominance that have arisen in other areas of North American economic and political life.

Stratification within Health Institutions

As members of the upper middle class, physicians occupy the highest stratum among workers in health institutions. Comprising about 7 percent of the health labor force, physicians receive a median net income (approximately $160,000 in 1995) that places them in the upper 5 percent of the income distribution of the United States. Under physicians and professional administrators are members of the lower middle class: nurses, physical and occupational therapists, and technicians. They make up approximately 29 percent of the health labor force, are mostly women, and early about $35,000. At the bottom of institutional hierarchies are clerical workers, aides, orderlies, and kitchen and janitorial personnel, who are the working class of the health system. They have an income of about $18,000 per year, represent 54 percent of the health labor force, and are 84 percent female and 30 percent black (13). The forces of racism, sexism, elitism, and professionalism divide health workers from one another and prevent them from realizing common interests. These patterns affect physicians, nurses, and technical and service workers who comprise the fastest growing segment of the health labor force (14).

Occupational Mobility

Class mobility into professional positions is quite limited. Investigations of physicians' class backgrounds in both Britain and the United States have shown a consistently small representation of the lower middle and working classes among medical students and practicing doctors (15). In the United States, historical documentation is available to trace changes in class mobility during the twentieth century. Despite some improvements for other disadvantaged groups like blacks and women, recruitment of working-class medical students has been very limited since shortly after publication of *The Flexner Report*. In 1920, 12 percent of medical students came from working-class families, and this percentage has stayed almost exactly the same until the present time.

In summary, class structure in the health system parallels the class structure of the entire society. Members of the corporate and upper middle class predominate in the decision-making bodies of North American health institutions. Within those institutions, workers are highly stratified. Mobility into the medical profession by individuals from working-class or lower middle-class families remains limited. As I consider later, strategies for changing the health-care system must take into account the broader class structure of the society.

MONOPOLY CAPITAL

During the past century, economic capital has become more concentrated in a smaller number of companies, the monopolies. Monopoly capital has emerged in essentially all advanced capitalist nations, where the process of monopolization has reinforced private corporate profit. Monopoly capital also has become a prominent feature of most capitalist health systems. Contributing to the problems of medical maldistribution and rising costs of care, monopoly capital manifests itself in several ways.

Medical Centers

Since about 1910, a continuing growth of medical centers has occurred, usually in affiliation with universities. Capital is highly concentrated in these medical centers, which are heavily oriented to advanced technology. Practitioners have received training where technology is available and specialization is highly valued. Partly as a result, health workers are often reluctant to practice in areas without easy access to medical centers. The nearly unrestricted growth of medical centers has heightened the maldistribution of health workers and facilities throughout the United States and within regions.

Emphasis on science and technology led to an industrialized economic base for modern medicine and a greater use of hospitals. A technologic imperative emerged, motivating the application of high technology to many health problems. *The Flexner Report* played a crucial part in the development of capital-intensive medical centers that increasingly relied on expensive machines and equipment, relative to human labor. The medical schools that remained open after the report's impact were those capable of attracting and maintaining a large enough capital base to support extensive laboratory facilities. Medical traditions that received disfavor and eventual disenfranchisement generally were not oriented to advanced scientific methods and did not require concentrated capital or technology (16)

Finance Capital

Monopoly capital also has been apparent in the position of banks, trusts, and insurance companies, the largest profit-making corporations under capitalism. For example, in the late 1990s, among private life and health insurance companies whose stock was publicly traded on the New York Stock Exchange, five companies (Metropolitan Life, CIGNA, Aetna, Nationwide, and Principal Financial Group) amassed 54 percent of the revenues accumulated by the top 26 of these companies. Among "mutual" life and health insurance companies, which technically are owned by policyholders, one company (Prudential) accumulated 31 percent of the revenues collected by the top 16 companies of this category. Metropolitan Life and Prudential each controlled more assets than General Motors, Standard Oil of New Jersey, or International Telephone and Telegraph (17).

Finance capital figures prominently in health reform proposals (18); most plans for national health insurance would permit a continuing role for the insurance industry. Moreover, corporate investment in managed care organizations has increased, partly because of the assumption that national health reform will continue to ensure the profitability of these ventures.

The "Medical-Industrial Complex"

The "military-industrial complex" has provided a model for industrial penetration into the health system, popularized by the term "medical-industrial complex." Investigations have emphasized that the exploitation of illness for private profit is a primary feature of the health systems in advanced capitalist societies. Many reports have criticized the pharmaceutical and medical equipment industries for advertising and marketing practices, price and patent collusion, and promotion of drugs before their safety is tested (19).

These industries have played a prominent role in developing and promoting expensive therapeutic innovations in cardiovascular disease (coronary care units and coronary artery bypass surgery), radiologic studies in hypertension and head trauma, fetal monitoring, computerized tomographic scanning, and so forth. The medical profession has tended to adopt technologically advanced diagnostic and treatment modalities without controlled trials demonstrating their effectiveness. Industrial growth in the health system comprises a rapidly expanding sector of the overall economy of the United States.

THE STATE

Because the state encompasses the major institutions of political power, its strategic importance is obvious. The state acts generally to repress revolutionary social change or political action that threatens the present system in any fundamental way. After socialist revolutions, the state apparatus persists, but with greatly modified functions. Before focusing on health care, a brief overview and definition of the state are necessary.

Marxist theories of the state emphasize government's crucial role in protecting the capitalist economic system and the interests of the capitalist class. The famous homily of *The Communist Manifesto* was: "the state is the executive committee of the bourgeoisie." Lenin concluded that the capitalist class would intervene forcibly to block any electoral victory that seriously threatened the private enterprise system. Other analysts have studied the structural patterns that preserve the dominance of the capitalist class over state policies, the mechanisms by which the state eases the recurrent economic crises of the capitalist system, and ideologic techniques by which the state reinforces popular acquiescence (20).

In this context the following definition, though limited by the subject's complexity, is appropriate. The state comprises the interconnected public institutions that act to preserve the capitalist economic system and the interests of the capitalist class. The definition includes the executive, legislative, and judicial branches of government; the military; and the criminal justice system—all of which hold varying degrees of coercive power. It also encompasses relatively noncoercive institutions within the educational, public welfare, and health-care systems. Through such noncoercive institutions, the state offers services or conveys ideologic messages that legitimate the capitalist system. Especially in periods of economic crisis, the state can use these same institutions to provide public subsidization of private enterprise.

The Private-Public Contradiction

The health system has two subsectors. The "private sector" is based in private practice and companies that manufacture medical products or control finance capital. The "public sector," as part of the state, operates through direct public expenditures and employs health workers in public institutions. Examples of institutions in the public sector of the United States are the Public Health Service, Indian Health Service, the Veterans Administration hospitals, county and municipal hospitals, public mental hospitals, and the Medicare and Medicaid systems. Despite the distinction between public and private sectors, the state frequently can channel public money or other capital into the private sector; this tendency creates a potential for abuse that I will discuss shortly.

Nations vary greatly in the private-public duality. In the United States, a dominant private sector coexists with a large public sector. The public sector is even larger in Great Britain and Scandinavia. In Cuba, the private sector essentially has disappeared.

The private sector, as mentioned in the last chapter, tends to drain public resources and health workers' time, to the benefit of private profit and to the detriment of patients using the public sector. This framework has helped explain some of the problems that have arisen in such countries as Great Britain and Chile, where private sectors persisted after the enactment of national health services. In these countries, practitioners have faced financial incentives to increase the scope of private practice, which they often have conducted within public hospitals or clinics. In the United States, the expansion of public payment programs such as Medicare and Medicaid has led to increased public subsidization of private practice, private hospitals, and the private insurance industry, as well as abuses of these programs by individual practitioners (21). This subsidization has heightened the problem of escalating costs for medical care.

Similar problems have undermined other public health programs (22). These programs frequently have obtained finances through regressive taxation, placing low-income taxpayers at a relative disadvantage. Likewise, the deficiencies of the Blue Cross and Blue Shield insurance plans have derived largely from the failure of public regulatory agencies to control payments to practitioners and hospitals in the private sector. Most proposals for national health insurance in the United States also would use public funds to reinforce and strengthen the private sector by ensuring payment for hospitals and individual physicians and possibly by permitting a continued role for commercial insurance companies.

Throughout the United States the problems of the private-public contradiction tend to worsen medical maldistribution. Private hospitals often transfer uninsured and low-income patients to public municipal or country hospitals. Although "dumping" of unstable patients from the private to the public sector is prohibited by federal legislation, stabilized patients can be transferred; this situation has created major financial burdens for public hospitals. Public hospitals in most large cities also have faced cutbacks, closure, or conversion to private ownership and control. The conversion of public hospitals to private control often has involved medical schools, which in many cases have assumed administrative and professional responsibility for these hospitals. Some medical schools have encountered financial difficulties in these arrangements; most schools, however, have benefited by public payment for low-income patients. In general, the public sector is weakened by the diverting of funds and professional resources to privately controlled facilities. Low-income patients face greater problems of access when public hospitals and clinics convert to private control, even when this conversion involves assumption of responsibility by medical schools (23).

General Functions of the State within the Health System

The state's functions in the health system have increased in scope and complexity. In the first place, through the health system, the state acts to legitimate the capitalist economic system based in private enterprise. The history of public health and welfare programs shows that state expenditures usually rise during periods of social protest and decrease as unrest becomes less widespread (24). For instance, in the early 1970s public opinion surveys uncovered a profound level of dissatisfaction with the role of business interests in government policies. Citizens who thought something was deeply wrong with their country and who expressed disenchantment with government became a national majority (25). Under such circumstances, the state's predictable response has been to expand health and other welfare programs. These incremental reforms, at least in part, reduce the legitimacy crisis of the capitalist system by restoring confidence that the system can meet people's basic needs. The cycles of political attention devoted to national health insurance in the United States appear to parallel cycles of popular discontent. Cutbacks in public health services to low-income patients in the 1980s and 1990s have followed the decline of social protest by low-income groups.

The second major function of the state in the health system is to protect and reinforce the private sector more directly. As previously noted, most plans for national health reform permit a prominent role and continued profits for the private insurance industry, particularly in the administration of payments, record keeping, and data collection. Corporate participation in new health initiatives sponsored by the state—including managed care organizations, preventive screening programs, computerized components of professional review organizations, algorithm and protocol development for paraprofessional training, and audiovisual aids for patient education programs—is providing major sources of expanded profit.

A third and subtler function of the state is the reinforcement of dominant frameworks in scientific and clinical medicine that are consistent with the capitalist economic system and the suppression of alternative frameworks that might threaten the system. The United States government has provided generous funding for research on the pathophysiology and treatment of specific disease entities. As critics even within government have recognized, the disease-centered approach has reduced the level of analysis to the individual organism and, often inappropriately, has stimulated the search for unifactorial rather than multifactorial causation. More recently, analyses emphasizing the importance of individual "life-style" as a cause of disease have received prominent attention from state agencies in the United States and Canada. Clearly, individual differences in personal habits do affect health in all societies. On the other hand, the life-style argument, perhaps even more than the earlier emphasis on specific cause, obscures important sources of illness and disability in the capitalist work process and industrial environment; it also puts the burden of the health squarely on the individual, rather than seeking collective solutions to health problems.

The issues that the state has downplayed in its research and development programs are worth noting. For example, based on available data, it is estimated that in Western industrialized societies environmental factors are involved in the etiology of approximately 80 percent of all cancers. There is now exhaustive documentation of common occupational carcinogens. Such findings are threatening to the current organization of capitalist production; they have received little attention or support from state agencies. Partly as a result, occupational and environmental health problems have persisted and deepened. A framework for clinical investigation that links disease directly to the structure of capitalism is likely to face indifference and active discouragement from the state.

Limits and Mechanisms of State Intervention

Although the state's activity in the health system has increased in all capitalist societies, state intervention faces certain structural limits. Simply summarized, these limits restrict state intervention to policies and programs that will not conflict in fundamental ways with capitalist economic processes based on private profit, or with the concrete interests of the capitalist class during specific historical periods.

"Negative selection mechanisms" are forms of state intervention that exclude innovations or activities that challenge the capitalist system (26). For example, agencies of the state may enact occupational health legislation and enforcement regulations. However, such reforms will not reach a level strict enough to interfere with profitability in specific industries. Nor will state takeover of industries responsible for occupational or environmental diseases occur to any major degree.

Negative selection also applies to the potential nationalization of the health system as a whole. In most capitalist societies, the state generally has opposed structural changes that infringe on private medical practice, private control of most hospitals, and the profitability of the pharmaceutical, medical equipment, insurance, and other industries operating in the health system. Therefore, the state's attempts to control health-care costs have been inconsistent and largely unsuccessful. While excluding nationalization through negative selection, the state sponsors incremental reforms that control excesses in each of these spheres, thus maintaining the legitimacy of the whole. As an example of negative selection, congressional deliberations in the United States systematically exclude serious consideration of a national health service (as opposed to national health insurance) that might question the appropriateness of private medical practice or the nationalization of hospitals. Another example is governmental regulation of the drug and insurance industries; aside from its erratic effects, state regulation rules out public ownership of these industries.

The state also can use "positive selection mechanisms" that promote and sponsor policies strengthening the private enterprise system and the interests of capital. As discussed earlier, positive selection has involved sponsorship of biomedical research that assumes unifactorial etiology or, more recently, the "life-style" analysis. Most important, state agencies tend to favor financial reforms, like health insurance, that would ensure the stability of the private sector in the health system. The state's positive selection of financial reforms contrasts sharply with the exclusion of organizational reforms that potentially might change the broader political and economic structures of the present system.

MEDICAL IDEOLOGY

Ideology is an interlocking set of ideas and doctrines that form the distinctive perspective of a social group. The events of history, in the Marxist perspective, emerge mainly from economic forces; this economic determinacy gives causal primacy to the sphere of production and class conflict. Ideology, however, helps sustain and reproduce the social relations of production and, especially, patterns of domination. Institutions of civil society, such as the educational system, family, mass media, and organized religion, promulgate ideas and beliefs that support the established order (27).

Along with other institutions, medicine fosters an ideology that helps maintain and reproduce class structure and social domination. Medicine's ideologic features do not diminish the efforts of individuals who use currently accepted methods in their clinical work and research; nevertheless, medical ideology has major ramifications beyond medicine itself. Studies of medical ideology have identified several key components:

Disturbances of Biological Homeostasis Are Equivalent to Breakdowns of Machines

Modern medical science views the human organism mechanistically. The health professional's advanced training permits the recognition of specific causes and treatments for physical disorders. The mechanistic view of the human body deflects attention from multifactorial origin, especially causes of disease that derive from the environment, work processes, or social stress; it also reinforces a general ideology that attaches positive evaluation to industrial technology under specialized control. This ideologic component helps justify costly and complex medical approaches that depend on advanced technology, as opposed to mundane but potentially more effective practices.

Disease Is a Problem of the Individual Human Being

The unifactorial model of disease contains reductionist assumptions, because it focuses on disruptions in individual biology rather than on the illness-generating conditions of society. A similar reductionist approach has emphasized sources of illness in life-style. In both cases, the responsibility for disease and cure rests at the individual rather than at the collective level. This orientation deflects attention from class structure and relations of production, even in their implications for health and illness.

Science Permits the Rational Control of Human Beings

The natural sciences have led to a greater control over nature. Similarly, it is often assumed that modern medicine, by correcting defects of individuals, can enhance their controllability. The quest for a reliable workforce has been one motivation for the support of modern medicine by capitalist economic interests. Physicians' certification of illness historically has expanded or contracted to meet industry's need for labor. Thus, medicine is seen as contributing to the rational governance of society, and managerial principles increasingly are applied to the organization of the health system (28).

Many Spheres of Life Are Appropriate for Medical Management

This ideologic assumption has led to an expansion of medicine's social control function; many behaviors that do not adhere to society's norms have become appropriate for management by health professionals. "Medicalization," as discussed earlier, creates ambiguities of caring and humanism. The medical management of behavioral difficulties, such as hyperactivity and aggression, often coincides with attempts to find specific biologic lesions associated with these behaviors. Historically, medicine's social control function has expanded in periods of intense social protest or rapid social change (29).

Medical Science Is Both Esoteric and Excellent

According to this ideologic principle, medical science involves a body of advanced knowledge and standards of excellence in both research and practice. Because scientific knowledge is esoteric, a group of professionals tend to hold elite positions. Lacking this knowledge, ordinary people are dependent on professionals for interpretation of medical data. The health system therefore reproduces patterns of domination by expert decision makers in the workplace, government, and many other areas of social life. The ideology of excellence helps justify these patterns, although the quality of much medical research and practice is far from excellent; this paradox has been characterized as "the excellent deception" in medicine (30). Ironically, a similar ideology of excellence has justified the emergence of new class hierarchies based on expertise in some countries, such as the former Soviet Union, that have undergone socialist revolutions. Other countries, such as the People's Republic of China, have cyclically tried to overcome these ideologic assumptions and to develop a less esoteric "people's medicine."

In the mass media, medical ideology appears in public statements by professional leaders and by state and corporate officials whose organizations regulate or sponsor medical activities. More important, health professionals also express ideologic messages in their face-to-face interaction with patients. The doctor-patient relationship as an arena for the transmission of ideologic messages is the subject of a later chapter.

INTERNATIONAL COMPARISONS

Structures of medical oppression gain greater clarity from international comparisons for several reasons. Of prime importance is the interdependency of nations.

From this perspective, economically advanced countries tend to dominate countries of the Third World. Imperialism, whether overt or subtle, is a cause of underdevelopment and maldistribution of medical resources. The health problems of underdeveloped countries in large part reflect international economic forces. Second, several countries that have passed through the transition to socialism from a position of underdevelopment have made dramatic changes in their health systems. These changes, and the political struggles that have accompanied them, are pertinent for strategy and policy making. Third, capitalist nations outside the United States have instituted health services or insurance programs. Comparative study clarifies the potential pitfalls of health reform proposals in the United States.

Health Care and Imperialism

Although it is a complex, multifaceted phenomenon, imperialism may be defined as capital's expansion beyond national boundaries as well as the social, political, and economic effects of this expansion. Imperialism has achieved many advantages for economically dominant nations. Marxist critiques have dealt with imperialist ventures of both advanced capitalist countries and socialist superpowers (including the "social imperialism" of the former Soviet Union). Health care has played an important role in several phases of imperialism.

One basic feature of imperialism is the extraction of raw materials and human capital, which move from Third World nations to economically dominant countries. The "underdevelopment of health" in the Third World follows inevitably from this depletion of natural and human resources (31). The extraction of wealth limits underdeveloped countries' ability to construct effective health systems. Many Third World countries face a net loss of health workers who migrate to economically dominant nations after expensive training at home.

Through imperialism, corporations also seek a cheap labor force. Workers' efficiency was one important goal of public health programs sponsored abroad, especially in Latin America and Asia, by philanthropies closely tied to expanding industries in the United States (32). Moreover, population-control programs initiated by the United States and other dominant countries have sought a more reliable participation by women in the labor force. At the same time, workers abroad who are employed by multinational corporations face high risks of occupational disease.

Another thrust of imperialism is the creation of new markets for products manufactured in dominant nations and sold in the Third World. This process, enhancing the accumulation of capital by multinational corporations, is nowhere clearer than in the pharmaceutical and medical equipment industries (33). The monopolistic character of these industries, as well as the stultifying impact that imported technology has exerted on local research and development, has led to the advocacy of nationalized drug and equipment formularies in several countries.

Imperialism reinforces international class relations, and medicine contributes to this phenomenon. As in the United States, medical professionals in the Third World most often come from higher-income families; even when they do not, they frequently view medicine as a route of upward mobility. As a result, medical professionals tend to ally themselves with the capitalist class—the "national bourgeoisie"—of Third World countries. They also frequently support cooperative links between the local capitalist class and business interests in economically dominant countries. The class position of health professionals has led them to resist social change that would threaten current class structure, either nationally or internationally. Similar patterns have emerged in some postrevolutionary societies. In the former USSR, professionals' class position, based on expertise, caused them to act as a relatively conservative group in periods of social change. Elitist tendencies in the postrevolutionary Cuban profession also have received criticism (34).

Frequently imperialism goes beyond economic domination to encompass military conquest. Despite its humanistic profile, medicine has contributed to the military efforts of European countries and the United States. For instance, health workers have assumed armed or paramilitary roles in Indochina and Northern Africa; health institutions also have taken part as bases for counterinsurgency and intelligence operations in Latin America and Asia (35).

Health Care and the Transition to Socialism

The number of nations undergoing revolutions against imperialism has increased, particularly in Asia and Africa, but also in parts of Latin America, the Caribbean, and southern Europe. Many of these revolutions have aimed toward the attainment of socialism. Socialism is no panacea; problems have arisen in all countries that have achieved socialist revolutions. The difficulties that have emerged in postrevolutionary countries are deeply troubling to Marxists and have been the subject of intensive analysis and debate.

On the other hand, socialism can produce major modifications in health-system organization, nutrition, sanitation, housing, and other services. Social structural change can lead, through a sometimes complex chain of events, to remarkable improvements in health. The morbidity and mortality trends that followed socialist revolutions in such countries as Cuba and China now are well known (36). The transition to socialism in every case has resulted in reorganization of the health system with emphasis on better distribution of health-care facilities and personnel. Local political groups in the commune, neighborhood, or workplace have assumed responsibility for health education and preventive medicine programs.

Class struggle continues throughout the transition to socialism. During Chile's brief period of socialist government, many professionals resisted democratization of health institutions and supported the capitalist class that previously and subsequently ruled the country (37). Countries like China and Cuba eliminated the major source of social class: the private ownership of the means of production. However, as mentioned previously, new class relations began to emerge that were based on differential expertise. Health professionals received larger salaries and maintained higher levels of prestige and authority. One focus of the Chinese Cultural Revolution was the struggle against the new class of experts that had gained power in the health system and elsewhere in the society. Later, after Mao's death, prior hierarchies reemerged. Other countries, including Cuba, have not confronted these new class relations as explicitly.

Improved health care remains linked to the general level of economic development (38). In some African nations, for instance, severe poverty hampers organizational and programmatic changes. Countries like Tanzania and Mozambique have undertaken health planning that ties general economic development to innovations in health care. Such planning is particularly important in postrevolutionary societies emerging from the prior deprivations of imperialism.

Contradictions of Capitalist Reform

While retaining the essential features of their capitalist economic systems, several nations in Europe and North America have instituted major reforms in their health systems. Some reforms have produced beneficial effects that policy makers view as possible models for the United States. Marxist studies, although acknowledging many improvements, have revealed shortcomings that appear inherent in reforms attempted within capitalist systems. These studies' conclusions are not optimistic about the success of proposed reforms in the United States. A crucial problem is that reforms attempted within the context of capitalism generally remain reformist in character; that is, they do not change broad structures of political and economic dominance. Nonreformist reforms seem much more difficult to achieve.

Great Britain's national health service has attracted great interest (39). Serious problems have balanced many of the undeniable benefits that the British health service has obtained; chief among these problems is the professional and corporate control that has persisted since the service's inception. Decision-making bodies contain large proportions of professional specialists, bankers, and corporate executives, many of whom have direct or indirect links with pharmaceutical and medical equipment industries.

The private-public contradiction has remained a source of conflict in several countries that have established national health services or universal insurance programs. Use of public facilities for private practice has generated criticism focusing on public subsidization of the private sector. In Britain, for example, this concern (along with more general organizational problems that impeded comprehensive care) was a primary motivation for several reorganizations of the national health service. In Chile, the attempt to reduce the use of public facilities for private practice led to crippling opposition from the organized medical profession. The private-public contradiction will continue to create conflict and limit progress when countries institute national health services while preserving a strong private sector.

The limits of state intervention also have become clearer from the example of

Sweden (40). Here, national health insurance has preserved some private practice and extensive corporate dealings in pharmaceuticals and medical equipment. Maldistribution of facilities and personnel has persisted, and costs have remained high. The accomplishments of Sweden's reforms cannot pass beyond the state's responsibility for protecting private enterprise. This observation leads to skepticism about health reforms in the United States that rely on private market mechanisms and that do not challenge the broader structures within which the health system is situated.

ILLNESS-GENERATING SOCIAL CONDITIONS

Structures of medical oppression are patterns within medicine that both mirror and reinforce oppressive conditions of society. While social contradictions impede the solution of major health problems, the social organization of medicine tends to reproduce the same broad contradictions. Social class, monopoly capital, the state, ideology, imperialism, and underdevelopment are structures of oppression that penetrate medicine and that medicine helps replicate. The interrelationships between medicine and social structure also include more direct destructive effects on health itself.

Social conditions that generate illness and early death comprise the focus of social epidemiology. The field's antecedents include the classic research of Engels, Virchow, and the nineteenth-century school of social medicine in Europe. Social epidemiology, sometimes called historical materialist epidemiology, relates patterns of death and disease to the political, economic, and social structures of society. The field emphasizes changing historical patterns of disease and the specific material circumstances under which people live and work. These studies try to transcend the individual level of analysis to find how historical and social forces, at least in part, determine health and disease. Several major findings are worth noting.

Social Class and Economic Cycles

The incidence and prevalence of mental illness follow periods of economic growth or recession. The relations are complex and differ by social class. There is also evidence which links economic cycles, particularly those that involve expanding or contracting employment, to general mortality and morbidity trends among various social classes and age groups (41).

Stress

Previous interest in stress usually has focused on the individual life cycle or family unit. Historical materialist epidemiology shifts the level of analysis to stressful forms of social organization connected to capitalist production and industrialization. Hypertension rates, for example, consistently have increased with the disruption of stable social communities and organization of work that is hierarchically controlled and time pressured. These observations apply to countries that have followed capitalist lines of development and socialist countries that have industrialized rapidly (42). Similar investigations have linked forms of social organization to coronary heart disease and cancer (43).

Work and Profit

Marxist studies in occupational health emphasize the contradiction between profit and safety. Beyond the studies discussed in the first chapter, specific research has clarified the illness-generating conditions of the workplace and profit system in reference to diseases such as asbestosis and mesothelioma, complications of vinyl chloride, drug abuse, and accidents (44). Observations of occupational health practices in socialist countries have shown that, although similar problems can persist, rapid improvements are possible when private profit is removed as a disincentive to change (45).

Racism and Sexism

Studies in this area focus on the interplay among race, sex, class structure, and work processes. Higher rates of hypertension among blacks and Hispanics in the United States, for example, have been attributed in part to the impact of racism. Genetic screening programs for such diseases as sickle-cell anemia have received criticism for implicitly racist assumptions resembling prior efforts in eugenics. The varying work experiences of women and men are related to their mortality rates and life expectancy. Historically, women's use of health facilities and the attitudes of medical practitioners toward women's problems have depended largely on women's class positions. This conclusion is especially evident from the history of the birth control movement, psychiatric diagnosis, and gynecologic surgery. The unique health hazards and difficulties that women face as housewives and paid workers are attracting greater attention (46).

One unifying theme in this field is modern medicine's limitations. Traditional epidemiology has searched for causes of morbidity and mortality that are amenable to medical intervention. Although it acknowledges the importance of traditional techniques, historical materialist epidemiology has found causes of disease and death that derive from social conditions. Structures of medical oppression encompass both the social organization of medicine and illness-generating conditions beyond the reach of health care alone. Because of the close linkages between medicine and society, attempts to reform medicine must be tied to wider strategies of change in the social order.

3

The Social Origins of Illness: A Neglected History

Conditions of society that generate illness and mortality are a central focus of social medicine, but a focus that has been largely forgotten and rediscovered with each succeeding generation. Now, when disease-producing features of the workplace and environment threaten the survival of humanity and other life forms, it is not surprising that such problems would receive attention. Social contradictions, especially the contradiction between profit and safety, foster illness and impede change. These issues, however, did not emerge recently; there is a long history of research and analysis that has been neglected, despite its relevance to the current situation.

Three people—Friedrich Engels, Rudolf Virchow, and Salvador Allende— made major early contributions to the understanding of social origins of illness (1). Although other writers also have examined this topic, the works of Engels, Virchow, and Allende are important in several respects. Engels and Virchow provided analyses of the impact of social conditions on health that essentially created the perspective of social medicine. Both men were writing about these issues during the tumultuous years of the 1840s; both took decisive—though quite divergent— personal actions which they saw as leading to the correction of the conditions they described. Allende's key work appeared during a later historical period, the 1930s, and a different geopolitical context. While Engels and Virchow documented the impact of early capitalism, Allende focused on capitalist imperialism and underdevelopment. Although little known in North America and Western Europe, Allende's studies in social medicine have exerted a great influence on health planning and strategy in Latin America and elsewhere in the Third World.

The writings of Engels, Virchow, and Allende explicitly or implicitly adopted a Marxist framework to investigate the social origins of illness. While they conveyed certain unifying themes, they also diverged in major ways, especially regarding the structures of oppression that cause disease, the social contradictions that inhibit change, and directions of reform. A look backward to these prior works gives a historical perspective to issues that today gain even more urgency.

55

FRIEDRICH ENGELS

Engels wrote his first major book, *The Condition of the Working Class in England*, under circumstances whose ironies now are well known (2). Between 1842 and 1844, Engels was working in Manchester as a middle-level manager in a textile mill of which his father was co-owner. Engels carried out his managerial duties in a perfunctory manner while immersing himself in English working-class life. The richness of Engels' treatment of working-class existence has attracted much critical attention, both sympathetic and belligerent (3). Engels' analysis of the social origins of illness, though central to his account of working-class conditions, has received relatively little notice.

In this book Engels' theoretical position was unambiguous. For working-class people the roots of illness and early death lay in the organization of economic production and in the social environment (4). British capitalism, Engels argued, forced working-class people to live and work under circumstances that inevitably caused sickness; this situation was not hidden but was well known to the capitalist class. The contradiction between profit and safety worsened health problems and stood in the way of necessary improvements.

Besides his own personal observations, Engels' work followed and made use of public reports to the Poor Law Commission in Britain. These reports appeared in the early 1840s and culminated in 1842 with the appearance of Chadwick's *Inquiry into the Sanitary Condition of the Labouring Population of Great Britain*. In this report, Chadwick documented the connections among economic deprivation, environmental pollution, disease, and mortality. Oriented partly to the philosophic tradition of Benthamite Utilitarianism, Chadwick emphasized such etiologic factors as unclean water supplies and the careless disposal of excreta and refuse. Correcting these problems, Chadwick argued, would enhance the common good of all groups in society (5). Engels analyzed problems similar to those Chadwick discussed. Engels' theoretical perspective, however, focused on the profound impact of class structure itself and the difficulties of change while the effects of social class persisted.

Engels first considered the effects of environmental toxins. He claimed that the poorly planned housing in working-class districts did not permit adequate ventilation of toxic substances. Workers' apartments surrounded a central courtyard without direct spatial communication to the street. Carbon-containing gases from combustion and human respiration remained within living quarters. Because disposal systems did not exist for human and animal wastes, these materials decomposed in courtyards, apartments, or the street; severe air and water pollution resulted.

Next Engels discussed infectious diseases caused in large part by poor housing conditions; tuberculosis, an airborne infection, was his major focus. He noted that overcrowding and insufficient ventilation contributed to high mortality from tuberculosis in London and other industrial cities. Typhus, carried by lice, also spread because of bad sanitation and ventilation.

Turning to nutrition, Engels drew connections among social conditions, nutrition, and disease. He emphasized the expense and chronic shortages of food supplies for urban workers. Lack of proper storage facilities at markets led to contamination and spoilage. Problems of malnutrition were especially acute for children. Engels discussed scrofula as a disease related to poor nutrition; this view antedated the discovery of bovine tuberculosis as the major cause of scrofula and pasteurization of milk as a preventive measure. He also described the skeletal deformities of rickets as a nutritional problem, long before the medical finding that dietary deficiency of vitamin D caused rickets.

Engels' analysis of alcoholism was an account of the social forces that fostered excessive drinking. In Engels' view alcoholism was a response to the miseries of working-class life. Lacking other sources of emotional gratification, workers turned to alcohol. Individual workers could not be held responsible for alcohol abuse. Instead, alcoholism ultimately was the responsibility of the capitalist class:

> Liquor is their [workers'] only source of pleasure. . . . The working man . . . *must* have something to make work worth his trouble, to make the prospect of the next day endurable. . . . Drunkenness has here ceased to be a vice, for which the victims can be held responsible. . . . They who have degraded the working man to a mere object have the responsibility to bear (6).

For Engels, alcoholism was rooted firmly in social structure; the attribution of responsibility to the individual workers was misguided. If the experience of deprived social conditions caused alcoholism, the solution involved basic change in those conditions rather than treatment programs focusing on the individual.

In this context Engels analyzed structures of oppression within the social organization of medicine. He emphasized the maldistribution of medical personnel. According to Engels, working-class people contended with the "impossibility of employing skilled physicians in cases of illness" (7). Infirmaries that offered charitable services met only a small portion of people's needs for professional attention. Engels criticized the patent remedies containing opiates that apothecaries provided for childhood illnesses. High rates of infant mortality in working-class districts, Engels hypothesized, were explainable partly by lack of medical care and partly by the promotion of inappropriate medications.

Engels next undertook an epidemiologic investigation of mortality rates and social class, using demographic statistics compiled by public health officials. He showed that mortality rates were inversely related to social class, not only for entire cities but also within specific geographic districts of cities. He noted that in Manchester childhood mortality was much greater among working-class children than among "children of the higher classes." In addition Engels commented on the cumulative effects of class and urbanism on childhood mortality. He cited data that demonstrated higher death rates from epidemics of infectious diseases like smallpox, measles, scarlet fever, and whooping cough among working-class children. For Engels, such features of urban life as crowding, poor housing, inadequate sanitation, and pollution combined with social class position in the etiology of disease and early mortality.

The social causes of accidents drew Engels' indignation. He linked accidents to the exploitation of workers, lack of suitable child care, and the consequent neglect of children. Because both husband and wife needed to work outside the home in most working-class families, and because no facilities for child care were available when parents were at work, children were subject to such accidents as falls, drowning, or burns. Engels noted that deaths from children's burns were especially frequent during the winter because of unsupervised heating facilities. Industrial accidents were another source of concern, especially the risks that industrial workers faced because of machinery. The most common accidents involved loss of fingers, hands, or arms by contact with unguarded machines. Infection resulting from accidents often led to tetanus.

In other sections of the book, Engels discussed diseases in particular types of industrial work. He provided early accounts of occupational diseases that did not receive intensive study until well into the twentieth century. Many orthopedic disorders, in Engels' view, derived from the physical demands of industrialism. He discussed curvature of the spine, deformities of the lower extremities, flat feet, varicose veins, and leg ulcers as manifestations of work demands that required long periods of time in an upright posture. Engels commented on the health effects of posture, standing, and repetitive movements:

> All these affections are easily explained by the nature of factory work. . . . The operatives . . . must stand the whole time. And one who sits down, say upon a window-ledge or a basket, is fined, and this perpetual upright position, this constant mechanical pressure of the upper portions of the body upon spinal column, hips, and legs, inevitably produces the results mentioned. This standing is not required by the work itself (8).

The insight that chronic musculoskeletal disorders could result from unchanging posture or small, repetitive motions seems simple enough. Yet this source of illness, which is quite different from a specific accident or exposure to a toxic substance, has entered occupational medicine as a serious topic of concern only recently.

Engels also singled out the eye disorders suffered by workers in textile and lace manufacturing. This work required constant fine visual concentration, often with poor lighting. Engels discussed such eye diseases as corneal inflammation, myopia, cataracts, and temporary or permanent blindness. After an exposition of ocular abnormalities, Engels returned to the passion of his social structural analysis:

> This is the price at which society purchases for the fine ladies of the bourgeoisie the pleasure of wearing lace; a reasonable price truly! Only a few thousand blind working-men, some consumptive labourers' daughters, a sickly generation of the vile multitude bequeathing its debility to its equally "vile" children and children's children.

... Our English bourgeoisie will lay the report of the Government Commission aside indifferently, and wives and daughters will deck themselves in lace as before (9).

For Engels the contradictions of class made themselves felt most keenly in symbolic paraphernalia like lace, which the capitalist class enjoyed at the expense of workers' eyesight.

Engels' exposition of pottery workers' "poisoning" was a clinical description of intoxication from lead and other heavy metals. His observations of occupational lead poisoning again are startling because this disease has evoked wide concern in modern industrial hygiene. He noted that workers absorbed lead largely from the finishing fluid that came into contact with their hands and clothing. The consequences Engels described included severe abdominal pain, constipation, and neurologic complications like epilepsy and partial or complete paralysis. These signs of lead intoxication occurred not only in workers themselves, according to Engels, but also in children who lived near pottery factories. Epidemiologic evidence concerning the community hazards of industrial lead has gained appreciation in environmental health mainly since 1970, again without recognition of Engels' observations.

Engels' discussions of lung disease were detailed and far reaching. His presentation of textile workers' pulmonary pathology antedated by many years the medical characterization of byssinosis, or brown lung:

In many rooms of the cotton and flax-spinning mills, the air is filled with fibrous dust, which produces chest affections, especially among workers in the carding and combing-rooms. . . . The most common effects of this breathing of dust are bloodspitting, hard, noisy breathing, pains in the chest, coughs, sleeplessness—in short, all the symptoms of asthma (10).

Engels offered a parallel description of "grinders' asthma," a respiratory disease caused by inhalation of metal dust particles in the manufacture of knife blades and forks. The pathologic effects of cotton and metal dusts on the lung were similar; Engels noted the similarities of symptoms experienced by these two diverse groups of workers.

Engels devoted even more attention to the ravages of pulmonary disorder among coal miners. He reported that unventilated coal dust caused both acute and chronic pulmonary inflammation that frequently progressed to death. Engels observed that "black spittle"—the syndrome now called coal miners' pneumoconiosis, or black lung—was associated with other gastrointestinal, cardiac, and reproductive complications. By pointing out that this lung disease was preventable, Engels illustrated the contradiction between profit and safety in capitalist industry:

Every case of this disease ends fatally. . . . In all the coal-mines which are properly ventilated this disease is unknown, while it frequently happens that miners who go from well to ill-ventilated mines are seized by it. The profit-greed of mine owners which prevents the use of ventilators is therefore responsible for the fact that this working-men's disease exists at all (11).

After more than a century, the same structural contradiction impedes the prevention of black lung.

For Engels, the analysis of the social origins of illness was part of a much larger agenda. *The Condition of the Working Class in England* resembled other Marxist classics in its scholarship, which the author intended mainly for the purpose of sociopolitical action. Engels quickly focused on other theoretical and practical concerns. Despite later writings on natural and physical sciences (12), he never returned to the social origins of illness as a major issue in its own right. Yet in a book that aimed toward a broad description of working-class life, Engels provided a profound analysis of the causal relationships between social structure and physical illness.

Engels interspersed his remarks about disease with many other perceptions of class oppression. His argument implied that the solution to these health problems required basic social change; limited medical interventions would never yield the improvements that were most needed. It is unfortunate that Engels' early work on medical issues has eluded later students and activists. As noted previously, however, Engels' analysis exerted a major influence, both intellectual and political, on one of the founders of social medicine, Rudolf Virchow.

RUDOLF VIRCHOW

Virchow's life spanned eighty years of nineteenth-century history, more than 2,000 publications, numerous major contributions in medical science and anthropology, and parliamentary activity as an elected member of the German Reichstag. His best known work is *Cellular Pathology* (13), which presented the first comprehensive exposition of the cell as the basic unit of physiologic and pathologic processes. Virchow's current reputation rests largely on his research in cellular pathology. Throughout this career, however, he tried to develop a unified explanation of the physical and social forces that cause disease and human suffering. His vision of the multifactorial and largely social origins of illness deserves more than the obscurity into which much of his work has fallen.

In his analyses of social medicine, Virchow acknowledged the impact of many sources, but particularly those of Bacon, Hegel, and materialists like Engels and Arnold Ruge. From Bacon, Virchow derived his commitment to an applied science that would be practically useful. Virchow quoted Bacon's aphorism that "knowledge is power" and claimed: "Knowledge which is unable to support action is not genuine—and how unsure is activity without understanding. This split between science and practice is rather new." After a lengthy critique of the defects of detached science pursued "for its own sake," Virchow concluded: "It certainly does not detract from the dignity of science to come down off its pedestal—and from the people science gains new strength" (14). From this perspective emerged Virchow's frequent assertion that the most successful science drew its problems largely from concrete social concerns. Science and scientific medicine, according to Virchow, should not be detached from sociopolitical reality. On the contrary, he argued, the scientist must seek to link the findings of research to political work suggested by that research.

Hegel was the main source of Virchow's dialectic approach to both biologic and social problems. On the biologic level, Virchow perceived natural processes as a series of antitheses, such as the humoral-solidistic or vitalistic-mechanistic dualities, that were resolved by syntheses such as cellular pathology. On the social level, Virchow also viewed historical processes dialectically. For example, in 1847, he anticipated the revolutions of 1848 by claiming that the apparent social tranquility would be "negated" through social conflict in order to reach "a higher synthesis" (15). Virchow used a similar dialectic analysis in tracing the process of scientific knowledge. Discoveries, he claimed, emerged from the "kernel of truth" in past observations that scientists initially interpreted erroneously. The dialectic of scientific knowledge therefore required the scientist's awareness of the concrete historical circumstances in which observations and interpretations were made (16).

While influenced by Hegel, Virchow rejected Hegelian idealism. Although the dialectic method, in Virchow's view, was applicable to biologic science, it needed grounding in specific material phenomena. Virchow argued for a new "materialism" in medicine that would replace dogma and spiritualism (17). In his attempts to construct a dialectic materialist approach in biology, Virchow studied the early work of Engels; he cited with approval Engels' approach in *The Condition of the Working Class in England* and used some of Engels' data to demonstrate the relationships between poverty and illness (18). During his early years, Virchow was influenced to perhaps an even greater degree by Arnold Ruge, who with Marx edited *Die Deutsch-Französischen Jahrbücher*. Virchow referred frequently to Ruge's writings and speeches, especially those on the ambiguities of political authority and on the need to discover "natural laws" of human society (19).

Virchow manifested these orientations—of applied science, dialectics, and materialism—in many ways, but most of all in his analyses of multifactorial etiology. In investigating the origins of specific illnesses, Virchow consistently studied a variety of social, political, economic, geographic, climactic, and physiologic factors that interacted with one another in the causation of disease. He emphasized the concrete historical and material circumstances in which disease appeared, the contradictory social forces that impeded prevention, and researchers' role in advocating reform. In the analysis of multifactorial etiology, Virchow claimed that the most important causative factors were material conditions of people's everyday lives. This view implied that an effective health-care system could not limit itself to treating the pathophysiologic disturbances of individual patients.

Based on study of a typhus epidemic in Upper Silesia, a cholera epidemic in

Berlin, and an outbreak of tuberculosis in Berlin during 1848 and 1849, Virchow developed a theory of epidemics that emphasized the social circumstances permitting spread of illness. He argued that defects of society were a necessary condition for the emergence of epidemics. Virchow classified certain disease entities as "crowd diseases" or "artificial diseases"; these included typhus, scurvy, tuberculosis, leprosy, cholera, relapsing fever, and some mental disorders. According to this analysis, inadequate social conditions increased the population's susceptibility to climate, infectious agents, and other specific causal factors—none of which alone was sufficient to produce an epidemic: "Don't crowd diseases point everywhere to deficiencies of society? One may adduce atmospheric or cosmic conditions or similar factors. But never do they alone make epidemics. They produce them only . . . where due to bad social conditions people have lived for some time in abnormal situations." From this perspective, for the prevention and eradication of epidemics, social change was as important as medical intervention, if not more so: "The improvement of medicine would eventually prolong human life, but improvement of social conditions could achieve this result even more rapidly and successfully" (20). Health workers deluded themselves to think that effects within the medical sphere alone would ameliorate these problems. The advocacy of social solutions thus became the necessary complement of clinical work.

The social contradictions that Virchow emphasized most strongly were those of class structure. He described the deprivations that the working class endured and linked disease patterns to these deprivations. For example, he noted that morbidity and mortality rates, and especially infant mortality rates, were much higher in working-class districts of cities than in wealthier areas. As documentation he used the statistics that Engels cited, as well as data he gathered for German cities. Describing inadequate housing, nutrition, and clothing, Virchow criticized the apathy of government officials for ignoring these root causes of illness. Virchow expressed his outrage about class conditions most forcefully in his discussion of epidemics like the cholera outbreak in Berlin:

> Is it not clear that our struggle is a social one, that our job is not to write instructions to upset the consumers of melons and salmon, of cakes and ice cream, in short, the comfortable bourgeoisie, but is to create institutions to protect the poor, who have no soft bread, no good meat, no warm clothing, and no bed, and who through their work cannot subsist on rice soup and camomile tea. . .? May the rich remember during the winter, when they sit in front of their hot stoves and give Christmas apples to their little ones, that the shiphands who brought the coal and the apples died from cholera. It is so sad that thousands always must die in misery, so that a few hundred may live well (21).

For Virchow, the deprivations of working-class life created a susceptibility to disease. When infectious organisms, climactic changes, famine, or other causal factors were present, disease occurred in individuals and spread rapidly through the community.

Virchow's understanding of the social origins of illness was the source of the broad scope that he defined for public health and the medical scientist. He attacked structures of oppression within medicine, particularly the policies of hospitals that required payment from the poor rather than assuming their care as a matter of social responsibility. He envisioned the creation of a "public health service," an integrated system of publicly owned and operated health-care facilities, staffed by health workers who were employed by the state. In this system, health care would be defined as a constitutional right of citizenship. Included within this right would be the enjoyment of material conditions of life that contributed to health rather than to illness (22). The activities of public health workers, to whom Virchow referred as "doctors of the poor" (*Armenärzten*), would involve advocacy as well as direct medical care; in this sense, health workers would become the "natural attorneys of the poor." Even with the best of motivations, he argued, doctors working among the poor faced continuous overwork and their own impotence to change the social conditions that foster illness. For these reasons, it was naive to argue for a public health service without also struggling for more basic social change.

Two other principles were central to Virchow's conception of the public health service: prevention and the state's responsibility to ensure material security for citizens. Virchow's stress on prevention again derived mostly from his observation of epidemics, which he believed could be prevented by fairly straightforward policies. For example, he found a major cause of the Upper Silesian typhus epidemic in several poor potato harvests preceding the epidemic; government officials could have prevented malnutrition by redistributing foodstuffs from other parts of the country. Prevention, then, was largely a political problem: "Our politics were those of prophylaxis; our opponents preferred those of palliation" (23). It was foolish to think that health workers could accomplish prevention solely by activities within the medical sphere; material security also was essential. The state's responsibilities, Virchow argued, included providing work for "able-bodied" citizens. Only by guaranteed employment could workers obtain the economic security necessary for good health. Likewise, the physically disabled should enjoy the right of public compensation (24).

Virchow's vision of the social origins of illness pointed out the wide scope of the medical task. To the extent that illness derived from social conditions, the medical scientist must study those conditions as a part of clinical research, and the health worker must engage in political action. This is the sense of the connections Virchow frequently drew among medicine, social science, and politics: "Medicine is a social science, and politics is nothing more than medicine in larger scale" (25). Virchow's analysis of these issues fell from sight largely because of conservative political forces that shaped the course of scientific medicine during the late nineteenth and early twentieth centuries. His contributions set a standard for current attempts to understand, and to change, the social conditions that generate illness and suffering.

SALVADOR ALLENDE

The practice of pathology was an ironic continuity between the lives of Virchow and Allende. Experience in autopsies exposed them to sources of illness and death in contradictions of society and oppressive social structures. Allende's political career is better known than Virchow's, partly because of the tragedy of its abrupt end. Social medicine, however, was a central concern for them both, and Allende recognized very early that the health problems of the Chilean people derived in large part from the country's economic and political conditions. Allende's understanding of the social origins of illness influenced his political activism, both within and outside the health sector. Writing in 1939 as minister of health for a Popular Front government, Allende presented his analysis of the relationships among social structures, disease, and suffering in his classic book, *La Realidad Medico-Social Chilena* (26).

La Realidad conceptualized illness as a disturbance of the individual that often was fostered by deprived social conditions. This conception implied that social change was the only potentially effective therapeutic approach to many health problems. After an introduction on the connections between social structure and illness, Allende presented some geographic and demographic "antecedents" necessary to place specific health problems in context. He devoted the next part of the book, following a similar emphasis as Engels and Virchow, to the "living conditions of the working classes." The last sections of the book presented an exhaustive review of health-care facilities and services and a plan for change based on socialist strategy.

The introduction of *La Realidad* explored the dilemmas of reformism and argued that incremental reforms within the health-care system would remain ineffective unless accompanied by broad structural changes in the society. Allende emphasized capitalist imperialism, particularly the multinational corporations that extracted profit from Chilean natural resources and inexpensive labor. He claimed that to improve the health care system, a popular government must end capitalist exploitation:

> Progress obtained in the output of national production has not yielded a sensible margin in well-being in the popular strata, because international capitalism—economic and financial master of the large centers of production—is interested only in producing to satisfy the demand of the market, and no more. For the capitalist enterprise it is of no concern that there is a population of workers who live in deplorable conditions, who risk being consumed by diseases or who vegetate in obscurity. . . . Therefore, the action of our government is not only the remedial task of transforming the people but moreover of defending against absorption and exploitation by the economic imperialists who encompass the earth. . . . [Without] economic advancement . . . it is impossible to accomplish anything serious from the viewpoints of hygiene or medicine . . . because it is impossible to give health and knowledge to a people who

are malnourished, who wear rags, and who work at a level of unmerciful exploitation (27).

Ill health, in Allende's analysis, was inextricably linked to underdevelopment and imperialism.

In his account of working-class life, Allende's analytic tone and statistical tabulations thinly veiled his outrage at the contradictions of class structure and underdevelopment. He focused first on wages, which he viewed as a primary determinant of workers' material condition. Many of his economic observations anticipated later concerns, including wage differentials for men and women, the impact of inflation, and the inadequacy of laws purporting to ensure subsistence-level income. He linked his exposition of wages directly to the problem of nutrition and presented comparative data on food availability, earning power, and level of economic development. Not only was the production of milk and other needed foodstuffs less efficient than in more developed countries, but Chilean workers' inferior earning power also made food less accessible. Reviewing the minimum requirement to ensure adequate nutrition, he found that the majority of Chilean workers could not obtain the elements of this diet on a regular basis. Allende linked malnutrition, illness, and low wages. He argued that high infant mortality, skeletal deformities, tuberculosis, and other infectious diseases all had roots in bad nutrition; improvements depended on better economic conditions.

Allende then turned to clothing, housing, and sanitation facilities. He found that working people in Chile were inadequately clothed, largely because wages were low and the greatest proportion of income went for food and housing. The effects of insufficient clothing, Allende observed, were apparent in rates of upper respiratory infections, pneumonia, and tuberculosis, that were higher than in any economically developed country. In his analysis of housing problems, Allende focused on population density. He noted that Chile had one of the highest rates of inhabitants per residential structure in the world; overcrowding fostered the spread of infectious diseases and poor hygiene. Again he cited comparative data that showed a correlation between population density and overall mortality. In a style reminiscent of both Engels and Virchow, Allende presented a concrete description of housing conditions, including details about insufficient beds, inadequate construction materials, and deficiencies in apartment buildings. He reviewed the provisions for private initiative in construction, found them unsatisfactory, and outlined the need for major public-sector investment in new housing. Allende then gave data on drinking water and sewerage systems for all provinces of Chile. He noted that vast areas of the country lacked these rudimentary facilities.

This view of working-class conditions laid the groundwork for Allende's subsequent analysis of medical problems. When he discussed specific diseases, he looked for their sources in the social and material environment. He expressed this unifying theme:

> The individual in society is not an abstract entity; one is born, develops, lives, works, reproduces, falls ill, and dies in strict subjection to the surrounding environment, whose different modalities create diverse modes of reaction, in the face of the etiologic agents of disease. This material environment is determined by wages, nutrition, housing, clothing, culture, and additional concrete and historical factors (28).

Because disease originated in part from social conditions, health programs could not succeed without changing the illness-generating conditions of society.

The medical problems that Allende considered were maternal and infant mortality, tuberculosis, venereal diseases, other communicable diseases, emotional disturbances, and occupational illnesses. He observed that maternal and infant mortality rates generally were much lower in developed than in underdeveloped countries. After reviewing the major causes of death, he concluded that malnutrition and poor sanitation, both rooted in the contradictions of underdevelopment, were major explanations for this excess mortality. In the same section Allende gave one of the first analyses of illegal abortion. He noted that a large proportion of deaths in gynecologic hospitals, about 30 percent, derived from abortions and their complications. Pointing out the high incidence of abortion complications among working-class women, he attributed this problem to economic deprivations of class structure. Again, after a statistical account of complications, Allende allowed his outrage to surface:

> There are hundreds of working mothers who, because of anxiety about the inadequacy of their wages, induce abortion in order to prevent a new child from shrinking their already insignificant resources. Hundreds of working mothers lose their lives, impelled by the anxieties of economic reality (29).

Allende designated tuberculosis as a "social disease" because its incidence differed so greatly among social classes. Writing before the antibiotic era, Allende reached conclusions similar to those of modern epidemiology—that is, the major decline in tuberculosis followed economic advances rather than therapeutic medical interventions. From statistics of the first three decades of the twentieth century, he noted that tuberculosis had decreased consistently in the economically developed countries of Western Europe and the United States. On the other hand, in economically underdeveloped countries like Chile, little progress against the disease had occurred. Within the context of underdevelopment, tuberculosis exerted its most severe impact on the working class.

In his discussion of venereal diseases, Allende emphasized socioeconomic problems that favored the spread of syphilis and gonorrhea. For example, he discussed deprivations of working-class life that encouraged prostitution. Citing the prevalence of prostitution in Santiago and other cities, as well as the early recruitment of women from poor families, he argued that social programs to eliminate prostitution must precede significant improvements in venereal diseases.

Regarding other communicable diseases, Allende turned first to typhus, the same disease that had shaped Virchow's views about the relations between illness and social structure. Allende began his analysis with a straightforward statement: "Some [communicable diseases], like typhus, are an index of the state of pauperization of the masses" (30). Like Virchow in Upper Silesia, Allende found a disproportionate incidence of typhus in the working class of Chile. He then showed that bacillary and amebic dysentery and typhoid fever occurred because of inadequate drinking water and sanitation facilities in densely populated residential areas. Similar problems fostered other infections, such as diphtheria, whooping cough, scarlet fever, measles, and trachoma. Allende's exposition of social factors in the etiology of infectious diseases antedated many emphases of modern epidemiology. His arguments transcended the search for specific etiologic agents and treatments—the dominant perspective of Western medicine at the time Allende was writing.

Addiction was another problem that troubled Allende deeply. He maintained a concern with addiction throughout his career; one priority of his health policies as president of Chile was a large-scale alcoholism program. In *La Realidad,* Allende analyzed the social and psychological problems that motivated people to use addicting drugs. Allende's analysis of the causes of alcohol intoxication was quite similar to Engels':

We see that one's wages, appreciably less than subsistence, are not enough to supply needed clothing, that one must inhabit inadequate housing . . . [and that] one's food is not sufficient to produce the minimum of necessary caloric energy. . . . The worker reaches the conclusion that going to the tavern and intoxicating oneself is the apparent solution to all these problems. In the tavern one finds a lighted and heated place, and friends for distraction, making one forget the misery at home. In short, for the Chilean worker . . . alcohol is not a stimulant but an anesthetic (31).

Rooted in social misery, alcoholism exerted a profound effect on health, an impact which Allende documented for a variety of illnesses, including gastrointestinal diseases, cirrhosis, delirium tremens, sexual dysfunction, birth defects, and tuberculosis. He also traced some of the more subtle societal outcomes of alcoholism; for example, he offered an early account of the role of alcohol in deaths from accidents.

In his account of occupational diseases, Allende recognized that the occupational causes of death and disability were among the most important that the country faced. The diseases of work revealed direct links between illness and oppressive social structures. Allende noted, however, that knowledge about occupational diseases remained at a rudimentary level. He reviewed such problems as industrial accidents and silicosis. But, reflecting the dearth of information that persisted at the time, he advocated "systematic study and planning of this aspect of our social pathology" (32).

Allende also analyzed monopoly capital and imperialist expansion by the pharmaceutical industry. In perhaps the earliest discussion of its type, Allende compared the prices of brand-name drugs with their generic equivalents:

> Thus, for example, we find for a drug with important action on infectious diseases, sulfanilamide, these different names and prices: Prontosil $26.95, Gombardol $20.80, Septazina $21.60, Aseptil $18.00, Intersil $13.00, Acetilina $6.65. All these products, which in the eyes of the public appear with different names, correspond, in reality, to the same medication which is sold in a similar container and which contains 20 tablets of 0.50 grams of sulfanilamide (33).

Beyond the issue of drug names, Allende also anticipated a later theme by criticizing pharmaceutical advertising: "Another problem in relation to the pharmaceutical specialties is . . . the excessive and charlatan propaganda attributing qualities and curative powers which are far from their real ones" (34). Throughout his career Allende maintained his concern with exploitation by multinational drug companies. As president, he helped developed a national generic drug formulary and proposed nationalization of the pharmaceutical industry that remained dominated by North American firms.

Allende concluded by setting forth the policy positions and plan for political action of the Ministry of Health within the Popular Front government. In considering reform and its dilemmas, he reviewed the social origins of illness and the social structural remedies that were necessary. Allende refused to discuss specific health problems apart from macro-level political and economic issues. He introduced his policy proposals with a chapter entitled, "Considerations Regarding Human Capital." Analyzing the detrimental economic impact of ill health among workers, he argued that a healthy population was a worthy goal both in its own right and also for the sake of national development. The country's productivity suffered because of workers' illness and early death, yet improving the health of workers was impossible without fundamental structural changes in the society. These changes would include "an equitable distribution of the product of labor," state regulation of "production, distribution, and price of articles of food and clothing," a national housing program, and special attention to occupational health problems. The links between medicine and broader social reality were inescapable: "All this means that the solution of the medico-social problems of the country would require precisely the solution of the economic problems that affect the proletarian classes" (35). Allende's insight was that health policy must transcend the health sector alone.

But he was not content to state this principle in abstract terms. Instead, he proposed specific reforms that he viewed as preconditions for an effective health system. These reforms called for profound changes in existing structures of power and finance. First of all, he suggested modifications of wages, which if enacted would have led to a major redistribution of wealth. Regarding nutrition, he developed a plan to improve milk supplies, fishing, and refrigeration, and suggested land reform provisions to enhance agricultural productivity. Recognizing the need for better housing, Allende proposed a concerted national effort in publicly supported construction as well as rent control in the private sector.

Since the major social origins of illness were low wages, malnutrition, and poor housing, the first responsibility of the public health system, according to Allende, was to improve these conditions. Allende did not emphasize programs of research or treatment for specific diseases; instead, he assumed that the greatest advances toward lowering morbidity and mortality would follow fundamental changes in social structure. This orientation also pervaded his proposed "medico-social program." In this program he suggested innovations including the reorganization of the Ministry of Health, planning activities, control of pharmaceutical production and prices, occupational safety and health policies, measures supporting preventive Medicine, and Sanitation programs. At the present time, the insight that the social origins of illness demand social solutions is not particularly surprising. Despite lip service paid to this concept, however, health-care analysts have contented themselves with limited reformism—often arguing that more basic structural change, though needed, is beyond their reach as political actors. Like Engels and Virchow before him, Allende saw major origins of illness in the structure of society. This vision implied that medical intervention without political activism would remain ineffectual and, in a deep sense, misguided.

CONVERGENCE, DIVERGENCE

Sensitivity to the social origins of illness emerged during the mid-nineteenth century and recently has deepened. In this field the lives and works of Engels, Virchow, and Allende were landmarks. Their varying analyses gave historical depth to these problems, which succeeding generations unfortunately have forgotten and later rediscovered. Engels' observations of illness and death caused by early capitalism made *The Condition of the Working Class in England* an overlooked classic. Although Engels maintained an interest in science which he developed in several later books, the breadth of his other theoretical concerns and the intensity of his political activism led him away from medical issues as a prime focus. Virchow's early studies of social etiology in medicine merged with his youthful political radicalism. Both these foci faded later, partly because of the reactionary environment of Western European intellectual life and partly because of Virchow's own reluctance to risk his prominent academic position. Working during a later historical period and in the much different context of imperialism and underdevelopment, Allende studied medicine as he became a leftist political leader. His commitment to changing the social origins of illness persisted throughout his later career. That he often subordinated health policy to broader social policy was consistent with his view that the most difficult medical problems had their roots in contradictions of class structure and underdevelopment. While they overlapped in many ways, the pathbreaking works of these individuals also diverged in crucial respects. These differences perhaps revealed even more than the similarities.

Engels, Virchow, and Allende held divergent, though complementary, views of the social etiology of illness. The divergences reflected more general differences in theoretical orientation. For Engels, economic production was primary. Even in his early work, Engels emphasized the organization and process of production. Disease and early death, in this view, developed directly from exposure to dusts, chemicals, time pressures, bodily posture, visual demands, and related difficulties that workers faced in their jobs. Environmental pollution, bad housing, alcoholism, and malnutrition also contributed to the poor health of the working class, but on balance these factors mainly reflected or exacerbated the structural contradictions of production itself. The principal contradiction which permitted illness-generating conditions, of course, was that between profit and safety. Engels noted that changes in the organization of work to prevent occupational illness and accidents, by increasing costs, usually would reduce profits. Engels' analysis of illness and mortality in the working class anticipated his later emphasis on the primacy of economic production in explaining many problems of capitalist society.

Rather than economic production, Virchow focused on inequalities in the distribution and consumption of social resources. Virchow shared Engels' view that the working class suffered disproportionately. In Virchow's analysis, however, the main sources of illness and early death were poverty, unemployment, malnutrition, cultural and educational deficits, political disenfranchisement, linguistic difficulties, inadequate medical facilities and personnel, and similar deficiencies that affected the working class. He believed, for example, that public officials could prevent epidemics by distributing food more efficiently. Disease and mortality, he argued, would improve if a public health service made medical care more available. Virchow did criticize profiteering by businessmen and the high fees of the private medical profession. But he did not emphasize the illness-generating conditions of production itself. Instead, he viewed unequal access to society's products as the principal problem of social medicine.

Allende also concerned himself with the impact of class structure, but chiefly in the context of underdevelopment and imperialism. The deprivations that the working class experienced in countries like Chile reflected the exploitation of the Third World by advanced capitalist nations. Allende attributed low wages, malnutrition, poor housing, and related problems directly to the extraction of wealth by international imperialism. He recognized that production itself could produce illness but, unlike Engels, devoted little attention to occupational illness per se. He did document distributional inequalities of goods and services which, as in Virchow's analysis, ravaged the working class. On the other hand, the most crucial social determinant of illness and death, in Allende's view, was the contradiction of development and underdevelopment. Economic advancement of the society as a whole, although impeded by imperialism, was the major precondition for meaningful improvements in medical care and individual health.

The contributions of Engels, Virchow, and Allende shared the framework of multifactorial causation. These writings conveyed a vision of multiple social structures and processes impinging on the individual. Disease was not the straightforward outcome of an infectious agent or pathophysiologic disturbance. Instead, a variety of problems—including malnutrition, economic insecurity, occupational risks, bad housing, and lack of political power—created an underlying predisposition to disease and death. Although these writers differed in the specific factors they emphasized, they each saw illness as deeply embedded in the complexities of social reality. To the extent that social contradictions affected individual disease, therapeutic intervention that limited itself to the individual level was both naive and futile. Multifactorial etiology implied social change as therapy, and the latter linked medical practice to political practice.

Another crucial divergence concerned policy, reform, and political strategy. Engels, Virchow, and Allende differed in their views of the strategies needed to achieve the policies they sought. They also held varying visions of the society in which these policies would take effect. Although their explanations of the social origins of illness complemented one another, the question of how to change illness-generating conditions evoked quite different strategic analyses.

Already present in his early work, Engels' strategy involved revolution, not reform. His documentation of the occupational and environmental conditions that caused illness and early death did not aim toward limited reform of those problems. Instead, as noted earlier, he intended his data to serve, at least in part, as propaganda. The purpose was to provide a focus of political organizing among the working class. Notably, Engels did not advocate specific changes in the conditions he described. While he detailed, for instance, the defects of housing, sanitation, occupational safety, maldistribution of medical personnel, and promotion of drugs, he did not explicitly seek reforms in any of these areas. The alternatives that he occasionally suggested, such as the cursory outlines of a public health service, were always speculations about how a more effective system might appear in a postrevolutionary society. The many deprivations of working-class life required fundamental change in the entire social order, rather than limited improvements in each separate sphere. Engels' later writings sometimes adopted a more flexible stance about reform in the context of capitalism. The companion piece of *The Condition of the Working Class in England,* however, was clearly *The Communist Manifesto.* The strategic implications of Engels' analysis of health problems were congruent with his role as a primary organizer of the First Internationale. From this perspective, reformism in health care made as little sense as any other piecemeal tinkering with capitalist society.

Virchow's strategic approach was quite different. Although he participated in the agitation of the late 1840s, and although he doubted that the ruling circles would permit needed changes in response to peaceful challenges alone, he ultimately opted for reform rather than for revolution. While the conditions he witnessed in the Upper Silesian typhus epidemic were horrifying, he believed that a series of reforms could correct the problem. The reforms he advocated transcended medicine to include rationalized food distribution, modifications in the educational system, political enfranchisement, and other changes at the level of social structure. He also adopted a broad view of the systematic reforms that were necessary in health care. An adequate health system, for example, demanded a public health service. In this service, health-care professionals would work as employees of the state and would act to correct maldistribution across class, geographical, and ethnic lines. As an overall political goal, Virchow favored a constitutional democracy that would reduce the power of the monarchy and nobility. He supported principles of socialism, particularly those that involved public ownership and rational organization of health and welfare facilities. However, Virchow argued against communism, mainly, he said, because of its naive view that a just society was feasible without a strong state apparatus. Virchow clearly believed that limited reforms within capitalist society were both appropriate and desirable, and he was optimistic that they would be effective. During his later life, the reformist slant of his strategic thinking became even clearer.

Allende's conceptualization of political strategy was more complex and differentiated than Engels' or Virchow's. In *La Realidad Medico-Social Chilena,* he stated unambiguously that the health problems of the working class were inherent in the contradictions of class structure and underdevelopment, and in the oppressive international relations of capitalist imperialism. Without basic modification of these structural problems, he argued, limited medical reform would prove futile. In Allende's view, revolutionary social change was necessary. But his revolutionary strategy remained that of the peaceful road. Throughout his life, Allende believed that progressive forces could achieve a socialist transformation of society through a sequence of peaceful actions within the framework of constitutional democracy. He and his co-workers based this position on a reading of prior socialist strategists, examples of other revolutions, and, most of all, a detailed analysis of Chile's concrete historical and material reality. From this viewpoint, the most important health-related reforms transcended medicine. Allende called for improvements in housing, nutrition, employment, and other concrete manifestations of class oppression. Such reforms were preconditions for reduced morbidity and mortality; without them, changes in health-care services could not succeed. On the other hand, structural reforms in the social organization of medicine, including a public health service and a nationalized pharmaceutical and equipment industry, were desirable goals en route to a socialist society. Allende did not accurately anticipate the violence of national and international groups about to be dispossessed on the peaceful road to socialism. The balance between reform and revolutionary alternatives remains a crucial and incompletely resolved problem in strategic planning.

The social origins of illness are not mysterious. Yet, many years after Engels' analysis first appeared, these problems have received remarkably little attention in research or political practice. Industrial hygiene has tended to accept as given the structures of the capitalist system; until recently, activities in occupational health and safety have focused on interventions that would ensure an efficient and profitable labor force. On the other hand, social medicine generally has adopted the medical model of etiology. In this model, social conditions may increase susceptibility or exacerbate disease, but they are not primary causes like microbial agents or disturbances of normal physiology. Since investigation has not clarified the causes of illness within social structure, political strategy—both within and outside medicine—seldom has addressed the roots of disease in society.

The social pathologies that distressed Engels, Virchow, and Allende remain with us. Inequalities of class, exploitation of workers, and conditions of capitalist production cause disease now as previously. Likewise, the constraints of profit and lack of societal responsibility for individual economic security still inhibit even incremental reforms. The links between social structure and disease become ever more urgent, as economic instability, unreliable food supplies, depletion of petroleum, nuclear and toxic chemical wastes, and related problems threaten humanity's very survival. Understanding these roots of illness also reveals the scope of reconstruction that is necessary for meaningful solutions.

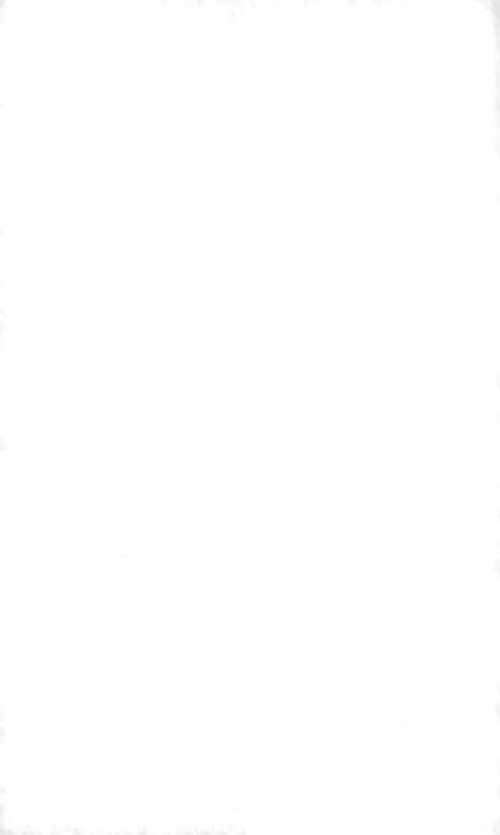

Part Two

Problems in Contemporary Health Care

4

Technology, Health Costs, and the Structure of Private Profit

In both advanced capitalist countries and underdeveloped nations, the financial burden of health care has become a major concern. Legislative and administrative maneuvers purportedly aim toward the goal of cost containment. New investigative techniques in health services research, based largely on the cost-effectiveness model, are entering into the evaluation of technology and clinical practices. The purposes of this chapter are to document the analytic poverty of these approaches and to offer an alternative interpretation which traces problems of costs to underlying social contradictions and to oppressive social structures within the organization of medicine.

From the Marxist perspective, costs cannot be divorced from the structure of private profit. As discussed earlier, the problem of diminishing returns in the face of rising costs emerges from several social contradictions. These contradictions include the corporate invasion of medicine, uneven socioeconomic development, ideologic patterns of medical science that presuppose the effectiveness of expensive technology, public subsidization of the private sector, and features of the medical labor force that impede humanistic care.

Incredibly enough, most non-Marxist analyses of costs either ignore the contradictions of capitalism or accept them as given. But the crisis of health costs intimately reflects the more general fiscal crisis that advanced capitalism is facing worldwide. In considering costs, it is foolhardy to overlook the connections between the health sector and the structure of the capitalist system. Wearing blinders that limit the level of analysis to a specific innovation or practice, while not perceiving the broader political-economic context in which costly and ineffective procedures are introduced and promulgated, will only obscure potential solutions to the difficulties that confront us.

The focus of this chapter is coronary care, a particularly revealing example of apparent irrationalities of health policy that make sense when seen from the standpoint of capitalist profit structure. However, the overselling of numerous other technologic advances—such as computerized axial tomography, new laboratory techniques, fetal monitoring, and many surgical procedures—reflects very similar structural problems.

THE EMERGENCE OF INTENSIVE CORONARY CARE

Early Claims

Intensive care for patients suffering heart attacks emerged rapidly during the 1960s, with the development of coronary care units (CCUs). The rationale for CCUs came from findings in pathology and physiology about the nature of heart attacks. When a person has a heart attack, or myocardial infarction (MI), a part of the heart muscle dies. For several days, this dying muscle is a source of electric instability that may cause serious irregularities in the heart's rhythm. If such an irregularity, or arrhythmia, occurs, the patient dies because the heart does not pump blood to vital organs. During the late 1950s and early 1960s, researchers in cardiology discovered techniques to control arrhythmias if caught in time. These techniques included intravenous drugs (such as lidocaine) and the application of electric shock to the chest wall (defibrillation).

The CCU's purpose is to provide continuous electronic monitoring of the heart's rhythm, through electrodes attached to the patient's chest and connected to electrocardiogram equipment. Through continuous monitoring, it is possible to start treatment, by drugs or electric shock, immediately when an arrhythmia begins. After an MI, a patient generally remains in a CCU during a critical period until the heart rhythm stabilizes. Medical practitioners have used CCUs for other problems, like congestive heart failure or blood pressure abnormalities, that sometimes follow an MI. The CCU's major rationale, however, is the monitoring and control of arrhythmias.

This rationale leads to a reasonable hypothesis: that CCUs would reduce morbidity and mortality from heart attacks. As reasonable as this hypothesis seems, it remains a hypothesis rather than a proven fact. A random controlled trial (RCT) is the only recognized way to confirm or disprove the effectiveness of CCUs, or any other new treatment. In an RCT, the experimental design would assign patients with MI randomly to CCU versus non-CCU treatment groups and then would compare the outcomes statistically. If patients with MIs showed improved survival or fewer complications in CCUs than in non-CCU settings, and if this difference reached statistical significance, the RCT would demonstrate the effectiveness of CCUs.

A controlled trial evaluating CCUs would be important for several reasons. In the first place, one can imagine some possible ways in which intensive care could interfere with recovery after an MI. Iatrogenic disease may arise, for example, because of disturbances in body chemistry stemming from intravenous solutions. Life-threatening infections also are more likely to occur in the hospital. In addition, the intensive care setting can be a fear-provoking experience. Emotional upset can be life-threatening after an MI; for example, patients in CCUs have died suddenly after witnessing other patients' deaths. Such technical and psychological problems need assessment before concluding that CCUs are effective. Second, although CCUs might improve short-term mortality in the hospital, they may have little effect on longer-term outcomes during the weeks and months after patients leave the hospital. The evaluation of intensive care properly would consider later survival and quality of life, beyond the acute period of hospitalization. Third, CCUs are enormously expensive. Capital expenditures for CCU equipment amount to millions of dollars for a single hospital. The daily costs of care in CCUs are two to three times more expensive than for hospitalization without intensive care.

A test of the hypothesis that CCUs are effective thus would seem appropriate. However, CCUs proliferated throughout the United States and around the world without any definite documentation of their effectiveness. Clinicians and investigators did not try to perform RCTs regarding the outcomes of CCU care. Instead, they advocated the adoption of the intensive care approach, with the unproven assumption that CCUs would improve survival by controlling early arrhythmias. Historically, high technology has conveyed an aura of scientific rigor, yet the promotion and acceptance of technology in such areas as coronary care have bypassed the scientific demonstration of effectiveness. Early arguments for CCUs showed an optimism unrestrained by the requirements of hypothesis testing.

The first major reports of CCUs were those written by Day, a cardiologist who developed a so-called coronary care area at the Bethany Hospital in Kansas City with financial help from the John A. Hartford Foundation (1). From these early articles until the mid-1970s, claims like Day's were very common in the literature. Descriptions of improved mortality and morbidity appeared, based totally on uncontrolled data from patients with MI admitted before and after the introduction of a CCU. The inconclusiveness of research designs that do not use randomization or a control group was at the time well recognized in medical research. The "before-after" approach adopted by Day and subsequent CCU advocates is designated in research methodology as the "one group pretest-posttest design" (2). This research design suffers from several sources of invalidity; problems include history (that is, changes outside the experimental situation that produce effects over time), maturation (processes inside the experimental situation that vary systematically with the passage of time), testing (the effect of the pretest itself), and a number of other issues. The RCT design solves all these problems of invalidity, but until the 1970s no major study of CCUs even attempted to include a randomized control group.

Day reached some grandiose inferences: "It is anticipated that 45,000 deaths [*sic*] occurring from acute MI could be prevented in the United States if the patients were treated in acute coronary areas." His reference here was "personal communication from Dr. J. P. Fitzgerald, Senior Surgeon, Department of Health, Education and Welfare, Washington, D.C." This unsubstantiated estimate of lives saved, presumably on an annual basis, reappeared frequently in policy-oriented justifications for CCUs, as noted later. Day's general conclusion was: "An acute coronary care area is the ideal location for the treatment of patients suffering from acute MI."

Day's enthusiasm spread to many others. In 1967, the classic descriptive study by Lown's group at the Peter Bent Brigham Hospital in Boston appeared. This study was supported by the U.S. Public Health Service, the Hartford Foundation, and the American Optical Company, which manufactured the tape-loop recall memory system that was being used in the CCU. The CCU's major objective, as the article pointed out, was to anticipate and to reduce early heart rhythm disturbances, thereby avoiding the need for resuscitation. The paper cited several other articles showing before-after decreases in mortality with a CCU, but never with randomization or other forms of statistical control introduced, and certainly never with a random controlled trial. Again, some grandiose goals concluded the article:

> Future goals include continuous monitoring of high risk patients outside the hospital while attending their daily chores. This information could be telemetered to special computers in the hospital preset to alert instantly both doctor and patient of any change in rhythm. The hospital would then have a new role not limited to treating illness, but would assume the much wider function of being a sentinel and guardian of community health. Thus the coronary care unit represents the first step in an exciting and still long journey which eventually must revolutionize the care of patients with coronary artery disease (3).

This publication led to a conference in 1968, sponsored by the Department of Health, Education, and Welfare (HEW), in which greater development and support of CCUs were advocated despite clear-cut statements within the conference that the effectiveness of CCUs had not been demonstrated. For example, at the conference the chief of the Heart Disease Control Program of the Public Health Service claimed:

> An attempt was made a few years ago to make some controlled studies of the benefits of CCU efforts, but it was not possible to carry out those investigations for many reasons, some of them fiscal. Therefore, we do not have proper studies for demonstrating the advantages of CCUs. But now that these opportunities and occasions to prevent heart rhythm disturbances have become a great deal more common, we can be assured that our efforts are worthwhile (4).

So, despite the lack of controlled studies showing effectiveness, there were many calls for the expansion of CCUs to other hospitals and increased support from the federal government and private foundations. In 1968 HEW also issued a set of *Guidelines for CCUs* (5). Largely because of these recommendations, CCUs grew rapidly in the following years. Table 4.1 showed the expansion of CCUs in the United States between 1967 and 1974 (6). Although some regional variability was present, a large increase in the proportion and an even larger increase in the absolute number of hospitals with CCUs occurred during this period—still, without demonstration of effectiveness.

Later Studies of Effectiveness

Serious research on the effectiveness of CCUs did not begin until the 1970s. As several critics pointed out, the "before-after" studies done during the 1960s simply could not lead to valid conclusions about effectiveness, since none of these studies had adequate control groups or randomization (7).

Later studies compared treatment of MI patients in hospital wards versus CCU settings (8). Patients were "randomly" admitted to the CCU or the regular ward, simply based on the availability of CCU beds. Ward patients were the "control" group; CCU patients were the "experimental" group. Table 4.2 reviews the findings of these studies, which are very contradictory. From this research it is unclear, at this late date, that CCUs improve in-hospital mortality.

Other research contrasted home versus hospital care (Table 4.3) (9). One major study was the prospective, random controlled trial by Mather and his colleagues in Great Britain. This was an ambitious and courageous study, of the type that was not considered possible by HEW in the 1960s. Although some methodologic problems arose concerning the randomization of patients to home versus hospital care,

Table 4.1   Growth of Coronary Care Units in the United States, by Region, 1967–1974

	Coronary Care Units (% of Hospitals)	
	1967	*1974*
United States	24.3	33.8
New England	29.0	36.8
Mid-Atlantic	33.8	44.2
East North Central	31.0	38.2
West North Central	17.0	25.3
South Atlantic	23.3	38.2
East South Central	13.4	30.1
West South Central	15.3	24.3
Mountain	21.4	29.3
Pacific	32.7	37.8

Source: Metropolitan Life Insurance Company, "Geographical Distribution of Coronary Care Units in the United States," Statistical Bulletin 58 (July–August 1977): 8.

Table 4.2   Studies Comparing Coronary Care Unit and Ward Treatment for Myocardial Infarction

	No CCU		CCU	
	N	*% Mortality*	*N*	*% Mortality*
Prospective				
Hofvendahl	139	35	132	17
Christiansen	244	41	171	18
Hill				
< 65 yrs	186	18	797	15
≥ 65 yrs	297	32	200	31
Retrospective				
Astvad	603	39	1108	41

Source: See studies cited in note 8, chapter 4.

the cumulative one-year mortality was not different in the home and hospital groups, and there was no evidence that MI patients did better in the hospital. A second random controlled trial of home versus hospital treatment tried to correct the methodologic difficulties of the Mather study by achieving a higher rate of randomization and strict criteria for the entry and exclusion of patients from the trial. The preliminary findings of this later study, conducted by Hill's group in Great Britain, confirmed the earlier results; the researchers concluded that for the majority of patients with suspected MI, admission to a hospital "confers no clear advantage." A third study of the same problem used an epidemiologic approach in the Teesside area of Great Britain. This investigation was not a random controlled trial

Table 4.3   Studies Comparing Hospital and Home Care for Myocardial Infarction

Prospective Randomized	Hospital		Home	
	N	*% Mortality*	*N*	*% Mortality*
Mather				
< 60 yrs	106	18	117	17
≥ 60 yrs	112	35	103	23
Total	218	27	220	20
Hill	132	11	132	13

Epidemiologic	Hospital CCU		Hospital Ward		Home	
	N	*% Mortality*	*N*	*% Mortality*	*N*	*% Mortality*
Dellipiani	248	13	296	21	193	9

Source: See studies cited in note 9, chapter 4.

but simply a twelve-month descriptive epidemiologic study of the incidence of MIs, how they were treated in practice, and the outcomes in terms of mortality. Both the crude and age-standardized mortality rates were better for patients treated at home.

In summary, these issues are far from settled even now. The thrust of available research indicates that home care is a viable treatment alternative to hospital or CCU care for many patients with MI. Early CCU promotion used unsound clinical research; more adequate studies have not confirmed CCU effectiveness. One other question is clear: if intensive care is not demonstrably more effective than simple rest at home, how can we explain the tremendous proliferation of this very expensive form of treatment?

From a Marxist viewpoint, these events cannot be chance phenomena. Nor are they simply another expression of the Pollyanna-like acceptance of high technology in industrial society. The enormously costly development of CCUs occurred without any demonstration of their effectiveness. Therefore, one must search for the social contradictions that fostered their growth and impeded their serious evaluation.

THE POLITICAL ECONOMY OF CORONARY CARE

The Corporate Connection

To survive, capitalist industries must produce and sell new products; expansion is an absolute necessity for capitalist enterprises. The economic surplus (defined as the excess of total production over "socially essential production") must grow continually larger. Medical production also falls into this same category, although it is seldom viewed in this way. The economist Mandel emphasizes the contradictions of the economic surplus: "For capitalist crises are incredible phenomena like nothing ever seen before. They are not crises of scarcity, like all pre-capitalist crises; they are crises of over-production" (10). This scenario also includes the health-care system, where an overproduction of intensive care technology contrasts with the fact that many people have little access to the most simple and rudimentary medical services.

Large profit-making corporations in the United States participated in essentially every phase of CCU research, development, promotion, and proliferation; many companies involved themselves in the intensive care market. Here I consider the activities of two such firms: the Warner-Lambert Pharmaceutical Company and the Hewlett-Packard Company. I selected these corporations because information about their participation in coronary care was relatively accessible and because they have occupied prominent market positions in this clinical area. However, many other firms, including at last eighty-five major companies, also have been involved in coronary care (11).

Warner-Lambert Pharmaceutical Company (W-L) was a large multinational corporation, with $2.1 billion in assets and over $2.5 billion in sales annually during the late 1970s. The corporation comprised a number of interrelated subsidiary companies. Warner-Chilcott Laboratories produced such drugs as Coly-Mycin, Gelusil, Anusol, Mandelamine, Peritrate, and Tedral. The Parke-Davis Company manufactured Caladryl lotion, medicated throat discs, influenza vaccines, Norlestrin contraceptives, Dilantin, Benadryl, Chloromycetin, and many other pharmaceuticals. Another division, Warner-Lambert Consumer Products, described its products as follows:

> The roster of Warner-Lambert consumer products reads like a page taken out of contemporary Americana. Listerine, Smith Brothers [cough drops], Bromo-Seltzer, Chiclets, DuBarry, Richard Hudnuts, Rolaids, Dentyne, Certs, Cool-ray Polaroid [sunglasses], and Oh! Henry [candy]—these are a few of the proper nouns that have become an integral part of the American language [*sic*]. They bespeak a culture of abundance, of leisure, of consciousness of personal care and personal appearance, and of the outdoors—a culture of which Warner-Lambert has made itself a part (12).

Warner-Lambert International operated in more than forty countries. Although several divisions of the W-L conglomerate participated actively in the development and promotion of coronary care, the most prominent division was the American Optical Company (AO), which W-L acquired during 1967.

By the early 1960s AO already had a long history of successful sales in such fields as optometry, ophthalmology, and microscopes. The instrumentation required for intensive coronary care led to AO's diversification into this new and growing area. The profitable outcomes of AO's research, development, and promotion of coronary care technology were clear from AO's 1966 annual report:

> Again, as in 1965, the market for instrumentation in cardiology and thoracic surgery continued to grow with an increasing shift towards complete systems in intensive and coronary care rather than procurement of individual instruments. In 1966, the number of American Optical Coronary Care Systems installed in hospitals throughout the United States more than tripled. Competition for this market also continued to increase as new companies, both large and small, entered the field. However, we believe that American Optical Company . . . will continue a leader in this evolving field (13).

After purchasing AO in 1967, W-L maintained AO's emphasis on CCU technology and sought wider acceptance by health professionals and medical centers. Promotional materials contained the assumption, never proven, that the new technology was effective in reducing morbidity and mortality from heart disease. Early products and systems included the AO Cardiometer, a heart monitoring and resuscitation device; the first direct current defibrillator; the Lown Cardioverter; and an Intensive Cardiac Care System that permitted the simultaneous monitoring of sixteen patients by oscilloscopes, recording instruments, heart rate meters, and alarm systems (14). In 1968 the company introduced a new line of monitoring instrumentation and implantable demand pacemakers. Regarding the monitoring systems, Warner-Lambert reported that "acceptance has far exceeded initial estimates" and that "to meet the increased demand for its products" the Medical Division was doubling the size of its plant in Bedford, Massachusetts (15). By 1969 the company introduced another completely new line of Lown Cardioverters and Defibrillators and claimed that "this flexible line now meets the requirements of hospitals of all sizes" (16). The company continued to register expanding sales throughout the early 1970s.

Despite this growth, W-L began to face a typical corporate problem: the potential saturation of markets in the United States. Coronary care technology was capital-intensive. The number of hospitals in the United States that could buy coronary care systems, though large, was finite. Without other maneuvers, the demand for coronary care products eventually would decline. For this reason, W-L began to make new and predictable initiatives to ensure future growth. First, the company expanded coronary care sales into foreign markets, especially in Third World countries. Subsequently W-L reported notable gains in sales in such countries as Argentina, Canada, Colombia, France, Germany, Japan, and Mexico, despite the fact that during the 1970s "political difficulties in southern Latin America slowed progress somewhat, particularly in Chile and Peru" (17).

A second method to deal with market saturation was further diversification within the coronary care field with products whose intent was to open new markets or to create obsolescence in existing systems. For example, in 1975 the AO subsidiary introduced two new instruments. The "Pulsar 4," a lightweight portable defibrillator designed for local paramedic and emergency squads, created "an exceptionally strong sales demand." The Computer Assisted Monitoring System used a computer to anticipate and control changes in cardiac patients' conditions and replaced many hospitals' CCU systems that AO had installed but that lacked computer capabilities. According to the 1975 annual report, these two instruments "helped contribute to record sales growth in 1975, following an equally successful performance in the previous year" (18).

A third technique to ensure growth involved the modification of coronary care technology for new areas gaining public and professional attention. With an emphasis on preventive medicine, AO introduced a new line of electrocardiogram telemetry instruments, designed to provide early warning of MI or rhythm disturbance in ambulatory patients. In addition, AO began to apply similar monitoring technology to the field of occupational health and safety. In 1970 W-L noted:

Sales of safety products were lower in 1970 than in 1969 as a result of cutbacks in defense spending, the general business slowdown, and the lengthy automobile industry strike. The outlook for the future, however, is encouraging because of the increased industry and government concern with safety on the job, as evidenced by the passage of the Federal Occupational Safety and Health Act late in 1970 (19).

During each subsequent year the sales of safety and health equipment, manufactured by the AO subsidiary and adopted partly from coronary care technology, continued to increase.

W-L was only one of many companies cultivating the coronary care market. Another giant was the Hewlett-Packard Company (H-P), a firm that in the late 1970s held more than $1.1 billion in assets and reported over $1.3 billion in sales. H-P was a less complex corporation than W-L since it controlled fewer subsidiaries. On the other hand, H-P's growth led to enormous wealth for a relatively small number of stockholders. For example, David Packard, chairman of the H-P board of directors and former assistant secretary of defense, as of 1978 owned H-P stock valued at approximately $562 million; the second highest holdings by a corporate executive in his own company were David Rockefeller's $13 million in shares of Chase Manhattan Bank (20).

Since its founding in 1939, H-P grew from a small firm, manufacturing analytical and measuring instruments mainly for industry, to a leader in electronics. Until the early 1960s H-P's only major product designated for medical markets was a simple electrocardiogram machine. Along with pocket computers, medical electronic equipment became the most successful of H-P's product groups. During the 1960s H-P introduced a series of innovations in coronary care (as well as perinatal monitoring and instrumentation for respiratory disease) that soon reached markets throughout the world.

Initially the company focused on the development of CCU technology. H-P promoted CCU equipment aggressively to hospitals, with the consistent claim that cardiac monitors and related products were definitely effective in reducing mortality from MI and rhythm disturbances. H-P's promotional literature made no reference at all to the problem of proving CCU effectiveness. Instead, such claims as the following were unambiguous: "In the cardiac care unit pictured here at a Nevada hospital, for example, the system has alerted the staff to several emergencies that might otherwise have proved fatal, and the cardiac mortality rate has been cut in half" (21). Alternatively, "hundreds of lives are saved each year with the help of Hewlett-Packard patient monitoring systems installed in more than 1,000 hospitals throughout the world. . . . Pictured here is an HP system in the intensive care ward of a hospital in Montevideo, Uruguay" (22).

Very early, H-P emphasized the export of CCU technology to hospitals and practitioners abroad. H-P anticipated the foreign sales that other companies like W-L also later enjoyed. In 1966 the H-P annual report predicted that the effects of a slumping economy would be offset by "the great sales potential for our products, particularly medical instruments, in South American, Canadian, and Asian markets. These areas should support substantial gains in sales for a number of years" (23). H-P developed an elaborate promotional apparatus, including "mobile laboratories" that could be transported by airplane or bus in foreign countries; by 1969 these exhibits had been "viewed by thousands of customers in Asia, Australia, Africa, and Latin America" (24). In materials prepared for potential investors,

HP made explicit statements about the advantages of foreign operations. For example, because H-P subsidiaries received "pioneer status" in Malaysia and Singapore, income generated in these countries remained essentially tax-free during the early 1970s: "Had their income been taxed at the U.S. statutory rate of 48 percent in 1974, our net earnings would have been reduced by 37 cents a share" (25). By the mid-1970s, H-P's international medical equipment business, as measured by total orders, surpassed its domestic business. More than 100 sales and service offices were operating in 64 countries.

Like W-L, H-P also diversified its products to deal with the potential saturation of the coronary care market. During the late 1960s the company introduced a series of complex computerized systems that were designed as an interface with electrocardiogram machines, monitoring devices, and other CCU products. Through the construction of computer-linked systems, as the company argued in its promotional activities, hospitals could achieve efficient data analysis for clinical decision making and CCU organization. For example, a computerized system to analyze and interpret electrocardiograms led to the capability of processing up to 500 electrocardiograms per eight-hour day: "This and other innovative systems recently introduced to the medical profession contributed to the substantial growth of our medical electronics business during the past year. With this growth has come increasing profitability as well" (26). Similar considerations of profitability motivated the development of telemetry systems for ambulatory patients with heart disease and battery-powered electrocardiogram machines designated for regions of foreign countries where electricity was not yet available for traditional machines.

In 1973 H-P provided a forthright statement of its philosophy of diversification and growth in the medical marketplace:

Hewlett-Packard's medical electronic instrumentation provides clinical tools for a great variety of medical disciplines. Much of this instrumentation did not exist as recently as ten years ago. When HP entered the medical electronics field in 1961, the electrocardiograph was the company's principal product. Today, HP provides many instruments and systems for monitoring the heart and its functions, as well as instrumentation to assist the medical profession in the areas of respiratory disease, internal medicine, and perinatal care. In 1961, the physician in private practice was the company's primary customer. Today, customer-users are in hospitals and clinics, in addition to private practice, and include a broad spectrum of physicians, surgeons, nurses, and technicians.

The ever-increasing need for technological assistance to improve both the quality and quantity of health care service is indicated by the continuing expansion of the company's medical business. Orders for medical instrumentation totaled $59.5 million in 1973, up 38 percent from the previous year. This was the third consecutive year that orders increased by more than 30 percent. Computerized systems added a substantial increment to the company's volume this past year, and will be an increasingly important segment in the years ahead. . . .

Health care expenditures, worldwide, will continue to increase significantly in the years ahead, and a growing portion of these funds will be allocated for medical electronic equipment. Interestingly, this growth trend offers the company—working in close collaboration with researchers, clinicians, and other hospital personnel—the unique opportunity to help shape the future of health care delivery (27).

From the corporate perspective, spiraling health-care expenditures, far from a problem to be solved, are the necessary fuel for desired profit.

The exploitation of illness for corporate profit will persist, much as H-P predicted, unless changes occur that limit the continuing commercialization of health care. Yet it is a mistake to assign too much responsibility to corporations. Private profits in coronary care and related fields would not be possible without the active support of clinicians and professionals who help create new technology of unproven effectiveness and put it into use.

The Academic Medical Center Connection

Academic medical centers have played a key role in the development and promotion of costly innovations like those in coronary care. Medical centers are a focus of monopoly capital in the health sector, yet they seldom have attracted attention in critiques of technology. New approaches generally receive their first clinical use in medical centers, before their adoption by practitioners in local communities and foreign countries. Both corporations considered here, W-L and H-P, obtained important bases at medical centers located in geographic proximity to corporate headquarters. Academic cardiologists participated in the proliferation of CCU equipment; their work doubtless derived in large part form a sincere belief that the new technologies would save lives and help patients, rather than greed or a desire for personal profit. Yet their uncritical support for these innovations fostered CCU's widespread acceptance without documented effectiveness.

Before its purchase by W-L, AO—with headquarters in Southbridge, Massachusetts—established ties with the Peter Bent Brigham Hospital in Boston. Specifically, the company worked with Bernard Lown, an eminent cardiologist, who served as an AO consultant, on the development of defibrillators and cardioverters. Lown pioneered the theoretical basis and clinical applications of these techniques; AO engineers collaborated with Lown in the construction of working models. As previously discussed, AO marketed and promoted several lines of defibrillators and cardioverters that bore Lown's name.

AO's support of technologic innovation at the Peter Bent Brigham Hospital was clear. The CCU developed in the mid-1960s received major grants from AO that Lown and his group acknowledged (28). AO also used data and pictures from the Brigham CCU in promotional literature distributed to the medical profession and potential investors. Lown and his group continued to influence the medical profession through a large number of publications, appearing in both the general medical and cardiologic literature, that discussed CCU-linked diagnostic and therapeutic techniques. In these papers Lown emphasized the importance of automatic monitoring. He also advocated the widespread use of telemetry for ambulatory patients and computerized data-analysis systems, both areas into which AO diversified during the late 1960s and early 1970s. AO's relationship with Lown and his colleagues apparently proved beneficial for all concerned. The dynamics of heightened profits for AO and prestige for Lown were not optimal conditions for a detached, systematic appraisal of CCU effectiveness.

H-P's academic base has been the Stanford University Medical Center, located about one-half mile from corporate headquarters in Palo Alto, California. For many years William Hewlett, H-P's chief executive officer, served as a trustee of Stanford University. In addition, as discussed later, a private philanthropy established by Hewlett was prominent among the University's financial benefactors.

More pertinent were H-P's links to the Division of Cardiology at Stanford. Donald Harrison, professor of medicine and chief of the Division of Cardiology, acted as H-P's primary consultant in the development of coronary care technology. Harrison and his colleagues at Stanford collaborated with H-P engineers in the design of CCU systems intended for marketing to both academic medical centers and community hospitals. H-P helped construct working models of CCU components at Stanford University Hospital, under the direction of Harrison and other faculty members. Stanford physicians introduced these H-P systems into clinical use.

Innovations in the treatment of patients with heart disease had a profound impact on the costs of care at Stanford. As documented in a general study of the costs of treatment for several illnesses at Stanford, the effects of intensive care technology were dramatic. In their conclusions Scitovsky and McCall stated:

> Of the conditions covered by the 1964–1971 study, the changes in treatment in myocardial infarction had their most drastic effect on costs. This was due principally to the increased costs of intensive care units. In 1964, the Stanford Hospital had a relatively small Intensive Care Unit (ICU). It was used by only three of the 1964 coronary cases. . . . By 1971, the hospital had not only an ICU but also a Coronary Care Unit (CCU) and an intermediate CCU. Of the 1971 cases, only one did not receive at least some care in either the CCU or the intermediate CCU (29).

Beyond the costs of intensive care beds, Scitovsky and McCall also observed rapid increases in expensive inputs of care that derived from the intensive approach, such as laboratory tests, electrocardiograms, intravenous solutions, X-rays, inhalation therapy, and pharmaceuticals. As the investigators noted, these changes occurred even while doubt remained about the overall effectiveness of CCUs in reducing morbidity and mortality.

During the late 1960s and early 1970s, many articles from the Harrison group described new technical developments or discussed clinical issues tied to intensive care techniques. Several papers directly acknowledged the use of H-P equipment and assistance. These academic clinicians also participated in continuing medical education programs on coronary care, both in the United States and abroad. The Stanford specialists thus played an important role in promoting technology in general and H-P products in particular.

Private Philanthropies

Philanthropic support figured prominently in the growth of CCUs. The motivations of philanthropic spending were complex. Humanitarian goals doubtless were present. On the other hand, profit considerations were not lacking, since philanthropic initiatives often emerged from the actions of corporate executives whose companies produced medical equipment or pharmaceuticals. Specific philanthropies enthusiastically supported the intensive care approach.

Primary among the philanthropic proponents of CCUs was the American Heart Association (AHA). The AHA sponsored research that led to the development of CCU products, especially monitoring systems. In addition, the AHA helped finance local hospitals establishing CCUs. The "underlying purpose" of these activities, according to the AHA's 1967 annual report, was "to encourage and guide the formation of new [CCU] units in both large and small hospitals." Justifying these expenditures, the AHA cited some familiar "data":

> Expansion of the Coronary Care Unit (CCU) program to communities throughout the nation was a prime objective of the Heart Association in 1967. Experience with the approximately 300 such specialized units already established, mostly in large hospitals, indicated that a national network of CCUs might save the lives of more than 45,000 individuals each year (30).

The source for this projected number of rescued people, though uncited, presumably was the same "personal communication" to which Day referred in his article appearing in 1963 (31).

Later in the 1960s, the AHA's annual number of estimated beneficiaries rose still higher, again with undocumented claims of effectiveness. According to the 1968 annual report, doctors were helpless to deal with MIs until well into the twentieth century, the era that "Dr. Paul Dudley White characterized . . . as 'B.C.' — Before Cardiology." Now, however,

> survival rates of hospitalized patients have been substantially increased by coronary care units. . . . Intensive coronary care units will be greatly expanded in hospitals treating acutely ill patients. At present, only about one third of hospitalized heart attack patients are fortunate enough to be placed in coronary care units. If all of them had the benefits of these monitoring and emergency service facilities, it is estimated that 50,000 more heart patients could be saved yearly (32).

This unsubstantiated estimate, raised from the earlier unsubstantiated figure of 45,000, persisted in AHA literature into the early 1970s. During this same period the AHA cosponsored, with the U.S. Public Health Service and the American College of Cardiology, a series of national conferences on coronary care whose purpose was "the successful development of the CCU program" in all regions of the United States.

Other smaller foundations also supported CCU proliferation. For example, the John A. Hartford Foundation gave generous support to several hospitals and medical centers during the early 1960s to develop monitoring capabilities. Two major recipients of Hartford wealth were Day's group in Kansas City and Lown's group in Boston. The Hartford Foundation's public view of CCU effectiveness was unequivocal; the Kansas City coronary care program "has demonstrated that a properly equipped and designed physical setting staffed with personnel trained to meet cardiac emergencies will provide prophylactic therapy which will materially enhance the survival of these patients and substantially reduce the mortality rates" (33). Another foundation that supported CCU growth, though somewhat less directly, was the W. R. Hewlett Foundation, founded by H-P's chief executive officer. The Hewlett Foundation earmarked large annual grants to Stanford University, which, after an undoubtedly fierce competitive evaluation of alternatives chose H-P equipment for its CCU and other intensive care facilities (34).

The commitment of private philanthropy to technologic innovations is a structural problem that transcends the personalities that control philanthropy at any specific time. The bequests that create philanthropies historically come largely from funds generated by North American industrial corporations that are highly oriented to technologic advances. Moreover, the investment portfolios of philanthropic organizations usually include stocks in a sizable number of industrial companies. These structural conditions encourage financial support for technical advances like those in coronary care. These same conditions tend to discourage philanthropic funding for new programs or organizational changes that would modify the overall structure of the health care system.

In addition, it is useful to ask which people made philanthropic decisions to fund CCU development. During the mid-1960s the AHA's officers included eight physicians who had primary commitments in cardiology, executives of two pharmaceutical companies, a metals company executive, a prominent banker, and several public officials (including Dwight Eisenhower). At the height of CCU promotion in 1968, the chairman of the AHA's annual Heart Fund was a drug company executive. During the 1960s and early 1970s, bankers and corporate executives also dominated the board at the Hartford Foundation. The Hewlett Foundation remained a family affair. Mr. and Mrs. W. R. Hewlett themselves made the decisions about grants until the early 1970s, when R. W. Heyns—former chancellor of the University of California, Berkeley, and also a director of Norton Simon, Inc., Kaiser Industries, and Levi-Strauss—assumed the Foundation's presidency. It is not surprising that philanthropic policies supporting CCU proliferation showed a strong orientation toward corporate industrialism.

The Role of the State

Agencies of government played a key role in CCU growth. The U.S. Public Health Service gave substantial financial support to clinicians for CCU development during the early 1960s. An official of HEW provided an "estimate" of potential lives saved by future CCUs (35); without apparent basis in data, this figure became a slogan for CCU promotion. Conferences and publications by HEW during the late 1960s specified guidelines for adequate CCU equipment, even though the effectiveness of this approach remained unproven by random controlled trial.

In these activities, as noted in chapter 2, three common functions of the state in capitalist societies were evident. First, in health policy the state generally uses positive selection to support private enterprise by encouraging innovations that enhance profits to major industrial corporations; the state does not enact policies that limit private profit in any serious way. Recognizing the high costs of CCU implementation, state agencies could have placed strict limitations on their number and distribution. For example, HEW might have called for the regionalization of CCU facilities and restrictions on their wider proliferation. Subsequently, studies of CCU mortality rates generally have shown better outcomes in larger, busier centers and have suggested the rationality of regionalized policies (36). HEW's policies supported just the opposite development. By publishing guidelines that called for advanced CCU technology and by encouraging CCU proliferation to most community hospitals, HEW ensured the profitability of corporate ventures in the coronary care field.

A second major function of the state is its legitimation of the capitalist political-economic system. The history of public health and welfare programs shows that state expenditures usually increase during periods of social unrest and decrease as unrest becomes less widespread. State spending in the health system enhances the legitimacy of government and corporations when much of the public no longer holds confidence in these institutions. The decade of the 1960s was a time of upheaval in the United States. The civil rights movement called into question basic patterns of injustice. Opposition to the war in Indochina mobilized a large part of the population against government and corporate policies. Labor disputes arose frequently. Under such circumstances, when government and corporations face large-scale crises of legitimacy, the state tends to intervene with health and welfare projects. Medical technology is a "social capital expenditure" by which the state tries to counteract the recurrent legitimacy crises of advanced capitalism (37). Technologic innovations like CCUs are convenient legitimating expenditures, since they convey a message of deep concern for the public health while they also support new sources of profit for large industrial firms.

Third, government agencies provide market research that guides domestic and foreign sales efforts. The Global Market Survey, published by the U.S. Department of Commerce, gave a detailed analysis of changes in medical facilities, hospital beds, and physicians throughout the world. The Survey specified those countries that were prime targets for sales of biomedical equipment. For example, the 1973 Survey pointed out that "major foreign markets for biomedical equipment are expected to grow at an average annual rate of 15 percent in the 1970s, nearly double the growth rate predicted for the U.S. domestic market" (38). The same report predicted that West Germany (which would emphasize CCU construction), Japan, Brazil, Italy, and Israel would be the largest short-term markets for products manufactured in the United States. According to the report, "market research studies identified specific equipment that present [*sic*] good to excellent U.S. sales opportunities in the 20 [foreign] markets"; "cardiologic-thoracic equipment" headed the list of products with high sales potential. Market research performed by state agencies encouraged the proliferation of CCUs and related innovations, whose capacity to generate profits overshadowed the issue of effectiveness in government planning.

Changes in the Health-Care Labor Force

Intensive care involves workers as well as equipment. Throughout the twentieth century, a process of deskilling has occurred by which the skilled trades and professions have become rationalized into simpler tasks that can be handled by less skilled and lower-paid workers (39). For instance, in the construction industry, apprentices have replaced many skilled carpenters. Deskilling of the health-care labor force, as noted earlier, has contributed to humanistic decline in the face of technologic progress. In medicine, paraprofessionals take on rationalized tasks that can be specified by algorithms covering nearly all contingencies. This deskilling process applies equally to CCUs and other intensive care facilities, where standard orders—often printed in advance—can deal with almost all situations that might arise. CCU work is glamorous, but as many health workers realize, much of this work can be quite routine. In some intensive care units, the term "automatic pilot" has appeared; this term refers to the preparation of routine intensive care orders, covering all anticipated possibilities, that subordinate health workers can follow. The term connotes the same process of deskilling that previously occurred in aeronautics.

The deskilling of the intensive care labor force was no accident. It was part of a policy of manpower development that received support from professional, governmental, and corporate planners. During the late 1960s and early 1970s, the training of allied health personnel to deal with intensive care technology became a priority of educators and administrators. According to this view, it was important to train a "cadre of health workers capable of handling routine and purely functional duties" (40). The linkage between allied health workers and new technology was a clear assumption in this approach. There were limits on "the extent to which a markedly greater delegation of tasks can be achieved without the introduction of new technology" that compensates for aides' lack of "decisional training" (41). The availability of monitoring equipment in CCUs made this setting adaptable to staffing partly by technicians who could receive lower wages than doctors or nurses. Paramedical training programs, focusing on intensive care, became a goal of national policy makers, even though they recognized the "built-in obsolescence of monitoring equipment" and the tendency of industrial corporations to "capitalize" in this field (42).

Intensive care work, though portrayed as challenging and exciting, often is boring. The turnover rate of nurses in CCUs is as high as or higher than in other areas; boredom is a major factor in nurses' decisions to leave intensive care (43). In the face of its unproven effectiveness, coronary care technology still requires workers to care for costly machines and the patients to whom they are attached. Trained in routinized tasks, allied health technicians have partially satisfied this need. Their deskilling, however, illustrates the same degradation of work that has affected the labor force outside the health sector.

COST CONTAINMENT UNDER CAPITALISM

The development, promotion, and proliferation of CCUs represented a complex historical process. Similar processes have occurred in the spread of many costly innovations and clinical practices. Straightforward tests of effectiveness seldom have guided policy decisions. Although not exhaustive, an overview helps clarify the history of CCUs and other medical "advances" (Figure 4.1).

Corporate research and development lead to the production of new technology, pharmaceuticals, and related innovations. The guiding motivation for corporations is profit; in this sense the commercialization of health care resembles that of non-

Figure 4.1   Overview of the Development, Promotion, and Proliferation of Coronary Care Units and Similar Medical Advances

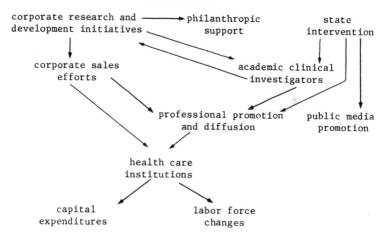

medical goods and services. Closely linked to corporations, philanthropies support research and clinical practices that enhance profits. Agencies of the state encourage innovations by grants for investigation, financial assistance to medical centers adopting new technology, and advocacy of new practices. While state intervention benefits private enterprise, it also enhances the faltering legitimacy of the capitalist political-economic system. Academic clinicians and investigators, based in teaching hospitals, help develop technology and foster its diffusion through professional publications and pronouncements in the public media. Corporate sales efforts cultivate markets in health institutions, both domestic and foreign. Technologic change generates the need for allied health workers who are less skilled than professionals. The cyclical acceptance of technologic innovations by medical institutions involves capital expenditures that drive up the overall cost of health care.

Cost-containment activities that do not recognize these dynamics of the capitalist system will remain a farce. Sophisticated methodologies to analyze costs and effectiveness have emerged in medical-care research; these techniques include clinical decision analysis and a variety of related methods. Ironically, economists first developed this type of analysis at the Pentagon in order to evaluate technologic innovations like new missiles (44). This methodology led to disastrous policy decisions in Indochina, largely because the cost-effectiveness approach did not take into account the broader, so-called imponderable context. This analysis did not predict accurately the political response of the Indochinese people to such technologies as napalm and mechanized warfare. Even more ironically, many of the same people who developed cost-effectiveness research at the Defense Department later moved into the health field, where this approach became quite fashionable (45).

In health care as in other areas, cost-effectiveness methodology restricts the level of analysis to the evaluation of specific innovations. Studies using this framework generally ignore, or make only passing reference to, the broader structures of capitalism. As a result, this approach obscures one fundamental source of high costs and ineffective practices: the profit motive. Apparent methodologic sophistication masks the analytic poverty of research that evaluates many different innovations while overlooking their common origins in the drive for profit. Because of this deficiency, cost-effectiveness analysis mystifies the roots of costly, ineffective practices in the very nature of our political-economic system.

Defects of research, however, are less dangerous than defects of policy. Cost containment has become a highly touted national priority. Services whose effectiveness is difficult to demonstrate by the new methodologies are prime candidates for cutbacks and therefore face a bleak future. Poor people and minority groups, historically victimized by the free-enterprise system, are the first to suffer from this purported rationalization of policy. Meanwhile, private profit in health care, a major fuel for high costs, continues unabated. Just as it eludes serious attention in research, the structure of profit evades new initiatives in health policy. Cost con-

tainment will remain little more than rhetoric, unless we begin to address the linkages between cost and profit. It is foolish to presume that major restrictions on
profit in the health system can succeed without other basic changes in the political-economic system.

In summary, the development and promotion of high technology in medicine
may seem irrational when analyzed in terms of proven medical effectiveness.
These trends appear considerably more rational when viewed from the needs of
the capitalist system. By questioning what capitalism does with our hearts, we get
closer to the heart of many of our other problems.

5

Social Medicine and the Community

The glamour and superficial luxuries of intensive care contrast with the realities of community medicine. Social contradictions that form the basis of problems in the health-care system are perhaps most glaring in local communities. While expensive technology of dubious effectiveness proliferates, services of the simplest kind remain inaccessible. Poor people and minorities historically have suffered most from these inequities. Despite some improvements in access since the initiation of public programs during the 1960s, regional and local maldistribution of health workers and facilities persists.

A series of social contradictions makes community medicine difficult. As noted in chapter 1, uneven economic development is a major determinant of the availability of both preventive and curative services. Geographic areas that face shortages of health workers and facilities tend to be the same areas that are most depressed economically. Monopoly capital in the health sector leads to a concentration of financial resources in a small number of medical centers and corporations. This concentration means that costly, technologically oriented medicine flourishes but low-income and minority communities lack needed services. Professional education, which emphasizes advanced technology and specialization, reinforces the effect of uneven development. After specialized training in medical centers, practitioners often are reluctant to work in areas without nearby hospitals and medical schools. Ideologic contradictions, like that between freedom and equality, add to the problems of community medicine. If health professionals remain free to decide the location of their practices and to control the conditions of their work, they tend to prefer the more lucrative and less demanding situations of practice. Increases in the supply of health-care professionals may motivate some practitioners to work in underserved areas, but the long-range impact of these trends is unclear. Meanwhile, inequalities in access to services continue to be rooted in patterns of geography, class structure, and racism; in many localities, these patterns impede the practice of community medicine.

The private-public contradiction is another impediment. The private sector is based in private hospitals, private practice, and companies that manufacture medical products or control finance capital. As part of the state, the public sector functions through public expenditures and employs practitioners in public institutions. Although nations vary greatly in the private-public contradiction, the private sector generally attracts public financing. Public subsidization of the private sector can diminish services that are accessible to low-income people and minorities. This effect can occur even though vast sums of public funds may be allocated for the care of these groups. In addition, one irony of expansion in the private sector involves public support for private hospitals and clinics. Such facilities tend to grow as public institutions contract. Although private expansion does little to assist clients who previously used the public sector, new hospital construction frequently has detrimental effects on needed housing and the quality of life in low-income and minority communities. This chapter explores private medical expansion, public medical contraction, and alternative systems that involve community clinics.

PRIVATE MEDICAL EXPANSION

Controlling private medical expansion is no easy task. In the past it has been difficult to argue against health-care facilities. Most people have accepted the notion that there is a need for more medical care that justifies new hospitals. This assumption has met several lines of criticism.

The most straightforward criticism of unrestricted expansion is that it leads to unnecessary duplication and overlap of facilities in certain geographic areas, while other areas remain underserved. New medical buildings and equipment appear where they are already highly concentrated. Such trends create grotesque paradoxes as expensive facilities remain underutilized because of duplication; meanwhile, clients from outlying areas find it difficult to gain access to services. Analysts of these trends argue for comprehensive and regionalized planning to improve distribution and coordination.

Another critique focuses on the problem of costs. Unused hospital beds ("overbedding") have contributed to the increased costs of health care. Questioning the benefits of more hospital beds relative to their costs, some health economists have advocated a general moratorium on hospital construction or expansion. Laws that require comprehensive planning, however, seldom apply abstract standards of rationality; the effects of such legislation often are more symbolic than real. For instance, laws in the 1970s requiring a "certificate of need" for new hospital construction achieved very little impact. While many hospitals' plans were modified, only a few applications were rejected. Hospital administrators and governing boards exerted great influence over the decisions of planning agencies responsible for controlling expansion (1). On the other hand, this failure of health-planning legislation does not dilute the criticism that private medical expansion is a major factor in the rising costs of medical care.

Hospitals and medical centers, of course, are not the only expanding institutions with which people in cities must contend. Urban renewal, with its emphasis on commercial development, has displaced millions of people form low-income housing. Banks, insurance companies, government office buildings, and highway construction have destroyed innumerable communities. The expansionary tendencies of medical centers have had a similar impact on urban neighborhoods.

The effects of private medical expansion in cities can be devastating. Hospital construction commonly involves hospitals' purchase and destruction of nearby low-income housing. Because such dwellings generally include rental units, evicted residents must seek housing in a tight rental market; frequently they must leave the neighborhoods where they and their families have lived for many years. Construction may lead to traffic congestion and parking problems. Noise and air pollution worsens, particularly when additional power plants are necessary. Unless expansion plans carefully consider local residents, new medical facilities threaten housing and living conditions.

Such outcomes become even harder when these facilities do not address residents' health-care needs. Private hospital construction often involves space for specialists, administrators, and research rather than for primary care services; expansion may not increase the health care actually available for people in surrounding communities. This paradox applies especially when low-income patients cannot afford private fees or when private practitioners do not accept patients with public insurance like Medicaid. In short, while private medical expansion can worsen living conditions, it does not necessarily improve services.

How common are such problems? During the late 1970s my co-workers and I conducted a survey of hospitals in the 20 largest cities of the United States (2). We found that in each city one or more medical centers expanded during the prior decade or had plans to expand in the near future (Table 5.1). One hundred ninety-two expansion projects, including at least one in every city, extended into residential areas; if completed, 125 would have led to the destruction of housing. One hundred twelve expansion plans encountered opposition from various sources; for 69 of these, opposition came from local residents' organizations.

From the survey it was possible to reach some conclusions about the dynamics of expansion. Although the tendency of medical centers to expand has modulated somewhat since the 1970s, medical expansion in cities has been quite common and has generated frequent opposition. Resistance to expansion has come from community organizations much more often than from government agencies. Because land use patterns have supported the needs of capital, medical expansion has interfered less with commercial or industrial facilities than with housing. Larger hospitals have been more likely to expand than have been smaller hospitals; they also encountered more opposition from local communities. Medical expansion provided space for administration, parking, and research; hospital growth therefore

Table 5.1   Medical Expansion in the 20 Largest Cities in the United States, Late 1970s

	Number of Hospitals[a]	Percent[b]
Actual or planned expansion	457	85
Purpose of expansion		
Patient care space	409	75
Support services	392	72
Parking	342	63
Administrative space	302	56
Research space	154	28
Other	21	13
Expansion into		
Residential areas	192	35
Commercial areas	93	17
Recreational areas	22	4
Industrial areas	20	4
Removal of		
Housing facilities	125	23
Commercial facilities	52	10
Recreational facilities	11	2
Industrial facilities	8	1
Any opposition to expansion	112	21
Opposition by		
Residents' organization	69	13
Comprehensive health planning agency	29	5
State government	16	3
City government	12	2
Environmental group	11	2
Community health organization	11	2
Federal government	7	1
Chamber of Commerce	2	0
Other	20	4

Source: H. Waitzkin, J. Wallen, and J. Sharratt, "Homes or Hospitals? Contradictions of the Urban Crisis," *Int. J. Health Serv.* 9 (1979): 407.

[a]Minimum figures, based on 549 respondents. Response rate = 549/662 = 83%.
[b]Denominator = 549 — noncodable responses.

responded to bureaucratic and other organizational needs in addition to patient care.

Private expansion thus has had many negative impacts. During the past three decades, one or more expanding private medical centers have destroyed low-income housing in every major city in the United States. Expansion generally has occurred in previously stable working-class communities; suitable replacement housing seldom has been available. Enlarging medical centers have worsened problems of traffic and pollution. Under these circumstances, medical expansion often has contributed to the deterioration of urban neighborhoods.

The success of community organizing against expanding medical institutions has varied. In several cities, private hospitals have simply destroyed nearby neighborhoods during expansion projects, despite the efforts of community activists. In New York City, Chicago, and San Francisco, medical centers have purchased low-income housing, evicted tenants, razed existing structures, and constructed new hospital facilities. In these cases, opposition by local residents has failed. Community organizers in other cities have been more successful. In Boston, for example, tenants resisted the expansion of a powerful, university-affiliated medical center. This struggle led to the construction of additional low-income and middle-income housing, the stabilization of a community, and the replacement of medical buildings in a manner that did not remove needed housing (3).

For those who control urban institutions, the human costs of private medical expansion sometimes are hard to understand. The attachments of working-class people to their neighborhoods generally are very strong. Fried has described these attachments: "A high degree of residential stability, deep commitment of people to their neighborhoods, and close-knit social organization are among the most striking features of working class community life" (4). When working-class people lose their homes because of medical expansion or other forms of urban redevelopment, they often suffer a deep and lasting grief that derives as much from the loss of their social networks as from the destruction of their homes.

One outcome of conflicts concerning medical expansion is a heightened consciousness about the nature of large urban institutions. By struggling against medical expansion, community residents learn that those who control policy in medical centers hold no special knowledge of the public good and have their own private interests as well. With this demystification, people who live in cities no longer will accept without criticism these institutions' claims for land, finances, or popular support. As people organize themselves to protect their communities, they come to believe that the destruction of urban housing to build private medical centers has little justification.

Private medical expansion also reflects political and economic processes that extend beyond the local level and the health-care system; control over the health-care system mirrors general patterns of class domination. As discussed in chapter 2, members of the corporate class, business middle class, and professional middle class hold the vast majority of positions on the governing boards of private medical centers. Board members tend to be bankers, executives, and professionals. They and the institutions with which they are affiliated often benefit, directly or indirectly, from construction loans, office space and laboratories, and sales of pharmaceuticals, equipment, and supplies that medical expansion generates. These corporate ties provide a structural basis for the "profit in non-profit hospitals" (5).

In addition, the expansion of private medical centers parallels general patterns of monopoly capital. During the twentieth century, control over capital has become more concentrated in a small number of organizations that dominate each sector of the economy, including the health-care system. Spatial arrangements in cities, especially the balance between housing and institutional land use, follow historical shifts in capital accumulation (6). Large private hospitals have expanded their capital, in the form of machines, equipment, and physical plant. Over time, the concentration of capital in private medical centers has resembled that in other economic sectors.

State intervention in private medicine further encourages expansion. "Social capital expenditures" by the state include public spending for welfare, health care, and similar programs. An underlying purpose of these expenditures is the public's restored confidence in the legitimacy of the capitalist system (7). Economic instability, inflation, stagnation, and unemployment lead to crises of legitimacy as people start to question current structures of political and economic domination. To reinforce its legitimacy, especially in times of social protest, the state increases social capital expenditures, including public subsidization of private medical expansion.

There are several forms of public subsidization. The most direct subsidy involves government grants for hospital construction. Historically, government in the United States has responded to economic and political pressures through massive spending to build hospitals. The Public Works Administration and Works Progress Administration provided much of this subsidization during the Depression of the 1930s, as did the Hill-Burton Program in the post–World War II period. Since 1946, when Congress passed the Hill-Burton legislation, this program contributed more than $3.5 billion to approximately 3,800 construction projects. By stimulating additional private and public investment, Hill-Burton's total financial impact exceeded $12.5 billion and helped build facilities for about 270,000 beds, more than half the total beds in private nonprofit hospitals in the United States. In general, the Hill-Burton program did not require coordinated planning. As a result, many of the approximately 2,300 hospitals receiving Hill-Burton money constructed overlapping and duplicated facilities. Overbedding and underutilized bed capacity increased costs.

Nonprofit status is another public subsidy for private expansion. Because of nonprofit status, private medical centers are exempt from many taxes on their income and property. Tax savings stimulate expansion in several ways. Contributions to hospitals from individuals, corporations, and foundations are tax deductible. Medical centers can sell bonds for construction; the purchasers of these bonds earn interest which is usually exempt from taxes. Most important, because nonprofit hospitals escape much of the burden of income and property taxes, they can reinvest a sizable portion of their revenues in new construction. Even when property held by private hospitals increases in value, property taxes remain low. The equity generated by property values that are largely nontaxable also allows these institutions to obtain loans at favorable interest rates. Such tax advantages foster expansion, even when added facilities may be unnecessary or detrimental to a community's needs for housing and public services.

A third public subsidization of private expansion involves the payment policies of public insurance programs like Medicare and Medicaid. Before the creation of these programs during the mid-1960s, insurance companies and Blue Cross had cooperated with private hospitals in the construction and maintenance of facilities. For example, in negotiating a reimbursement formula with "third-party" insurers, a hospital could receive payment for the depreciation of equipment and physical plant. This arrangement meant that a proportion of insurance payments for hospitalized patients would cover the estimated deterioration of a hospital's physical facilities, over and above the actual costs of medical care for those patients. Medicare and Medicaid allowed a variety of formulas for depreciation, including accelerated depreciation payments during the first few years after completion of construction. Depreciation payments from public insurance programs became an impetus for private medical expansion.

Medicare and Medicaid also have permitted private hospitals to request reimbursement for interest payments on bank loans and for unspecified "hidden" expenses of patient care. The latter, so-called plus factor was an extra payment under public insurance programs that was calculated as a fixed percentage, usually between 2 and 5 percent, of a hospital's annual operating costs. Although such agreements vary among hospitals and states, they all tend to reduce the financial risk of new construction. In short, the subsidies that public insurance programs provide through depreciation, interest payments, and the plus factor create powerful incentives for private medical expansion.

Public funds have become a major source of income for many, if not most, private hospitals. Aside from subsidies that foster construction, direct public funding of patient care provides a large proportion of hospital revenues. In some geographical areas, private hospitals receive more patient-care revenues from the public-sector Medicaid and Medicare programs than do the local public hospitals.

What difference does public subsidization of the private sector make? If private institutions provided accessible services of high quality, it could be argued that public support is warranted. The growth of public subsidies for private medicine, however, has corresponded to an erosion of public health services and institutions. Private hospitals often are not accessible to low-income and minority patients. These private facilities tend to refuse services to such clients, or to transfer them to public hospitals at the earliest opportunity. Public hospitals and programs also have suffered cutbacks and closures at the same time that private institutions have attracted greater public funding. Inaccessible private services, "patient dumping" from the private to the public sector, and the contraction of public facilities—which are all detrimental effects of the private-public contradiction—now deserve attention.

PUBLIC MEDICAL CONTRACTION

The contraction of public hospitals and services is the grim underside of private expansion. While private facilities enlarge with the aid of public subsidies, public health-care institutions tend to deteriorate. Public medical contraction varies widely. It has affected some communities more than others and occurs at a different pace in various parts of the United States. The decline of public medical facilities also goes hand in hand with cutbacks of other public services. The general instability of the economy contributes to the recurrent financial crises of many cities and counties. With these crises it becomes more difficult to maintain public services of all kinds. Contraction of public medical care is only one manifestation of the general fiscal crisis in the public sector.

Public hospitals in the United States have a long history that dates back at least to the eighteenth century. They arose originally in major cities along the East Coast. The motivations of their founding were complex. An important goal was the control of infectious diseases. Tuberculosis, typhus, syphilis, and other infections periodically swept through urban areas. Epidemics frequently arose first among the poor, who suffered from inadequate housing, nutrition, and sanitation and who could not afford the fees of private physicians. Contagion among the poor also threatened the wealthy; infections often spread from poor neighborhoods to wealthier ones, and large-scale epidemics interrupted commerce. One rationale for public hospitals was to provide free or inexpensive medical services to the poor, as a method to prevent the spread of infections.

Humanitarian goals also influenced the founding of public hospitals. Ethical norms in the medical profession called for physicians to devote a specific, though small, proportion of their time to the care of indigent patients. Professional leaders encouraged doctors to offer charitable services within public hospitals and clinics. Patients who used these facilities traditionally provided teaching material for medical students and doctors in training. Participation by the poor in medical education was seen as an appropriate exchange for free or inexpensive services. Wealthier clients generally received care from practitioners who had obtained training in charitable institutions. Incentives for the formation of public hospitals, then, included a variety of practical and ethical considerations (8). Similar institutions later opened in the South, Midwest, and West, usually as a responsibility of local governments. By the early twentieth century, public hospitals existed in most major cities or counties of the United States.

The decline of public hospitals did not begin until the mid-1960s, with the passage of Medicare and Medicaid legislation. These laws provided publicly financed insurance for indigent patients, who could use their benefits to obtain services from private practitioners and private hospitals in addition to public institutions. The organized medical profession, especially the American Medical Association, had opposed such legislation for several decades. However, the money that these laws provided led to an abrupt and ironic reversal in professional attitudes. Within three years after the passage of Medicare and Medicaid, a majority of physicians in the United States switched from opposition to support for public financing of indigent patients (9). As noted in chapter 1, public expenditures for health care increased drastically after the mid-1960s, and these funds increasingly went to private practitioners and private hospitals. With public insurance, charity medicine in theory was no longer necessary; poor patients could be "mainstreamed" into the private sector. Other motivations for public hospitals also were less keen than previously. With better sanitation and antibiotics, epidemics were not important public health problems. Medical education could take place in private hospitals affiliated with medical schools, where indigent patients now would bring with them their public insurance benefits. In short, by the early 1970s several prior rationales for public hospitals weakened.

The deepening fiscal crisis of cities and counties, coupled with the availability of public insurance, has led to a gradual contraction of public hospitals, clinics, and services. Contraction has manifested itself in several ways. The most common form involves cutbacks in facilities and services. Outpatient clinics associated with public health departments, for instance, have reduced their hours and staffing. Preventive and outreach programs have been phased out. Regarding inpatient care, many public hospitals have reduced the number of beds available for patients needing hospitalization. As a result, the emergency rooms of these hospitals may turn away seriously ill patients who in prior years would have been admitted. Such reductions have occurred in cities and counties throughout the United States.

What happened to patients who previously would have used such hospitals and clinics? It is commonly thought that the private sector has taken over the care of these patients. As noted earlier, the income of private hospitals from public insurance programs has increased markedly. Clearly, private hospitals do provide services to some indigent patients with Medicare and Medicaid funding. However, there is also evidence that many clients who previously would have obtained care from public hospitals are not receiving adequate attention in the private sector.

Several groups of patients typically cannot afford private fees, do not hold private insurance, and are not eligible for public insurance programs. For instance, many of the "working poor" have incomes that place then slightly above the poverty level and yet disqualify them from Medicaid eligibility. Members of minority groups, especially those who do not speak English, often face extreme difficulties in using private hospitals, which historically have made little effort to hire minority workers or to provide bilingual services. Private hospitals often are located in wealthier neighborhoods that are distant from urban and rural areas with low-income and minority populations. Geographic inaccessibility hinders the use of these private facilities, even when patients qualify for public funding. Legally, individual doctors and private hospitals may refuse care to patients covered by Medicare and Medicaid; in some areas of the country, practitioners and hospitals either decline to see publicly insured patients or limit such patients to a fixed proportion of total visits. Many states have restricted their financial contributions to the Medicaid program.

Both Medicaid and Medicare frequently pay less than prevailing professional fees; in these situations, patients often receive bills for the uncovered portion. In short, a series of obstacles hinder patients form utilizing services in the private sector.

Before the passage of Medicare and Medicaid, "patient dumping" from the private sector to the public sector was a common phenomenon. Uninsured patients who arrived at the offices of private practitioners or at the emergency rooms of private hospitals generally were refused service and referred to the local public hospital. Although Medicare and Medicaid modified this pattern somewhat, a study in the early 1970s found that dumping persisted to a large degree (10). In Alameda County, California, a follow-up study in the early 1980s concerned transfers of patients from private hospitals to the county hospital's emergency room (11). The county hospital had faced declining bed capacity and staffing. Nevertheless, during the first seven months of 1981, private hospitals throughout the county transferred 458 patients to the emergency room of the public hospital. As expected, a sizable proportion of these patients, 43 percent, had no insurance coverage. Surprisingly, many patients did have either private or public insurance; about 36 percent had MediCal or were MediCal eligible, 12 percent had Medicare, and 2.6 percent held private insurance policies. Many of the transferred patients were quite sick; 66 percent of them were transported to the public hospital by ambulance, and 69 percent were admitted for inpatient care. The racial characteristics of transferred patients were noteworthy. Thirty percent of them were black; among blacks who were transferred, 43 percent had MediCal insurance, while this figure was only 14 percent for whites. In other words, transfers affected blacks more than whites, regardless of their eligibility for public insurance.

Beyond this apparent effect of racial criteria, patients' ability to pay seemed the most important factor in transfer policy. As the study concluded:

> The remarkably low percentage of transferred patients who had private insurance coverage—14 times lower than the percentage in the county as a whole—suggests that a powerful selection mechanism is operating in transfer policy. This mechanism appears to be ability to pay. In short, our study supports the conclusion of previous analyses: patient dumping is extensive and almost exclusively limited to the poor and minorities (12).

Despite the weakening of public hospitals, the dumping of uninsured patients—as well as insured patients who may be undesirable for a variety of reasons—from the private sector to the public sector persisted. Other studies in the 1980s found dumping in other urban areas (13). Eventually national legislation prohibited the transfer of medically unstable patients. After the stabilization of patients' conditions, hospitals continued to dump patients to the public sector (a phenomenon known as "second day dumps").

The availability of public insurance for indigent patients at private hospitals, then, has not met the needs of many patients who formerly used public hospitals.

Although gaps in services arise when the staffing and bed capacity of public hospitals decline, such problems become even more severe when public hospitals actually close. Municipal or county hospitals have closed in New York City, Philadelphia, Detroit, and several other large cities across the United States. The same process has occurred in smaller cities and rural areas. In some cases, the planned closure of public hospitals has led to protests by community residents that occasionally have prevented the disappearance of these facilities. In other cases, protests have failed. The likelihood of closing public hospitals is directly related to the fiscal crises of cities and counties. Wealthier communities with a stronger tax base tend to keep public hospitals open and sometimes even enlarge them. When cities and counties encounter greater economic difficulties, especially in the East and Midwest, public hospitals close more frequently (14).

In addition to closure, another change affecting public hospitals involves the privatization of ownership and control. Privatization refers to the purchase of public hospitals by private corporations or the assumption of administrative responsibility by private management firms. Under either arrangement, city or county funding continues to flow into the hospital for health services, but the control of day-to-day operations changes from a public agency to a private entity. A common justification for the conversion to private control is that private management is less bureaucratic and more efficient than public administration. Another rationale, especially when medical schools take over public hospitals, is that the quality of care improves because of closer supervision of interns and residents by faculty members. There is little substantiation for these assumptions. In fact, studies of private management show costs that are equal to or greater than those of public management and negligible improvements in quality (15).

After public hospitals are privatized, uninsured patients are supposed to receive services with financial subsidies from city or county governments. Investigations of several counties in California where privatization occurred show that many fewer uninsured patients used privatized facilities than those who formerly used the hospitals when they were publicly owned and controlled. What happened to these patients is not entirely clear, but available evidence indicates that uninsured patients frequently are unaware that they can obtain care at privatized hospitals which receive county or municipal funding (16). The public funds available for uninsured patients at privatized hospitals seldom are publicized. For this reason, it appears that indigent patients tend not to turn to privatized hospitals except under dire emergencies.

Privatization has occurred throughout the United States. Occasionally, political organizing in local communities and among workers in public hospitals prevents or delays privatization. In rare instances, the failures of private management result in a later return to administration by public agencies. Coupled with a trend toward closure, however, privatization has drastically affected the nature of services that poor people and minorities can obtain. These changes are especially detrimental when patients are not eligible for public insurance programs like Medicare and Medicaid.

To summarize, public medical contraction has taken place in many parts of the United States. This trend has been intimately tied to the general economic crisis of local governments, most apparent in communities with more severe financial difficulties. Despite the availability of public insurance under Medicare and Medicaid, private hospitals have tended to dump uninsured or otherwise undesirable patients into public hospitals. Public hospitals themselves have been weakened by cutbacks in facilities and staffing; frequently, they have closed altogether. Some public hospitals have converted to private ownership and/or control. Although this arrangement presumably allows payment for poor and uninsured patients from city or county funds, such patients often have not understood their eligibility for these services and consequently have not used privatized facilities. Resistance by community residents and public-sector workers has occurred in several localities; in some instances these struggles have stopped or delayed cutbacks, closures, and privatization. In many communities, however, the gradual erosion of public-sector medicine has continued, and the detrimental effects of public contraction have become clear.

AN ALTERNATIVE: THE MULTISERVICE COMMUNITY CLINIC

Community clinics have appeared in many parts of the United States. They now exist in rural and urban areas that previously lacked regular and accessible services. These clinics differ in their clienteles, organizational structure, and political orientation. Many of them have created remarkable accomplishments, and most suffer from commonly shared problems.

The private-public contradiction has been an incentive for the formation of community clinics. Private medical centers have expanded while leaving the health-care needs of the poor and minorities largely unmet. Public hospitals, which formerly provided services to these groups, have contracted. While community clinics are a partial response to the deficiencies that the private-public contradiction fosters, they remain a fragile and incomplete solution.

The history of community clinics in the United States goes back to the late nineteenth century and in Europe even earlier. In North American cities, they began as an extension of settlement houses. These organizations, usually located in poor and immigrant neighborhoods, offered charitable relief and assistance in housing and employment. Medical programs received financial support from private philanthropy and public health departments. As in the case of public hospitals, an important motivation for the formation of community clinics was the prevention of infectious diseases that could spread to wealthier neighborhoods and interfere with commercial activities. Later, during the first two decades of the twentieth century, community clinics became stronger, reflecting the social reformism of the Progressive Era and an emphasis on uplift of the poor. Medical reformers of this period saw the local clinic as a focus of community life and an institution that, along with other charitable services, would help people over-come the effects of poverty. Some clinics employed community residents in paraprofessional roles, and some adopted procedures of democratic policy mak-ing by residents and clinic workers. Although community clinics formed in many North American cities, they were short-lived. With the Depression, fund-ing dwindled, and most of the clinics that opened during the Progressive Era ceased to exist (17).

The political turbulence of the late 1960s and early 1970s was a major factor in the reemergence of community clinics. The civil rights movement led to a grow-ing recognition that inadequate health care was one of many manifestations of racism in North American society. Several militant organizations started medical programs to serve the needs of minority groups. For instance, the Black Panther Party opened clinics in Chicago, New York, Boston, and other cities. These clin-ics offered primary care and preventive services. Volunteers usually staffed the clinics; the party organized community-based governing boards to make policy decisions. Services were given free or with nominal charge. While the Black Pan-ther clinics responded to black communities, the Young Lords Party started health-care programs to serve mainly Latinos. Organizing in several cities also led to the formation of clinics serving Native American, Asian, and other racial minorities.

There were additional political movements during this period that motivated new clinics and health-care programs. The women's movement in particular revealed gaps and insensitivities in obstetrics and gynecology. Sexism in medi-cine, as noted in chapter 2, was a structure of oppression that excluded women from professional training and that fostered practices that women perceived as degrading. In both urban and rural areas, feminist organizations began to form health-care agencies to address these problems; women practitioners generally served women clients. Most feminist clinics developed educational programs, so that laypersons could learn diagnostic procedures and treatments. Again, these programs frequently used volunteers, who provided services with no or minimal expense to clients.

The countercultural movement also was an impetus for community-based clin-ics. A critique of modern medicine was one component of a more general criticism of technologically oriented culture. From this standpoint, specialization and tech-nology were dehumanizing features of medicine that required resistance. Advo-cates of the countercultural approach correctly pointed out that alternative healing traditions—including homeopathy, chiropractic, herbal remedies, and non-West-ern methods like acupuncture and meditation—had been suppressed in the United States, even though their effectiveness had not been evaluated systematically. In several cities and rural areas, countercultural clinics started to provide alternative forms of healing. These "free clinics" often gave services without cost to clients, but the symbolism of free care also extended to the notion of freedom from stifling qualities of mainstream medicine.

Minority-group organizers, the women's movement, and the countercultural movement usually favored voluntary services and self-sufficiency. During the same period, however, a major expansion of government and philanthropic financing for community medicine occurred. Funding policies acknowledged that poverty, racism, and geographic isolation were associated with inaccessible medical care and higher rates of morbidity and mortality. New medical programs often followed urban riots that focused worldwide attention on social class deprivation and racism in the United States. Many health initiatives during the late 1960s and early 1970s led to the creation of community clinics. Local clinics received funds from the Office of Economic Opportunity, the Model Cities programs, the Department of Health, Education, and Welfare, the Department of Housing and Urban Development, revenue-sharing moneys, the National Health Service Corps, and other federal sources. Private philanthropies also made contributions. In large part a response to political unrest, public and philanthropic spending encouraged the growth of clinics in size and number. By the mid-1970s, more than 1,000 community clinics were serving clients throughout the United States.

Although community clinics show enormous variety (as discussed later), they share certain characteristics (18). In general, they emphasize family care and primary services. This emphasis responds to the difficulties of specialized and technologically oriented practice based in hospitals and medical centers. At community clinics, clients and their families can consult a primary practitioner who acts as a generalist caring for most problems and referring patients to specialists only as required. The clinics also encourage new roles for health workers. "Mid-level" practitioners—including physicians' assistants, nurse practitioners, midwives, and allied paraprofessionals—take on greater responsibility for patient care. Although these practitioners work under the supervision of physicians, they generally see patients on their own, develop a regular group of clients, and consult with a supervising doctor at their discretion. Similarly, the clinics offer training and employment for community residents. People without formal professional education can obtain jobs as medical assistants, outreach workers, receptionists, laboratory aides, and related roles. In addition to employment opportunities, the education that clinics provide helps some workers later to enter professional schools of medicine, nursing, and allied health-care disciplines.

Community clinics usually improve the accessibility of medical care. Many clinics have opened in urban or rural areas that previously lacked services. In addition, most clinics charge low fees on a sliding scale for clients who do not have private or public insurance. The clinics seek external funding to supplement payments from patients, so that financial barriers do not prevent clients form receiving needed care. Clinics rarely if ever turn away patients who are unable to pay, even though this policy creates continuing problems of financial stability for the institutions.

The clinics' policy-making structures usually foster accessibility and responsiveness. A governing board, composed largely of "consumers" elected by the local community, sets formal policy for most clinics. The actual power exercised by these boards varies. Coupled with the employment of local residents as staff members, however, community boards offer a mechanism by which clients can make their needs felt and achieve greater accountability.

Despite these common characteristics, community clinics are quite diverse. Many of them serve specific minority groups. Others are women's clinics. In most large cities, one of two "free" clinics focus on alternative medicine; their clients usually are young people with countercultural concerns. Some clinics have organized to deal with the needs of the elderly and disabled. Funding comes from different sources. Most clinics adopt a sliding fee schedule for clients with low incomes; if patients have third-party coverage, the clinics usually submit bills to Medicare, Medicaid, and private insurance companies. Grants from government agencies and foundations often support clinics with indigent clients. There is also diversity in governance and policy making. Some clinics have formed as one of several projects started by minority organizations, women's groups, community associations, unions, and similar organizations whose purposes go beyond health care alone. Such clinics generally have strong governing boards that set policy. Other clinics have emerged from the initiative of government or philanthropic agencies. Although consumers usually sit on the boards of these institutions, major directions of policy frequently come from the external funding agencies.

In many urban areas the diversity of clinics is startling. By the mid-1970s, for example, ten community clinics had formed in Alameda County, California. This county includes Oakland, Berkeley, and several other cities on the eastern side of San Francisco Bay. Although the county government has operated local clinics, many groups have felt the need for health-care services beyond those the county has provided. Table 5.2 shows some of the community clinics' characteristics. Specific clinics serve predominantly black, Latino, Asian, and Native American minorities; others reach clients who are principally women, the elderly, or young people oriented to counterculture. All the clinics have governing boards composed mainly of nonprofessionals who represent clients in policy decisions. In addition, some of the clinics have adopted formal principles that encourage participation by professional and nonprofessional workers in policy making. The clinics differ widely in size and finances. Some have a small paid staff and depend on volunteers, while other clinics have hired a greater number of workers. Larger institutions have provided a spectrum of services that include primary medical care, hospitalization, dentistry, optometry, mental health, social work, nutrition, and child care. Annual budgets range from approximately $2.9 to $10.3 million. Some clinics rely on personal contributions and voluntary work, while others receive a combination of payments from clients, third-party insurers, government agencies, and philanthropies.

Despite the clinics' diversity, they have formed a cooperative network, the Alameda Health Consortium. The Consortium tries to coordinate funding, equipment, and staffing for the ten clinics. These efforts foster mutual support among clinics that otherwise might compete for scarce resources. The Consortium encourages regular meetings that include the clinics' administrators and staff members; close communication supports cooperation rather than competition. Through the Consortium, the clinics can identify common needs, can consult with one another about planning and fund-raising, and can share expertise. This arrangement permits the coordination of services throughout a large geographic area and avoids fragmentation.

While such cooperative links are helpful, community clinics face typical and chronic problems. The roots of many of these problems are the same social contradictions discussed earlier. For example, the private-public contradiction means that public support for community clinics is constantly tenuous. Although government funding may increase temporarily, especially in response to political unrest, public money is always subject to cutbacks and therefore is undependable. During the late 1960s and early 1970s, public financing for community medicine grew rapidly. However, during the late 1970s these allocations began to level off and eventually to decrease. Major cuts affected the budgets of federal programs. Grants initiated by the Department of Health, Education, and Welfare (later, the Department of Health and Human Services) and revenue-sharing programs declined. The National Health Service Corps, which had provided salaries of professionals working in many community clinics, faced drastic cutbacks. Because of these cutbacks, most community clinics had to reduce services, and many closed altogether. Meanwhile, the public subsidies of private hospitals and private practice—including grants for construction, tax advantages from nonprofit status, and reimbursement under public insurance programs—continued more or less unabated. The financial insecurity of community clinics is not simply a matter of

Table 5.2   Participating Clinics in the Alameda Health Consortium, Alameda County, California, 1997

Clinic	Annual Encounters	Annual Budget ($)	Location
Asian Health Services*	43,160	4,580,398	O
Berkeley Community Health Project	10,348	3,549,289	B
East Bay Native American Health Center	31,992	3,549,289	O
La Clínica de la Raza*	84,053	10,323,622	O
Lifelong Medical Care*	40,950	4,971,026	B, O
Planned Parenthood Golden Gate*	43,669	2,900,370	O, H, F, P
Tri-City Health Center*	22,676	3,423,946	F
Tiburcio Vásquez Health Center*	34,824	4,822,727	UC, H
Valley Community Health Center*	57,808	4,076,192	P, L
West Oakland Health Center*	50,289	9,431,198	O, B
Consortium Total	419,769	51,628,057	

Source: Alameda Health Consortium, 1999.
*Includes data for multiple sites. Key to location codes: O = Oakland, B = Berkeley, H = Hayward, F = Fremont, UC = Union City, P = Pleasanton, L = Livermore.

short-term fluctuations in political climate or economic conditions. Instead, this problem is an inherent feature of the private-public contradiction that affects not only community clinics but also the health-care system as a whole.

Uneven development is another social contradiction that perpetuates the community clinics' financial problems. The provision of services to poor people is usually one of the clinics' explicit goals. To increase accessibility, clinics usually are located in communities with a large proportion of minority and indigent residents. The communities most in need of accessible and inexpensive care are least able to provide direct financing for these services. Indigent communities lack medical facilities in large part because they lack financial resources. To a great extent, funds must come from outside these communities if local clinics are to survive. This dilemma means that community clinics are highly dependent on external funding sources and that financial self-sufficiency is extremely difficult to achieve. While wealthier communities can continue to support private practitioners and hospitals, economic underdevelopment leads to chronic insecurities for clinics in low-income communities.

Financial dependency and insecurity are evident even in clinics that have attracted external funding and that have operated over long periods of time. An example is La Clínica de la Raza, a member of the Alameda Health Consortium. This clinic opened in 1971 to serve a largely indigent and Spanish-speaking population in East Oakland. The clinic grew rapidly since its founding. Eventually it has provided medical, dental, optometry, nutrition, and psychiatric services, with about 84,000 patient visits per year. It has employed over 250 professional and nonprofessional workers (many of whom live in the surrounding community) and has maintained an annual budget of about $16 million.

Despite its successes, this clinic has remained highly dependent on outside funds and vulnerable to cutbacks. Table 5.3 gives a breakdown of the clinic's funding sources in 1998–1999. Only about 48 percent of the clinic's annual income has derived from patient-generated revenues, including both private and public insurance. Many of the clinic's clients have been among the working poor, who lack private insurance yet do not qualify for public programs. Other patients have come to the United States illegally. Although the precise proportion of "undocumented" clients at the clinic is not known, these patients rarely can obtain insurance and usually are extremely poor. The clinic's board has adopted a sliding fee schedule that enables indigent patients to obtain needed care. Under such conditions, however, it has been impossible to maintain the level of services without financial support from external sources. Fifty-two percent of annual revenues have come from outside funding agencies, which include federal, state, and local government, as well as private philanthropies. By obtaining grants from different sources, La Clínica has protected itself from the dangers of dependency on any single agency. On the other hand, most of these grants have had a term of two years or less and have been subject to cuts based on the changing policies of government and philanthropic agencies.

In short, fund-raising becomes a constant struggle for clinics that serve low-income and minority communities. This struggle involves not only seeking financial support but also meeting the demands of agencies that do provide funds. Almost all external funding is contingent on the preparation of extensive reports documenting the services provided. Many agencies require audits of clinical practices, high standards of "productivity" (in numbers of patients seen per unit of time), evaluation procedures, and data collection. Such requirements differ by funding agency. To meet these provisions, clinics must use the time and energy of staff members in activities that funding sources demand but that may not be related to clients' needs. Financial dependency implies major administrative responsibilities, both to obtain funds and to meet funding agencies' requirements.

Administrative tasks add to the inherent difficulties of providing clinical services to clients who are poor and of minority background. Patients who use community clinics often present medical problems that are challenging, both technically and in their social dimensions. Because clients frequently have had little prior access to medical services, their problems tend to be complex and severe. The challenges that clients raise are both exciting and exhausting. The demand for accessible, inexpensive, and culturally sensitive services leads to arduous workloads. Because patients need attention from different disciplines, primary care practitioners coordinate the efforts of clinic workers who act in clients' behalf. Poverty and language barriers interfere with clients' ability to use transportation, educational facilities, and welfare benefits for which they are eligible; workers at community clinics therefore take on advocacy roles to help clients meet their

Table 5.3   Funding Sources, La Clínica de la Raza, Oakland, California, 1998–1999

Source	Amount ($)	Percent of Total
Federal	3,207,045	20
State	946,180	6
County	2,613,127	16
City	198,794	1
Patients & Third Party*	7,659,307	48
Other Agencies**	941,368	6
Foundations/Corporations	399,935	3
TOTAL	15,965,756	100

Source: La Clínica de la Raza, Planning Office, 1999. Funding differs from Table 5.2 because of grants for capital improvements and related nonoperating costs.

*Patient and third-party revenues include self-pay, Medi-Cal, California Department of Health Family PACT, Alameda Alliance for Health, Medicare, Cal Kids, Healthy Families, Access for Infants and Mothers (AIM), Private Insurance, and California Child Health and Disability Prevention program.

**Other agencies include pharmacy and X-ray revenues, management revenues, registration fees, interest income, donated services, and other miscellaneous revenues.

needs. Clinics also organize educational and outreach activities that emphasize prevention and participation in policy making. There are few financial rewards for working in community clinics; tight budgets and insecure funding constrain salaries. For workers committed to the goals of community clinics, their activities in patient care can be gratifying. But the burdens of administration, technically complex problems, harsh working conditions, and low pay can be wearing. Even aside from other sources of instability, the nature of work in these clinics makes it hard to maintain continuity of staffing. "Burnout" of professional and nonprofessional workers is a common phenomenon.

The most important problem of community clinics, however, is that they do not achieve a unified health-care system. A well-organized and responsive clinic can make an enormous difference in a specific community. There are many examples of clinics that have created remarkable achievements with limited resources. Whether a clinic forms in a given geographic area, on the other hand, depends largely on the initiative of local residents. Although clinics have started in some parts of the United States, many areas still lack rudimentary facilities. Even when clinics establish cooperative links such as consortiums, the clinics themselves remain quite diverse in coverage and rarely can provide comprehensive services to all residents of a locality. Clinics formed at local initiative inevitably leave gaps in care for large parts of the population. Community clinics do not substitute for a comprehensive system of health care that would ensure services regardless of geography, income, or race. As discussed in the last part of the book, other countries have integrated community clinics into a national health system. Although several proposals have called for a similar approach in the United States, there has been little progress toward this goal so far. Without a unified health system, clinics will remain isolated and vulnerable.

Despite their problems, community clinics offer a potential for politicization and organizing that go beyond health care alone. Under certain circumstances, clinics can be a focus of nonreformist, social change, in both medicine and the broader society. In the first place, health programs can be an important part of local community development. Historically, community clinics have suffered from financial dependency on external funding agencies and the uncertainties of cutbacks. Self-sufficiency is a difficult goal when a clinic aims to serve low-income clients. Yet some clinics have struggled toward self-sufficiency by linking health services to other efforts in developing the community's economic base. For example, community organizations have undertaken a comprehensive approach to housing, land trusts, food distribution, small enterprises that produce marketable goods and services, credit unions, and health-care programs. Cooperatively owned housing and productive enterprises, as well as credit unions that accumulate savings, can generate funds to support local clinics.

Although clinics are insecure financially when they operate in isolation, they gain strength when linked to other institutions that create revenues. Several clinics in different parts of the United States have reduced their dependency and vulnerability by such efforts in cooperative community development. It is doubtful that development strategies can lead to clinics' full financial self-sufficiency while they continue to serve predominantly poor clients. Community development also cannot be seen as an end in itself. Some communities are better able than others to undertake development strategies, and local successes still will not substitute for a unified national health system. On the other hand, the integration of health-care programs with wider community development can lead to shifts in power and finances that may foster clinics' longer-term survival.

A second direction of politicization and organizing that involves community clinics is the emergence of community-worker control. Most clinics have governing boards with nonprofessional members who represent clients in policy decisions. The activism of board members varies widely. In clinics formed at the initiative of government agencies, administrators often appoint people to serve on the board, which then usually ratifies the policies that the administrators favor. When the initiative to start a clinic comes from local residents, however, people generally join the board through election by other clients. Elections focus attention on a clinic's activities and policies. Elected boards tend to be more active and critical in evaluating a clinic's services and in advocating new directions. In addition to community participation through the governing board, some clinics have adopted procedures that encourage workers' participation in policy making. These procedures require workers' discussion and ratification of policy decisions, as well as regular channels of communication between workers and the governing board. In some clinics, both professional and nonprofessional workers elect a council that cooperates with the board in setting policies. In other clinics, a union serves a similar purpose as a workers' council. Although community-worker control differs among clinics, it usually fosters responsiveness to the needs of both clients and workers.

Such links between health workers and the communities they serve are especially important when cutbacks in funding threaten clinics' survival. Community-worker coalitions have taken a crucial role in political action against cutbacks and in fund-raising efforts. The struggle toward financial self-sufficiency, including the strategy of community economic development, requires cooperative action by workers and local residents. Reduced public funding can create destructive antagonisms that community-worker coalitions help overcome. For instance, public hospitals and community clinics have received funds from government agencies that are subject to cuts. Both types of institution provide needed services. However, workers who face job loss, or who fear the effects of cutbacks on services, previously have competed with one another when funds become scarce. Workers at county and municipal hospitals sometimes have opposed the continued public funding of community clinics when funding agencies threaten cutbacks. Likewise, workers and clients of community clinics have not always been sensitive to the weaknesses of public hospitals. In several cities community-worker coalitions have expanded to include participation by clients and workers at both public hospitals and local clinics. Frequently these coalitions have involved unions of public-sector workers, as well as major community organizations. Although they have not stopped all cutbacks, community-worker coalitions have bridged prior divisions based partly on material interests. As instability of the economy persists, these coalitions promise to continue as a focus of political organizing.

When the latest round of community clinics began to open in the 1960s, some leaders called attention to their broader political significance. From this perspective, the medical problems of poor people and minority groups were deeply embedded in social structures of oppression. These structures included poverty, racism, and political powerlessness. Besides attending to unmet medical needs, community clinics could become a tool for organizing and empowerment.

Some organizations started clinics as one phase of political strategy. For instance, the Black Panther Party hoped that its clinics would attract support and new members. Black Panther organizers worked as paraprofessionals and advocates within the clinics. They gave information and education to clients and encouraged participation in policy decisions. Similarly, during the early 1970s, the United Farm Workers Union opened a system of five community clinics. The clinics were one of many services that the union provided to farmworkers who became members. Political education and organizing within the clinics were regular activities. The union saw the health problems of its members as inseparable from poverty and political disenfranchisement. The clinics sought not only to improve members' health but also to build a stronger union (19). For a number of complex reasons, the clinics of the Black Panther Party and the UFW declined over time. In particular, they suffered from the same problems of financial insecurity and staff burnout that community clinics face more generally.

The viewpoint that clinics can and should be a focus of organizing and politicization, however, has persisted. In some localities, this orientation has stimulated the formation of community-worker coalitions that address many issues other than health care alone. Aside from providing needed services in deprived communities, and despite their many problems, clinics can be a tool for wider organizing. Intertwined with medical care, this organizing is one of community clinics' most important contributions.

6

The Micropolitics of the Doctor-Patient Relationship

The last two chapters have dealt with problems of social medicine at fairly broad levels of analysis—the international proliferation of costly technology and the difficulties of health care in local communities. Although these problems may seem diverse, they derive in large part from similar underlying social contradictions. Corporations and medical professionals promote technologic innovations of unproven effectiveness and take actions that undermine public health services. Monopoly capital in the health-care system fosters expensive technology and the expansion of private facilities. The state generally provides legitimation and public subsidization for private initiatives, while community-based institutions in the public sector face severe obstacles to survival. Dominant ideologies reinforce an uncritical acceptance of high technology and private medicine.

This chapter moves to a more limited level of analysis: the doctor-patient relationship. The interpersonal relationship between doctor and patient has been a topic of endless speculation; like other issues in medicine, this relationship has received attention mainly as a problem in itself, rather than as a problem within a social and historical context. Larger social contradictions, however, penetrate the intimacy of professional-client interaction. In addition, what transpires between doctor and patient may reinforce oppressive structural arrangements beyond the encounter itself.

The focus on the interpersonal level returns to a theme raised earlier; the ambiguities of medical humanism. Few would deny the importance of a caring relationship between doctor and patient. Yet, within the rubric of caring, numerous areas of personal and social life have fallen under medical control. The medicalization of social problems is a subject of growing concern.

How, and to what extent, do micro-level encounters between individuals maintain and reproduce macro-level structural patterns of domination and oppression? The purpose here is to explore these connections between micro-level processes and macro-level contradictions in the face-to-face interaction of doctors and patients. Professional service is an anomalous process. On the one hand, doctors provide intervention and advice that people who are physically sick, or who are at risk of sickness, want and need. A recurring argument in this book is that social contradictions which impede equitable services should change. On the other hand, certain features of doctor-patient encounters do medicalize, and thereby depoliticize, the social structural roots of personal suffering. This phenomenon is subtle, and its nuances are sometimes difficult to recognize. The critique of medicalization holds that medicine has become an institution of social control and that the health-care system helps promulgate the dominant ideologies of a society.

THEORETICAL AND PRACTICAL ISSUES

Medical Ideology

As noted in chapter 2, ideology (although difficult to define simply) is a social group's distinctive set of ideas and doctrines. In classic Marxist theory, the events of history emerge chiefly from economic forces. The principle of economic determinancy attaches great importance to production and to the conflicting relations of social class. From this viewpoint, economic forces profoundly affect the ideologies of a specific historical period. Despite the primacy of economic forces, ideology is crucial in sustaining and reproducing the social relations of production, and especially patterns of domination. Marx called attention to the mechanisms by which ideology reinforces capitalist relations of production and the interests of the capitalist class (1). Ideologies arise in many different areas, including religion, ethics, aesthetics, and politics (2). Early Marxist analyses did not discuss in depth the ideologic components of medicine. Medical science and practice, however, contain major ideologic features that deserve to be examined (3).

First, it is helpful to consider other theories in the Marxist tradition that have extended this framework. According to Gramsci, the capitalist class uses two types of sociopolitical control to maintain and reproduce relations of production. In the first place, there is direct domination or physical coercion; by holding the legal means of violence—in the armed forces, police, prisons, courts, and related institutions—the state protects the established order partly through force and repression. However, Gramsci argues, no regime can survive for long periods of time strictly by authoritarian rule. Ideologic hegemony is a second and ultimately more important mechanism of control. Such institutions as the schools, churches, mass media, and family inculcate a system of values, attitudes, beliefs, and morality that permeates a society. This ideologic system supports the established order and the class interests that dominate it. The same ideologic forces achieve acquiescence and mute resistance from groups who are oppressed (4).

Influenced by Gramsci, Althusser extends the analysis of the structures that exercise control of the population in capitalist society. Although Althusser's interpretation resembles Gramsci's, Althusser considers in more detail the interrelationships among repressive and ideologic institutions, as well as their positions within the capitalist state. Repressive state apparatuses (RSAs), he argues, include the army, policy, prisons, courts, and other institutions that maintain control through violence or repression. Ideologic state apparatuses (ISAs) are institutions that instill dominant ideologies in the population. ISAs include the family, legal system, electoral politics, mass media and communication systems, and cultural systems. RSAs are not purely repressive, nor are ISAs purely ideologic. Ideologies often legitimate the actions of RSAs. For example, justice and equality are ideologic notions that legitimate the functioning of the courts. Similarly, ISAs may use punishment for discipline, such as physical force or other forms of sanctioning that occur in the family or school system (5). Althusser argues that ISAs are especially important in reproducing class structure and the relations of economic production:

> [The] reproduction of labour power requires not only a reproduction of its skills, but also, at the same time, a reproduction of its submission to the rules of the established order, i.e., a reproduction of submission to the ruling ideology for the workers. . . . *It is in the forms and under the forms of ideological subjection that provision is made for the reproduction of the skills of labour power* (6; emphasis in original).

According to Althusser, many social institutions—particularly the educational system—promulgate ideologies that ensure the population's acquiescence and participation in capitalist relations of production.

Althusser's interpretation of the capitalist state is open to criticism. In particular, he includes essentially all major social institutions within the state apparatus, through these institutions' repressive or ideologic effects. For this reason, the state seems to merge into the rest of society. The state's far-reaching impact is undeniable, but the inclusion of such a wide variety of social institutions as formal components of the state apparatus is misleading. Althusser's categories of RSA and ISA gloss over important differences between the state apparatus and specific social institutions involved in repression and promulgation of ideology, as well as differences among these institutions.

On the other hand, Althusser and Gramsci clarify the wide-ranging repressive and ideologic effects of many institutions in society. Both writers emphasize the impact of ideology in controlling the population. These analyses have stimulated much critical debate, whose complexities are outside the intended scope of this chapter. Neither Gramsci nor Althusser considers the institution of medicine as contributing to ideologic hegemony and reproduction. This issue is a major focus here.

Another theoretical approach contributes to an understanding of medical ideology. The "critical theory" of Habermas and other analysts of the "Frankfurt School" provides a link between ideology and science—and, by extension, scientific medicine (7). Although critical theory and Althusser's structuralism both have major roots in classical Marxism, these two schools of thought diverge in fundamental ways. In particular, critical theory assumes that individuals have the capacity to reflect critically about society and to take "purposive" political action. Althusser's structuralism diminishes the potentiality for effective criticism and political action by individuals. Both approaches, however, emphasize the impact of ideology. While Althusser focuses on ideologic effects of various social institutions in reproducing the relations of production, Habermas stresses the ideologic components of science.

For Habermas science is ideology par excellence because it claims to be above ideology, that is, objective and value-neutral. As discussed in chapter 1, Habermas argues that scientific ideology has defined an increasing range of problems as amenable to technical solutions. For this reason, science tends to depoliticize these issues by removing them from critical scrutiny. According to Habermas, science legitimates current patterns of domination, including the class relations of production. Science has become "an apologetic standard through which these same relations of production can be justified as a functional institutional framework." Seen in this way, science no longer is "the basis of a critique of prevailing legitimations in the interest of political enlightenment," but instead is itself "the basis of legitimation" (8). Scientific ideology, Habermas claims, pervades society and legitimates class structure:

> Technocratic consciousness is, on the one hand, "less ideological" than all previous ideologies. For it does not have the opaque force of a delusion that only transfigures the implementation of interests. On the other hand today's dominant, rather glassy background ideology, which makes a fetish of science, is more irresistible and farther-reaching than ideologies of the old type. For with the veiling of practical problems it not only justifies a *particular class's* interest in domination and represses *another class's* partial need for emancipation, but affects the human race's emancipatory interest as such (9; emphasis in original).

What are the specific processes by which scientific ideology provides legitimation? One problem in Habermas' account is that it remains on an abstract level and rarely grounds theoretical claims in empirical reality. Habermas conveys an impression that scientific ideology creates legitimation through cultural symbols in the mass media, educational system, and technical organization of the workplace. He also argues that ideology and domination appear in the face-to-face interaction of individuals. "Distorted communication" arises in both the macro-level realm of politics and the micro-level realm of interpersonal relationships. Domination creates distortion in communication, and undistorted communication is impossible, according to Habermas, under conditions of domination (10). Undistorted communication thus becomes a goal of critical theory. Creating the potential for undistorted communication involves a struggle against both societal and interpersonal domination (11). Concrete examples of scientific ideology rarely appear in Habermas' work; for this reason, his account remains abstract and utopian regarding directions of change. The analysis, however, causes one to search for specific instances of scientific legitimation and for strategies to achieve undistorted communication.

These considerations lead to an appraisal of medical encounters. Doctor-patient interactions predictably may convey ideologic messages that legitimate current structures of oppression in society. These encounters may manifest components of distorted communication and may suggest standards of undistorted communication. Doctor-patient interaction may be one arena for the promulgation of scientific ideology. Empirically, one can ask how and to what extent such processes occur in actual doctor-patient encounters.

Social Control and Ideology

Social control refers to mechanisms by which agencies of society achieve people's adherence to norms of appropriate behavior. Ideologic manipulation is one form of social control. In medicine, ideology and social control are closely related. As previously noted, the medicalization of social problems involves the expansion of health professionals' activities to include the control of many areas of life.

Several studies have presented theoretical analyses of social control in medicine, at both the macro level of social structure and the micro level of the doctor-patient relationship (12). Regarding economic production, Brown argues that modern medicine has tended to define health as the ability to work. Professional leaders, corporate executives, and government officials have promoted this definition of health, the ideologic impact of which has been important in enforcing workers' discipline under twentieth-century capitalism. Regarding the family, Parsons depicts the sick role as a "safety valve" which eases periodic strains and which doctors regulate. While increasing in scope, professional control of family life also has received heightened criticism. Relatively repressive institutions like prisons and the military, which I observed in my own research, often expand access to the sick role to prevent more disruptive social protest. Zola and Illich maintain that medicine is growing as an agency of social control because complex technologic and bureaucratic systems foster reliance on professional experts. As Freidson points out in his analysis of professional dominance, doctors may be more effective in enforcing societal norms than are other social control agents; doctors are less accountable to the public and therefore freer to inject class and professional biases into their relationships with clients. Medical social control thus has extended to economic production, the family, and other major institutions.

Medicalization, as pointed out previously, is one ambiguity of medical humanism. Social control in medicine is often an unintended process, dimly perceived by the participants in doctor-patient encounters. With the holistic purpose of caring for the totality of a client's needs, health professionals assume control over wide facets of social and personal life.

Drawing from these perspectives, one can postulate that social control in medicine largely involves the transmission of ideologic messages. These messages, voiced with the symbolism of medical science, arise at the micro level of professional-client interaction. Such ideologic communication tends to be distorted, because it occurs within an asymmetric interpersonal relationship. The professional holds technical knowledge that is not only a major reason for the client's seeking help but is also a basis of inequality between professional and client. Predictably, actual doctor-patient relationships may vary in doctors' assumption of a dominant role, or in patients' initiative to overcome this dominance. The expected variability, however, does not reduce the relationship's inherent asymmetry.

From a position of relative dominance, doctors can make ideologic statements that convey the symbolic trappings of science. These messages reinforce the hegemonic ideology that emanates from other institutions—the family, educational system, mass media, and so forth—and that pervade a society. The same messages tend to direct clients' behavior into safe, acceptable, and nondisruptive channels; this is the essence of social control in medicine. Ideologic utterances within the doctor-patient relationship seldom are repressive. That is, health professionals rarely compel clients to take specific actions or forcefully restrain them from taking other actions. Within medical encounters, ideologic communication takes much of its forcefulness from the symbolism of medical science and the asymmetry of the doctor-patient relationship.

Medical social control also involves the management of potentially troublesome emotions. Doctors, for instance, regularly deal with patients' anger, anxiety, unhappiness, social isolation, loneliness, depression, and other emotional distress. Often these feelings derive in one way or another from patients' social circumstances, such as economic insecurity, racial or sexual discrimination, occupational stress, and difficulties in family life. Such emotions, of course, are one basis of political outrage and organized resistance. How health professionals manage these sentiments is a question of great interest. One of medicine's most profound effects may be the defusing of socially caused distress.

The transmission of medical ideology goes beyond the control of individual behavior. Like science and technology more generally, medicine also helps legitimate and reproduce class structure and the relations of capitalist production. Medicine is not the only institution in which these processes occur, nor do these processes necessarily occupy a major part of medical encounters. Still, it is worth asking how such micro-level processes take place.

Empirical Studies of Doctor-Patient Interaction

During the last three decades, many empirical studies have examined the doctor-patient relationship. Researchers have found major interactional problems and communication gaps (13). In general, this research portrays doctor-patient interaction as a frequently dismal process, filled with misunderstandings, insensitivity, and frustration. Patients often leave the medical encounter with their perceived needs for information unmet. Even when highly motivated, doctors tend to underestimate patients' desire for information and to overestimate their own communicative skills. Communication barriers seem greatest when professionals and clients of different class background, sex, or race try to interact.

Methodologically, these studies have used a variety of techniques, with varying success. Most researchers have selected a sample of doctors and patients, usually from the outpatient department of a teaching hospital but occasionally from private practice. To study communication, investigators have used such methods as participant observation, retrospective questionnaires and interviews, the case-study method, experimental communication, and the direct recording and analysis of doctor-patient interaction. Each approach has strengths and weaknesses. Cumulatively, this research has documented the enormous difficulties of communication that arise in medical encounters.

On the other hand, most research in this area suffers from an atheoretical stance that views the doctor-patient relationship as a phenomenon without social and historical context. The documentation of communication difficulties within the relationship is worthwhile, but it is also important to consider theoretically the social context in which doctor-patient interaction occurs. As argued throughout this book, medicine ultimately is inseparable from the wider society. Problems in medical care derive from and reinforce social contradictions. Distorted communication in medical encounters both reflects and supports the institutional context in which doctors and patients participate. The study of ideologic reproduction and social control in medicine must link concrete medical encounters with this wider context.

The next part of the chapter presents a contextual analysis of three medical encounters. These doctor-patient interactions come from a large random sample of doctor-patient interactions. The overall research project is described in other writings (14). In brief, 336 randomly selected interactions were studied. Interactions were tape-recorded and questionnaires were administered to doctors and patients. Several quantitative measures of communication were related to characteristics of the doctors, patients, and social situations in which they interacted. Quantitative data for the full sample were used for purposes other than the theoretical questions of this chapter; the findings are reported elsewhere (15). To study medical ideology and social control, complete transcripts were prepared for 50 interactions randomly selected from the larger sample; at least two observers listened to each tape and agreed on the final version of the transcript. Although the transcripts do not convey many nuances, particularly nonverbal, of the tape-recorded interactions, they do permit a contextual analysis of ideology and social control. The following passages illustrate recurring themes in the encounters.

THREE MEDICAL ENCOUNTERS

Some personal background about the participants sheds light on the social context of their interaction. The data about the doctors and patients are from questionnaires that they answered after the tape-recorded encounters; a brief summary of these personal data precedes an interpretation of the transcribed interaction. The transcripts, which report the full verbal interaction recorded, appear in figures that are printed in tandem with the interpretive analysis. This format permits verification or alternative interpretations. (Although the transcript can be read selectively, the interpretation probably can be evaluated best by a full reading.) The line numbers noted on the transcripts are used in the analysis. Ellipsis points (. . .) indicate pauses, and slashes (/) denote interruptions. To protect confidentiality, blanks (_____) substitute for proper names.

The patient in Encounter A is a 55-year-old white male high school graduate who works as a radial drill operator. He is Protestant, Irish, married, and the father of an 18-year-old child. He reports that he wants to be told all the details of his medical condition and that he is "very well satisfied" with the explanation he receives. There is no information available about the patient's wife, who accompanies him during part of the encounter. The doctor is a 38-year-old white male specializing in internal medicine and gastroenterology. He is Protestant and states that his ethnic background is English. The doctor has known the patient for five and one-half years and believes that the primary diagnoses are "coronary artery disease" and "severe recurrent depression." The encounter takes place in a private practice near Boston.

What is the patient's main concern in this encounter? The patient begins with a long discussion of smoking, his unsuccessful attempts to stop, and guilt regarding his failure. The background understanding for this worry is the fact of a prior heart attack. Having learned that smoking exacerbates heart disease, he expresses distress about inhaling (lines 1–20). Although the doctor changes the subject, the

Encounter A (Code 05/048/01)

```
 1 Doctor: What's the problem?
 2 Patient: Huh . . . I don't know if it's running.
 3 D: Yeah, now it's running. What's the problem?
 4 P: I'm having a terrible time trying to stop smoking.
 5 D: Is that right?
 6 P: Yeah.
 7 D: Real withdrawal symptoms?
 8 P: Yeah (sigh). Gee, I, I realize of course I don't smoke
 9    cigarettes.
10 D:              /Yeah/
11 P:                      /Smoke cigars.
```

patient's wife returns to the smoking as a major source of the patient's distress (ll. 36–45). Again the doctor moves to other topics, although he does voice a brief question about the type of cigar the patient smokes (ll. 69–73). Later the doctor tries to reassure the patient and/or his wife that smoking probably does less harm than worrying about it (ll. 200–206).

The doctor concludes his remarks about smoking with a religious image and implies that the patient's best efforts will never be good enough: "We can't get you to the point that we can canonize you, we just want to keep you going" (ll. 232–234). The doctor conveys this pastoral utterance with good humor and concern for this patient's frustrated aspirations. The implication of the doctor's message, cloaked in scientific medicine, is that the client's attempts to stop a self-destructive habit are unnecessary and—to the extent that they create emotional tension—dangerous. Since the patient cannot become a saint, the doctor implies, attempts to attain a more perfected life-style are unwarranted. The patient's primary expressed concern receives intermittent and ultimately arbitrary attention, while the doctor's communication, uttered as a judgment of scientific medicine, contains heavy symbolic and ideologic overtones. Meanwhile, the physician expresses clear concern for the patient's happiness and well-being, and the patient claims to be quite satisfied.

Control of the patient's role in economic production, largely through messages of medical ideology, is another striking feature of this encounter. The doctor asks about the patient's work situation early in the interaction and needs to be reminded that the patient has not returned to work (ll. 74–100). Several interrelated issues then arise. Although details are incomplete, it is clear that the patient is receiving disability payments, apparently because of his heart disease. The doctor previously has certified that this disability would end by a specific date (ll. 118–131). A second problem is an impending strike that the patient anticipates may begin shortly after the disability period ends (ll. 96–97). The patient worries about a potential scenario in which his disability payments stop, he goes back to work, but then he must go out on strike, thus losing income. Perhaps because the patient does not elaborate, the doctor does not acknowledge this issue explicitly. Instead, he focuses on a third concern, the postulated association between the client's emotional distress and unemployment. According to the doctor, the patient's depression will become worse if he does not return to work ("I tell you if this guy stays home, he's going to curl up in a ball and be, you know, unreachable," ll. 129–131). Later the physician reiterates his view that getting back to work will be "the best thing in the world for you" (ll. 173–179, 217–220, 225–226). Whether the doctor is oblivious to the financial problems that may arise if the patient returns before the strike, or whether he consciously chooses to ignore the issue, remains unclear. The overall implication is that working is good for this patient specifically and perhaps for workers in general. In this sense, health is subtly defined as the capacity to work.

This passage illustrates medicine's social control over labor, and the transmis-

12 D: How many a day do you smoke?
13 P: Oh, about two or three of those small Tijuana smalls.
14 D: If you smoke two or three does that keep you from getting
15   withdrawal symptoms?
16 P: Yeah, but I inhale 'em. You're not supposed to.
17 D: Even so, two or three I think is better than having to go off
18   the deep end with uh certainly a lot better than a pack
19   of cigarettes.
20 P: Yeah but I should cut 'em out completely. I know that.
21 D: How do you feel physically?
22 P: Oh, physically I'm all right.
23 D: Other than a sore finger.
24 P: Oh, that finger's coming along beautiful.
25 Wife: He's so frustrated that he really doesn't
26   know what to/
27 D: /Any chest pains?
28 P: Uh, yeah I have some.
29 W: He made this face the other night at the
30   dinner table./
31 P: /Yeah/
32 D: Pressure pains or/
33 P: /No it's/
34 W: /tension with the uh . . . /
35 P: /Probably tension, I don't know.
36 W: He'll go to bed at quarter of eight at night.
37   He seems to feel better if he goes to bed.
38   It's almost as though he stops concentrating on
39   the cigarettes/
40 D: /He runs away, runs away from the problem.
41 P: Run away from it, yeah.
42 W: He said this morning he wanted to be in accepting the
43   fact that he hadn't ought to smoke and he shouldn't.
44 D: It's difficult to accept it, uh
45 W: Mmm after 40 years.
46 D: Uh, what do you weigh today, Mr. _____?
47 P: 149.
48 D: 149, Uh, uh what are you taking for medication now?
49 P: Well I don't know. I'm right at a point now I don't
50   know if I should take Mellaril, Librax/
51 W: /Librium
52 P: um, Librium . . . or poison.
53 D: You're just all wound up now. . . . You want to take poison?
54 P: Jeepers I don't know what, I don't know what to take.
55   I'm right at a point now, I don't know what would do
56   any good.
57 D: Do you have any trouble sleeping?
58 P: Yeah/
59 W: /Umm

sion of ideologic messages about work, at the level of the doctor-patient relationship. The doctor controls the patient's work life by withholding the continued certification of illness. Despite some attempts to communicate concern about the timing of his return to work, the patient does not participate actively in this decision.

With benevolence, the doctor expropriates the decision-making process regarding both health and work. The patient explicitly states that returning to work in the face of an impending strike "seems to bother me." The doctor invalidates this concern and implies that the strike will be settled by "mid-June," although he could not know this with any certainty. If the patient returns during mid-June, the doctor argues, "it . . . won't bother you." The patient feebly replies, "No" (ll. 96–100). Beyond the decertification of illness and loss of decision-making power, the patient receives a strong ideologic message that work is beneficial for his health. This ideologic position is an ambiguous one. In many people's lives, work does contribute to emotional stability and feelings of personal worth, even if work is alienating and conflictual. The point here, however, is that a professional assumes directive control over the patient's occupational behavior; with medical authority, the doctor mediates the worker's role in production. Despite the pressures of work and contract negotiations, the doctor argues, the worker will feel better, mentally and physically, if he is working than if he is idle. Such micro-level communications, which tend to reproduce macro-level relations of production, are quite common in doctor-patient interaction, although the participants rarely perceive that these messages may have broader social import.

The medical management of emotional distress also occurs in this interaction. At the outset, it is important to recognize that the encounter involves a patient with heart disease and a doctor specializing in internal medicine with a subspecialty in gastroenterology. Although the doctor is not a psychiatrist, a major part of the encounter focuses on the patient's emotional problems. In his verbal behavior, the patient gives no evidence of psychosis; his statements seem appropriate, grounded in reality, and without bizarre or incomprehensible features. On the other hand, the patient is clearly upset and perhaps suicidal, although he expresses his feelings laconically. One revelation is the patient's terse comment on his medications: "I'm at a point right now I don't know if I should take Mellaril, Librax, um, Librium . . . or poison" (ll. 42–59). This danger signal leads to two brief questions by the doctor, apparently intended to assess the patient's suicide potential. Quickly, however, the issue of suicide disappears from the conversation.

The doctor does not attempt to explore the patient's distress in depth. Instead, three professional interventions occur, none of which encourages the patient to seek the roots of his depression in psychodynamics or in the social environment. First, the doctor offers technologic assistance in the form of drugs. To manage the patient's emotional problems, the doctor uses polypharmacy—a variety of medications without clear-cut pharmacologic rationale. Prescriptions include (a) Mellaril, a major tranquilizer whose indication is schizophrenia or other serious psychosis; (b) Librium, a minor tranquilizer intended for relief of anxiety and/or neurosis; (c) Librax, a combination of Librium and an antispasmodic for emotion-

60 P: /I have a hard time getting to sleep and wake up
61   quite a bit in the night.
62 D: Have you had to take any nitroglycerin or anything
63   under your tongue at all/
64 P: /No
65 D: /for pain?
66 P: No, no.
67 W: You haven't been taking Nembutal either, have you?
68 P: No, I haven't been taking Nembutal either.
69 D: You have . . . there's two or three of those little, uh
70   those little, what are they? They're like cigars
71   aren't they, those little/
72 P: /Yeah, Tijuana smalls, white.
73 W: With a little filter on the end. And a white . . .
74 D: How are things coming at work?
75 W: He hasn't been to work yet.
76 P: Well they, you know, they prolonged it, they've
77   extended the contract for 10 days.
78 D: Yeah.
79 P: Which is a good sign.
80 D: Yeah.
81 P: From what I heard that's a good sign.
82 D: So when would you be able to, when would they be
83   ready to go if they approve a contract?
84 P: Oh, it'd probably be, well the contract runs out
85   the 26th.
86 D: Of this month, that's this Saturday.
87 P: That's this Saturday.
88 D: And it's prolonged . . .
89 P: It'll be a week and a half.
90 D: Yeah, so if they arrange something, they'll know
91   by mid-June.
92 P: They should.
93 D: Is that bugging you? The idea of going back to work?
94 P: Well . . . actually I think I want to go back.
95 D: Yeah, I think you should go back you know.
96 P: Actually I think I want to go back, but then go back
97   and go on strike? That seems to bother me.
98 D: Yeah. But if you go back mid-June it won't,
99   won't bother you.
100 P: No.
101 D: I think if you're going to take anything,
102   you ought to take the Mellaril. We ought to
103   maybe add some Elavil. 'Cause I think most of
104   your symptoms are depression and frustration
105   right now.
106 W: He doesn't want to eat either/
107 D: /Yeah, that goes with/

108 W: /gag, just a few mouthfuls.
109 D: I think that as far as the gut is concerned, you know,
110   I think a lot of those symptoms, you know the gagging,
111   bellyaches and so forth are secondary to the depression.
112   Uh, but he sounds like his heart's doing OK. Not having
113   troubles there. . . . Let's take a look at you. You know
114   where the room is./
115 P: /Yeah.
116 D: Just strip down to your waist, Mr. _____.
117   [door opens and closes]
118 D: [to wife] What did I say on that form last time,
119   I don't remember. Did I say first of June? For
120   returning to work.
121 W: On one of the forms you did, you said the first
122   of June . . .
123 D: I thought that's what we decided on, the first
124   of June . . .
125 W: We thought perhaps he could go back, yeah,
126   around the first.
127 D: I think he's gotta go back.
128 W: He is, I told him/
129 D: /I tell you if this guy stays
130   home, he's going to curl up in a ball, you know,
131   unreachable.
132 W: Well, he feels it's all the cigarettes.
133   But if it isn't one thing/
134 D: /it's something else.
135   Knock down one soldier and another one pops up.
136   Gotta carry this with me so
137   [tape off, then on in other room]
138 D: I'll break this and than we'll be
139   [blood pressure being tested]
140 D: 120/70. Does that slip off easy or does it
141   look funny to you?
142 P: Yeah, looks good. You can take it off, if
143   you want to.
144 D: Yeah, must be interesting, you're lucky.
145   That tube gauze is nice stuff, isn't it?
146 P: Yeah. Yeah I got some of this at home.
147 D: Did you?
148 P: Called "Surgitube."
149 D: Yeah, same stuff.
150 P: And uh, they told me down there, you might
151   lose that nail; more than likely you will
152   lose the nail. You'll be better off to let
153   that nail come off and let the new nail grow over.
154 D: If you pull them off then you get those horny,
155   lousy looking nails, huh. . . . Good . . . that looks fine . . .
156   want to lay back [loud noises and pause]. . . . Don't

157 breathe . . . good . . . breathe . . . in . . . out . . . don't
158 breathe . . . good . . . that sounds great. Do you have
159 any cramps or diarrhea?
160 P: Not too much diarrhea.
161 D: When did you have your heart attack? It'll be
162 awhile . . .
163 P: November 29.
164 D: November 17. I think that we'll check the cardiogram
165 today, but I think, stay on the Mellaril four times a day
166 and we'll add another drug called Elavil.
167 P: One four times a day or two?
168 D: One. One and I'm going to add another medication
169 called Elavil. Stay off the Librium, cause I think
170 it's just going to aggravate the symptoms.
171 P: I'm getting to a point that I just don't know
172 what to take.
173 D: I'll check the cardiogram. I would think that
174 maybe we would plan on getting you back, say
175 mid-June, you know, to work, which I think is
176 the best thing in the world for you, to get
177 back to work. Your heart's strong enough, your
178 blood pressure's good, there's no reason why we
179 can't get you back in the middle of things.
180 P: Well, what do you think about going to Maine,
181 down and back in one day?
182 D: How long a drive would it be?
183 P: Be 12 hours and 15 minutes, 12 and a half.
184 D: So long as you stop the car every hour and get
185 out and take a little walk around, keep the
186 circulation going, fine, no problem.
187 P: Yeah.
188 D: Come on in after you get dressed. Right?
189   [tape off and on]
190 D: That's not unusual, just, you get light-headed/
191 P: /Yeah
192 D: Yeah, lots of people get that. Just laying down,
193 lay down a few minutes. That's positional, doesn't
194 mean anything. [to wife] I asked him to stay on
195 Mellaril four times a day.
196 W: One or two?
197 D: Uh, one. And then I asked him to take this Elavil,
198 which is, in addition, twice a day. Stay away from
199 the Librium, OK? Think the bulk of his symptoms are
200 due to his depression and worry over things. I
201 think as far as I can see, he's going to do less harm
202 to himself by smoking those three little gizmos a
203 day than he is worrying to death, you know?
204 W: That's what I said, ask the doctor about it,

related gastrointestinal disturbances; and (d) Elavil, an antidepressant (ll. 48–68, 101–111, 165–172, 194–199). The literature of psychopharmacology sheds doubt on the usefulness of any of these agents for this patient, whose distress seems to derive in large part from the social situation, especially work, and from concern about heart disease. Moreover, when suicide is a possibility, the danger of over-dose from these drugs, especially in combination, is severe (16). Despite these concerns, polypharmacy converts a socioemotional problem to a technical one. Drug treatment objectifies a complex series of psychological and social questions. Symbolically, scientific medicine shifts the focus to the physical realm, depoliti-cizes the social structural issues involved, and mutes the potential for action by the patient to change the conditions that trouble him.

A second intervention, already discussed, also aims to reduce emotional dis-tress. The doctor's reassurances about smoking address the principal problem that the patient and his wife express. According to the doctor, the patient's worry about smoking is worse than smoking itself. The doctor combines the symbolism of reli-gion ("We can't get you to the point that we can canonize you," ll. 232–233) with that of criminal justice ("Yeah, you incriminate yourself," ll. 237–238) in per-suading the patient not to feel bad. One might doubt that smoking is in fact the major determinant of the patient's suicidal fantasies, despite the emphasis this topic receives from all three participants in the encounter. The doctor uses weighty imagery to ease the patient's guilt, but ultimately the problem remains unanalyzed and mystified.

The third intervention concerning emotional distress, also mentioned earlier, involves the medicalization of work. A rosy picture of work's psychic benefits diverts attention from its physical, socioemotional, and economic hazards. The patient voices concern (though not too articulately) about these hazards, but the doctor portrays idleness as a root of psychic disaster and reemployment as a mode of adjustment if not cure. Voiced with the authority of medical science, this ideo-logic message reproduces the worker's place in the relations of production. The professional's words also convey the false promise of happiness, or at least rela-tive happiness, in work as currently organized.

While the medical encounter reinforces the structure of work, it patterns leisure as well. In this interaction, the doctor decides not only how and when the patient should work but also under what conditions the patient may relax, travel, and enjoy himself. The doctor argues that too much leisure time is bad for physical and men-tal health. On the other hand, the patient and his wife carefully seek permission to travel (ll. 180–186). Just as the doctor states the date for return to work, the patient questions whether a trip to Maine would be acceptable. The patient does not ask for a long vacation, just a one-day excursion. In response, the doctor requests information about how long a drive this will involve. The doctor then approves a twelve- to thirteen-hour trip, as long as the patient stops every hour to walk. Per-haps the physician's concern here is the possibility of blood clots in the patient's legs if he remains seated for too long. It is worth noting, however, that the patient is more assertive about his desire for this drive to Maine than any other stated goal

205   I said, here you're beating yourself up one side
206   and down the other. . . . Now is it all right for him
207   to, he thought he might like to take a trip to
208   Maine/
209 D: /To Maine, yeah/
210 W: /Yeah?/
211 D: Sounds fine as long as you stop the car every
212   hour, let him get out and walk around a bit.
213   Uh, let's have him get a cardiogram today/
214 W: /Mmm mmm
215 D: let me see him again in uh six weeks/
216 W: /Uh huh/
217 D: and uh, let's plan on say mid-June getting him
218   back, OK? . . . Like to hear from him just about the
219   time he's ready, it's time for him to go back to
220   work, just give me a progress report.
221   [to P] I gave your wife a prescription, Mr. _____,
222   and uh, and uh so you can go down and get a
223   cardiogram, and uh, I'll see you in six weeks, and
224   maybe you can give me a call in about three weeks,
225   let me know how things are going, which would be
226   just about the time you'd be going back to work.
227   I think from the standpoint of what's going to do
228   more harm to you, it's going to do more harm to
229   you worrying over those three cigarettes a day than it
230   is smoking them. I think. So I think that this
231   would probably uh three a day, certainly even though
232   you inhale them is not, let's face it. We can't
233   get you to the point that we can canonize you, we
234   just want to keep you going.
235 P: Yeah, when I do smoke them, I get all nerved up
236   about it, I get so mad at myself/
237 D: /Yeah, you
238   incriminate yourself/
239 W: /The doctor feels it's better.
240 D: Yeah, well I still think that you're going to be
241   better off to have those few cigarettes, than to
242   sit around and mope and hope and grope around and/
243 W: That's all he thinks about, that's all I think
244   about from the time I open my eyes until I close
245   them at night.
246 D: Listen, after you get the cardiogram, do me a
247   favor. This will add only a few more minutes to
248   your stay here today. Fill this out if you would.
249   This is a confidential form. There's a young
250   lady out there with long blond hair, and uh give
251   this to her. She's uh from the Massachusetts

in the encounter except reduction of smoking. His wife reiterates the patient's request later and again receives conditional approval (ll. 206–212). This couple do not indicate what other activities give them pleasure. The leisure they do seek, however, is subject to medical regulation.

This encounter also maintains an uncritical stance regarding family relations. Participation by the patient's wife in the encounter is striking but not unusual. The interaction allows certain inferences about family dynamics and the doctor's reinforcement of them. While the patient is the economic breadwinner, he emerges as a relatively helpless person, unable to care for, or even speak for, himself without his wife's assistance. The wife elaborates at length on the patient's emotional disturbances (ll. 34–39, 129–135, 204–206, 239–245), sleep problems (ll. 57–68), disability certification (ll. 118–128), and desire for a pleasure trip (ll. 206–212). She and the doctor hold side conversations between themselves, both in and outside the patient's presence. Although the doctor encourages the patient to become more active by returning to work, he subtly colludes with the wife in retaining the patient's day-to-day helplessness within the family. This collusion extends from agreement about the emotional impact of idleness, to diminishing the patient's concern about smoking, to instructions about drug dosages (ll. 194–206). Further, the patient himself voices no objection to this pattern of communication. Although the doctor recognizes depression as one of the patient's two major medical diagnoses, he does not explore the possibility that family life may be part of the problem. To whatever extent that psychological problems in the family exist, the medical encounter reinforces the status quo.

Throughout the interaction, technical knowledge occupies a minor place, in comparison to the ideology and symbolism of scientific medicine. The doctor asks a few questions from the standpoint of cardiology (regarding chest pain, ll. 27–32), inquires about the use of a cardiac medication (nitroglycerine, ll. 62–66), discusses gauze and nail care (ll. 140–155), performs a brief physical exam, and orders an electrocardiogram. Otherwise, it is difficult to find evidence in this encounter of scientific medicine per se. On the other hand, the doctor offers a series of pronouncements about smoking, work, leisure, and emotional difficulties. These utterances contain little or no scientific rationale, yet their impact derives from the symbolism of scientific knowledge and technique. Carrying the authority of medical science, the doctor dominates the interaction. In this sense the communication remains distorted, as the professional assumes control over major areas of life inside and outside the medical realm.

252   General Hospital. Everything is confidential in
253   this form. It's just going to go to the study
254   people, and, uh, be very truthful in your answers.
255 W: OK.
256 D: OK. Thank you.

The discourse in this encounter does not empower or provide autonomy for the client in any apparent way. The doctor gives little technical information but many ideologic messages. Much of the communication mystifies the social roots of distress with the symbolism of scientific medicine. The professional assumes decision-making control over wide areas of the patient's existence; the dialogue obviates the possibility of independent action or resistance directed against social conditions that the client may find oppressive. In all this, the patient acquiesces. The doctor truly cares for the patient, the patient appreciates the doctor's concern, and for all the participants' conscious intents and purposes, this is probably an excellent doctor-patient relationship. That the encounter may reinforce the social sources of discontent and suffering escapes notice entirely. Such are the puzzling anomalies of a caring relationship between doctor and patient in this society.

In Encounter B the patient is 50 years old, white, married, Roman Catholic, and "English-Irish-French" in ethnic background. She attended some college, has four children, and reports her occupation as "wife." She states that she wants to know all the details about her medical condition and that she is satisfied with the doctor's explanation. The doctor is a 39-year-old white male, with a German background and Episcopalian religious preference. The doctor's specialty is general internal medicine. According to the doctor, the patient—whom he has known for five years—has "rheumatic heart disease with mitral insufficiency" and "menopausal syndrome." The encounter takes place in the doctor's private office.

The highly technical orientation of Encounter B distinguishes it from the non-technical orientation of Encounter A. In fact, Encounter B contains more content based in scientific medicine than any other of the thirty transcripts randomly selected from the larger sample of doctor-patient interactions. The patient suffers from rheumatic heart disease that affects principally the mitral valve. In the past she has endured episodes of congestive heart failure and irregularities of heart rhythm. She takes at least two cardiac medications—hydrochlorothiazide (Hydrodiuril) to reduce fluid accumulation and propranolol (Inderal) to control rhythm disturbances. Although the patient has been able to manage fairly well with limited physical exertion, her heart disease is serious enough that the doctor is contemplating heart surgery with valve replacement. In addition, the patient has menopausal and hearing problems.

A large part of the interaction deals with technical issues of diagnosis and treatment (ll. 1–170, 235–467). The doctor asks questions about exercise tolerance, compliance to medication schedule, symptoms of heart failure (pain, shortness of breath, ankle swelling), menstrual symptoms, and ear symptoms. He does a partial physical exam and an electrocardiogram. He then spends considerable time explaining his notion about the relation between the patient's symptoms and her irregular heart rhythm. Because he apparently believes that her rhythm abnormality may have returned because she decided on her own to reduce her medication, he requests her to use the prescribed dose and to check with him before making further changes.

Encounter B (code 09/092/01)

1 Doctor: OK, so, what's happened since February?
2 Patient: Well, I've been pretty good for a couple of months
3   and uh started to have trouble.
4 D: What sort of trouble?
5 P: Well, you know, it just doesn't seem that I can do
6   what I used to. I mean what I had built up to doing,
7   now, you know, just being exhausted, losing my breath,
8   just walking, you know.
9 D: Yeah, have you, did you notice any change in your
10   rhythm that uh/
11 P: /Well, it's difficult to say, because,
12   yes I have. It's much, well, when I had trouble with
13   the period being slow so that when I do anything, it
14   would make it go faster, and that would just seem
15   normal fastness to counting. But, you know, it just
16   knocked me out.
17 D: Yeah.
18 P: So I decided to you know try to rest. Maybe I had done
19   something or something had gone wrong. My daughter had
20   been home one weekend and I, maybe there had been a
21   conflict, emotional conflict/
22 D: /Yeah, yeah/
23 P: /because, I don't
24   know why it would do it so suddenly, but I felt/
25 D: /Would
26   you notice that it came on you all of a sudden?/
27 P: /Well,
28   [inaudible] then all of a sudden next day, it uh . . .
29 D: Did you change the medication, stop the Inderal or
30   anything?
31 P: Not/
32 D: /Or/
33 P: /Not really. I think I took instead of just
34   taking a pill in the morning and afternoon, I
35   think I took it a little oftener, but then I cut it
36   back since that didn't seem to help/
37 D: /How much are you
38   taking now?
39 P: All I've had now is one this morning about an hour ago.
40 D: But you take one three times a day/
41 P: /I'd been taking/
42 D: /normally?/
43 P: /No, I've cut back/
44 D: /You've cut down?/
45 P: /to one in the morning or one in the morning and
46   one in the afternoon, just depending on how it, so

47   then I wondered if maybe I didn't really need it
48   and the one in the morning was doing something,
49   but it's just, it's better, but it's never been
50   seemed quite right again, and . . .
51 D: Yeah.
52 P: And a couple of weeks ago I decided to come see you
53   and then checked and found out I had an appointment
54   in a couple of weeks, so/
55 D: /Uh huh. Ok, well, um.
56   Did you have any pain associated with it?
57 P: No.
58 D: Not at all. But shortness of breath you felt was
59   really a significant feature?
60 P: Why yes. It is, and it pounds.
61 D: Mmm hmm.
62 P: And to me it pounds to the effect, extent that I
63   feel like it's going through.
64 D: Yes.
65 P: But if you really feel my pulse, it's not uh,
66   it just seems like a normal pattern.
67 D: Is it fairly regular? Or does it seem to be skipping?
68 P: Well, if I'm doing anything at all, it gets irregular.
69 D: Mmm hmm.
70 P: I can cook the dinner and wash the clothes, but you
71   know, any sweeping, cleaning that I do, that kind of
72   sounds like an excuse, but it really isn't.
73 D: [laughs] Yeah. No, I . . .
74 P: It's just when I used to do it, like in 15 or 20 minute
75   intervals, and then sit and relax for 5 or 10 minutes,
76   then I could carry on. Now I can't do that. It's sort
77   of maddening, because/
78 D: /Can you lie flat in bed at night?
79 P: I think I, I don't know because my husband pointed out
80   that when he wakes, when I wake up in the morning I
81   have doubled over the pillow, so maybe I'm not
82   lying flat.
83 D: But at least there hasn't been a dramatic change, that
84   you're getting up in the middle of the night to uh
85   gasping for air . . .
86 P: Oh no, no there's nothing like that, just when I'm doing
87   something.
88 D: How about the ankles, are they swelling up?
89 P: I've been taking more fluid pills, but my period has
90   come oftener.
91 D: Mmm hmm.
92 P: It was regular until about the last time. The time
93   before that then it was. . . . I have more, more fluid in
94   the middle, middle of the period I guess.

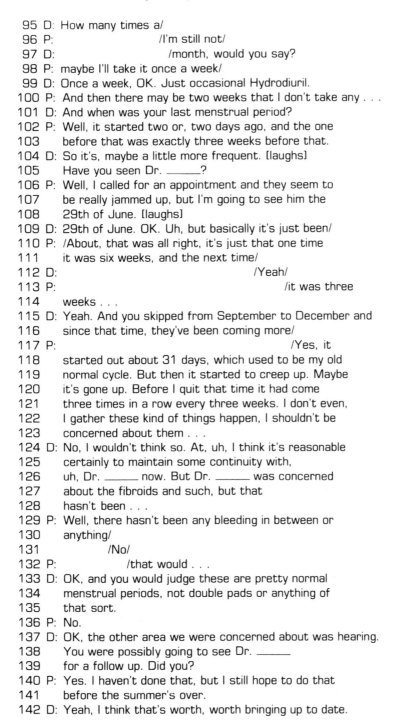

95 D: How many times a/
96 P: /I'm still not/
97 D: /month, would you say?
98 P: maybe I'll take it once a week/
99 D: Once a week, OK. Just occasional Hydrodiuril.
100 P: And then there may be two weeks that I don't take any . . .
101 D: And when was your last menstrual period?
102 P: Well, it started two or, two days ago, and the one
103   before that was exactly three weeks before that.
104 D: So it's, maybe a little more frequent. [laughs]
105   Have you seen Dr. _____?
106 P: Well, I called for an appointment and they seem to
107   be really jammed up, but I'm going to see him the
108   29th of June. [laughs]
109 D: 29th of June. OK. Uh, but basically it's just been/
110 P: /About, that was all right, it's just that one time
111   it was six weeks, and the next time/
112 D: /Yeah/
113 P: /it was three
114   weeks . . .
115 D: Yeah. And you skipped from September to December and
116   since that time, they've been coming more/
117 P: /Yes, it
118   started out about 31 days, which used to be my old
119   normal cycle. But then it started to creep up. Maybe
120   it's gone up. Before I quit that time it had come
121   three times in a row every three weeks. I don't even,
122   I gather these kind of things happen, I shouldn't be
123   concerned about them . . .
124 D: No, I wouldn't think so. At, uh, I think it's reasonable
125   certainly to maintain some continuity with,
126   uh, Dr. _____ now. But Dr. _____ was concerned
127   about the fibroids and such, but that
128   hasn't been . . .
129 P: Well, there hasn't been any bleeding in between or
130   anything/
131   /No/
132 P: /that would . . .
133 D: OK, and you would judge these are pretty normal
134   menstrual periods, not double pads or anything of
135   that sort.
136 P: No.
137 D: OK, the other area we were concerned about was hearing.
138   You were possibly going to see Dr. _____
139   for a follow up. Did you?
140 P: Yes. I haven't done that, but I still hope to do that
141   before the summer's over.
142 D: Yeah, I think that's worth, worth bringing up to date.

143   Uh, have you felt that that's continued to decrease/
144 P: /It's
145   been/
146 D: /Or has that been stable?
147 P: It's been absolutely beautiful. [laughs]
148 D: OK.
149 P: In fact, quite better than it has been for a
150   long time until late yesterday, then, all of a
151   sudden boom, it's almost cut off. And, uh, I
152   wonder if the atmosphere . . .
153 D: Well, it may be. Yeah.
154 P: It's the first time I felt that happen, and then
155   sometime when I was sleeping, the room was air
156   conditioned, and all of a sudden I heard it pop
157   or do something, you know, then I wished it hadn't
158   because it was even louder . . .
159 D: Yeah, yeah, OK. But the question of that certainly
160   is not the otosclerosis problem.
161 P: No, that isn't what it is, but there must be
162   something else . . .
163 D: It must be atmospheric, and it's probably just that,
164   you know that the middle ear gets blocked off, uh,
165   with the changes in atmosphere. Do you have a head
166   cold or any congestion?
167 P: No.
168 D: No. OK.
169 P: Not at all. Except I always have this, you know,
170   a nasal drip.
171 D: Yeah, OK. The areas of pressure and stress. Your
172   husband is, now . . .
173 P: He's employed and he's in state/
174 D: /He's employed now/
175 P: /and as far as/
176 D: /And . . . liking it better?
177 P: Well, he makes anything interesting. He really does
178   it all out, you know, better than anybody else could
179   do it.
180 D: Yeah, yeah, sure.
181 P: Um, but his comment on it is, "Any high school kid
182   could do it." Well I don't think they really could.
183 D: No, no.
184 P: They might basically understand some of it, but
185   they couldn't meet with the engineers and/
186 D: /Well, he
187   takes a lot of pride I think in the fact that, you
188   know, that he can, obviously is pretty competent.
189 P: And he always cuts himself down [laughs], so . . .
190 D: Yeah, OK, right. How about the kids?

191 P: They're all doing fine right now, and . . .
192 D: So the stresses and pressures that you've/
193 P: /They're/
194 D: /felt earlier are/
195 P: /Yeah/
196 D: /alleviating. What are the
197   summer plans? Are they going to be away or how many
198   will be home?
199 P: Well, uh, my daughter's going to be home, after
200   school. She's been away for three weeks, and she's
201   coming back this weekend to do lifeguarding and
202   teaching at the pool in town.
203 D: Mmm hmm.
204 P: And I'll take that when it comes. [laughs]
205 D: OK.
206 P: Uh, the oldest boy has been home, but he's going
207   to be away for a month. He's going to take some
208   ROTC county training.
209 D: Mmm hmm. So, will you get away this summer?
210 P: I don't know, cause _____ had hoped, he thought
211   he should see his mother. She's about 79, and it's
212   been several years, but driving to St. Louis might
213   be prohibited by gas and . . .
214 D: Mmm hmm.
215 P: Too much. I tried to talk him into flying, but
216   he wouldn't go without me. [laughs]
217 D: Why, you don't want to fly or . . .
218 P: Well, we couldn't finance it/
219 D: /Oh, I see/
220 P: /flying two.
221 D: Well, I wonder if it isn't almost, in terms of the
222   time it takes you to drive, and motels and so forth,
223   that if you/
224 P: /Well, we go to Pittsburgh and spend the day
225   with my family, and then go to St. Louis in one hop.
226 D: So it is obviously/
227 P: /I've tried to talk him into doing
228   it some other way many times, but it's um, you know . . .
229 D: That's a long haul. Yeah.
230 P: For me, but um it's the only way to do it.
231 D: So you're not at least, going to be lolling on the
232   beach this summer anywhere?
233 P: He's not a beach loller. [laughs] He would be, I
234   guess, but he sunburns easily. That's why.
235 D: OK. Let's see what your weight is today. . . . OK, 144.
236   And that's four pounds down from uh/
237 P: /Oh yeah, I've
238   been working on that.

239 D: Yeah, but that also suggests that you're not
240   retaining that much fluid either.
241 P: Oh, I had a pill yesterday, but I, it's been,
242   I can tell because it jumps five pounds . . .
243 D: Uh huh.
244 P: Boom, just like that.
245 D: Uh, huh, yeah.
246 P: And at first I thought, well I've just gained
247   weight, but after I got, you know, in trouble,
248   with tension and the like, but then I discovered
249   that when I took a pill it dropped five pounds
250   just like that.
251   [sound of blood pressure being taken]
252 D: 130/80, and it's quite regular and quite slow.
253   Not dramatically slow, but uh, you took just one
254   Inderal this morning?
255 P: Yes, and I think it's, you know, either it's just
256   beginning to take, it tends to be, after a while,
257   more sensitive, [inaudible] if I do anything.
258 D: OK, we'll check it out here. Deep breath . . . OK.
259   Could I have you lie back . . . it's interesting
260   because it's irregular now. Are you aware of it?
261 P: Yes/
262 D: /Yeah, But it's/
263 P: /But it's not like it was with
264   the kidney . . .
265 D: OK, I'm going to have Mrs. _____ just get a
266   rhythm strip on this just to see. [beep beep]
267   I'd like to know a little bit more what it's doing,
268   'cause it was perfectly regular in, uh, in February.
269   We'll see what we see. [tape off, then on]
270   . . . I guess that showed it as being absolutely regular,
271   and what we'll do is, I'm just going to have you
272   exercise a little bit and let's just run the uh,
273   run the machine. OK. Could you do some sit-ups
274   for me? Just put it on, you're on lead two.
275 Nurse: Yes.
276 D: Just, do them a little faster. You can stop it
277   now and then. And, uh, OK. Just do about, uh,

This patient takes an active role in the technical discussion. When confused about the doctor's explanation or instruction, she asks frequent questions. The doctor confirms her competence: "I know you're sensitive and a good observer" (ll. 344–345). Despite this compliment, he suggests that she not modify her medication independently. That the patient does understand is clear from her response to a question in the interview after the medical encounter. The questionnaire asks: "Did Dr. _____ say that anything was wrong with you? What did he say?" She replies: "Bigeminy beat has returned with exercise. We will attempt to control it with increased medication." Regarding the technical basis of the encounter, the doctor seems eager to share full information with the patient and to encourage her autonomous participation. Although the doctor's professional knowledge remains a basis of asymmetry in the relationship, in comparison to Encounter A the doctor communicates this knowledge in a straightforward way. He thus reduces the inherent inequality of the relationship and avoids domination in the encounter. Interestingly, these positive features of the interaction seem to stem in part from its focus on predominantly technical issues relating to the patient's physical illness.

Against this background, the messages of ideology and social control that the physician does convey are noteworthy. Although the interaction in Encounter B appears more equalitarian than in Encounter A, the overriding goal is still the client's adequate functioning in work—in this case, the occupation of "wife." The patient's physical symptoms are problematic mainly insofar as they interfere with this occupation. Exertion in housework triggers the patient's symptoms of irregular heart rhythm. This experience makes her unhappy and even guilty: "I can cook the dinner and wash the clothes, but you know, any sweeping, cleaning that I do, that kind of sounds like an excuse, but it really isn't. . . . It's sort of maddening" (ll. 70–77). The doctor has several options at this point. He could try to explore and to ease the patient's guilty feelings about her physical limitations; he could also suggest alternative social arrangements, including greater division of labor in housework. Instead, he opts for a pharmacologic solution, increasing the dose and frequency of a medication to suppress irregularities in heart rhythm. He views this technical intervention as a desirable alternative in dealing with physical demands (ll. 366–375). An extraordinary expression of this attitude is the doctor's encouraging comment as he instructs the patient to exercise more strenuously during the electrocardiogram: "Could you do some sit-ups for me? . . . Just do about, uh, try to get yourself a little bit short of breath. . . . Try again. . . . Just scrub one more room" (ll. 273–279).

The implicit ideologic message is that the woman's occupational role in housework is worthwhile, desirable, and necessary. Again, the ideologic position is ambiguous. Struggling against sexism perhaps would be too much to expect in such an encounter. Questioning or challenging the patient's work at home might upset her deeply; on some level the doctor may be aware of this dilemma, yet the doctor reinforces this woman's household activities and even her troubled feelings about them. As many commentators have pointed out, such work by women is crucial in reproducing the relations of economic production. Here a well-intentioned doctor contributes to this socioeconomic arrangement. There is no critical appraisal of any aspect of the woman's role, even those physical demands that exacerbate symptoms of heart disease.

That the woman's continuing ability to reproduce her husband's economic role

278   try to get yourself a little bit short of breath. . . .
279   Try again. . . . Just scrub one more room.
280 P: [laughs] All I have to do is lie down and
281   everything flips. [laughs]
282 D: OK. Let's try it now. Just lie back.
283   [aside] Put on two.
284   All right. Yeah. So what we see again goes back
285   into that pattern of the extra beats. It's what's
286   called bigeminy. You know, remember you used to
287   have that all the time, and uh, and this is sort
288   of infrequent. All right . . .
289 P: Now it's doing it.
290 D: Yes. OK, but it's starting to settle down.
291   And there are a couple of different . . . OK. Fine.
292   That's good. 'Cause that at least documents what
293   you're feeling. I'm sure this is what happens
294   when you, when you exert and exercise. That,
295   two things happen, that the rate becomes a little
296   irregular, although it doesn't go back to your
297   fibrillations. But you do have these extra . . .
298   [aside] Can you show me the . . .
299   You see each time one of these extra beats comes
300   in, see this different complex here is when
301   you're, uh, notice the thumping.
302 P: Yeah.
303 D: Because it uh/
304 P: /When I did that, what that happens at
305   much closer intervals when I/
306 D: /Well, well/
307 P: /just sweep,
308 P: sweep the/
309 D: /I would think/
310 P: /floor. [laughs]/
311 D: /that uh,
312   basically the way to suppress that will be, uh,
313   I'm not sure that cutting back to one or two of
314   the Inderal a day was, uh, I don't think that's
315   your problem. I think it's probably that you
316   need a little more of it.
317 P: You think I need more . . .
318 D: Yeah, we had you on two three times a day/
319 P: /That was
320   a lot/
321 D: /That was, yeah. But uh, the time action of
322   the drug is not that great, so I would think that
323   uh that you can suppress the tendency to the extra
324   beats, but this is not heart failure or anything of
325   that sort at all.

326 P: Is, is there anything in the Inderal that could
327   possibly react, it just seems to me that the reason
328   I cut down to one was because it would slow my
329   my heart action down to the point where you know
330   I'd just/
331 D: /You felt it was that/
332 P: /Yes/
333 D: /uh, slow.
334 P: It was like being hit with something. You just sat
335   and tried to move, it was moving like, I guess, just
336   turned to sleep. As I remember it was almost like
337   the reaction I had to the digi . . .
338 D: Digitalis.
339 P: The digoxin.
340 D: The digoxin slowed you too much/
341 P: /Yeah. Except that
342   not that extreme. But it would just get very very
343   feathery and very very tired.
344 D: Yeah, well I know you're sensitive and a good
345   observer, I/
346 P: /And when I cut it back to one, every-
347   thing seemed to be so much better/
348 D: /Except when you/
349 P: [inaudible] for a long period. Until I almost cut
350   it out, sometime last summer, or during the fall I
351   got back into a more regular pattern/
352 D: /Well in February
353   you were on three a day.
354 P: Yeah, but at that time I had cut it back to two
355   instead of, and I had cut back to one and one and
356   one, three a day, but one each time.
357 D: Yeah, well it seems that the irregularity is when
358   you place, you know, when there is either increased
359   tension or increased stimulation to your heart or
360   more demands on it because you're starting to work
361   more. And that/
362 P: /What worries me is that the demand
363   is such a little thing/
364 D: /Yes.
365 P: That I, I cut out so many things, that you have to do.
366 D: Oh, absolutely. And you see what we wanted you to do
367   is allow you to do those things without, without having
368   the tendency to the irregularities or the poundings,
369   and if we can suppress, you know, the intent of the
370   Inderal, uh, or propranolol, is to, it blocks, if you
371   will, some of the extra, you know, some of the extra
372   beats. So that when your heart is being pushed by
373   any sort of external or internal influence, this can

374 slow that down. Now, obviously we don't want to put
375 you. . . . Where are you checking your pulse, at the wrist
376 or the chest?
377 P: Well
378 D: Over the chest/
379 P: /At the time, at the time, yes, I see,
380 because you had said it doesn't always get to the/
381 D: /No.
382 P: And, but when this happens, lots of times you can't
383 even feel . . .
384 D: Mmm hmm, OK. It may be, you see, that it's just so
385 regular. I'm sure it's not stopping.
386 P: [laughs] I'm sure it isn't either. Uh, I mean, if
387 I ever felt like that I would call. [laughs]
388 D: Yeah, if it stops, tell me, would you. [P. laughs]
389 Um, I would think that, um, I would think that the
390 Inderal, I would, it's still a very low dose, of uh/
391 P: /Well, I'll increase it.
392 D: To go back to three a day, and let's see how it's,
393 see how you're doing and maybe we'll see you a little
394 sooner to see what/
395 P: /Well, what you said that if I feel
396 any, you know, reactions to it I should come and have
397 you check it.
398 D: Yeah, give me a call rather than sort of worrying it
399 out. Come in and just call, and we'll see you and
400 say, OK, this is what's happening and we've got to do
401 something differently or not/
402 P: /Well, this is really
403 the first time, in two months, really the first
404 time that it's happened, that it really didn't respond/
405 D: /But it seems to me/
406 P: /I mean, since I started.
407 D: Yeah, yeah. It seems to me this is a, is a rhythm
408 situation rather than in any way implying heart failure
409 or anything of that sort, and uh you know the decision
410 that's always sort of rolling around in the back of the
411 mind is well, you know, when do we make a decision that
412 maybe that valve should be replaced and such, but with
413 your other problems that you've had with the kidney and
414 such, [she laughs] I think we're hesitant to be too
415 cavalier about, about saying, you know, if those were
416 not the cases/
417 P: /You don't have a couple of machines
418 to put me on. [laughs]
419 D: Well, if those were not the case, you know obviously
420 many years ago, you know, I'm sure that they would

is a major goal also is clear from the doctor's inquiry about life stress. This topic would seem a reasonable one for a concerned physician to initiate. Notably, the doctor's question about stress addresses the work of the patient's husband: "The areas of pressure and stress. Your husband is, now . . ." (ll. 171–172). The brief conversation that follows implies that the husband has found a job after a period of unemployment, is happier than he was previously, works hard, yet feels dissatisfaction because his work lacks challenge. Although the doctor praises the husband's competence, the patient reports that her husband denigrates himself. After hearing that the children are "fine right now," the doctor concludes that the "stresses and pressures that you've . . . felt earlier are . . . alleviating" (ll. 192–196). One cannot fault the physician here for his concern about life stress. The revealing feature of this concern, however, is that it focuses first and foremost on the economic role of the patient's husband. The caring doctor hopes that such stress will not take its toll on the patient, and also that the patient's physical condition will not impede her ability to maintain the breadwinner's home. Doctor and patient seem mutually to desire these outcomes; alternatives escape critical scrutiny. The encounter subtly affirms that stress related to the husband's occupational role is a necessary part of social life and that medicine's goals include satisfactory adjustment to this stress.

Similarly, the physician tries to learn about and to manage other tension-laden experiences in the family. Early in the interaction, the patient mentions a possible relation between irregular heart rhythm and emotional conflict with her daughter (ll. 18–21). The doctor drops the subject but returns to it later, when he asks about the children. Again the patient alludes to problems she anticipates when her daughter returns to work as a lifeguard. That the daughter's presence is a source of anxiety is clear from a laughing claim that the patient is trying not to worry now: "I'll take that when it comes" (ll. 199–204). Also in response to the doctor's question whether the children will be home, the patient briefly refers to her oldest son's military training in ROTC but does not elaborate (ll. 206–208). The reasons for the doctor's concern about family life are not entirely evident. Apparently he wants to do what he can to reduce, or at least to investigate, sources of emotional stress that may affect the patient's physical health; perhaps because no acute problems seem present, he does not offer concrete suggestions.

One cannot argue that the inquiry about family life is inappropriate in itself. On the other hand, the structure of the doctor-patient encounter does not encourage a critique of ongoing social relations in the family. The medical management of psychic distress generally involves an intervention—medication, advice, or even the permitting of negative comments and emotional catharsis concerning family members—that facilitates the client's adjustment to troublesome circumstances. The medical encounter rarely elicits a critical analysis of distressing social patterns within the family, let alone strategies for structural change. (Although psychotherapy may lend itself to a more critical appraisal, many have noted that traditional psychiatry and clinical psychology tend to foster adjustment rather than

421   have considered putting another valve in, but, uh,
422   and it may still come to that, somewhere along the
423   way, and uh, if we can't manage you well medically,
424   then uh, then I think that's a reasonable alternative
425   to consider.
426 P: I just realized that the six months that I wasn't having
427   a period I had a lot less problems [laughs] than I
428   have. I think that's/
429 D: /I suspect, certainly hormonal
430   factors can be playing a feature here too. And uh,
431   you know, you are in that sort of menopausal period,
432   where your periods are still stuttering around.
433 P: Yeah.
434 D: And it might be that that would change a great deal
435   after/
436 P: /Yeah, I forgot about that, you know, realizing
437   that yesterday and today, before the heat, too. I
438   mean heat/
439 D: /Mmm hmm.
440 P: I don't move very well, but it, you know, would, may
441   make a difference.
442 D: Yeah, OK. Well, I think, let's push back to the
443   Inderal. You keep on the, if you notice you're holding
444   onto more fluid, the Hydrodiuril can be used more
445   than once a week without any trouble, you know, not
446   just in reference to the menstrual period, but rather
447   in reference to/
448 P: /Well, I've cut way back on salt and
449   things like that too, I did, for you, not use it, and
450   I started using it again. I decided to cut back on
451   that, I think maybe that will help.
452 D: OK, I'm sure.
453 P: I hope that my weight . . .
454 D: Yeah, OK. So let's um, keep in touch on this. I
455   think what we can do is this. I'd like to see you
456   in about three months. But if during this interval,
457   as you're adjusting the Inderal, you feel that there's
458   something that I'm just not understanding about how
459   your heart's working, call and we'll see you sooner.
460 P: OK, now you said go back to two, three times a day?
461 D: One.
462 P: One.
463 D: One, three times a day. I don't think we have to
464   jump into the other, I'd like to see if we can't
465   suppress those extra beats.
466 P: I would too. [laughs]
467 D: OK, fine. OK.

change.) The health professional may ask questions about family life and may make limited suggestions, but major structural alternatives—sexual equality in housework and child care, women's employment outside the home, divorce, children's emancipation, and so on—seldom are suitable recommendations. Thus the ideologic impact of the medical encounter tends to be conservative. Although reduction of stress may seem desirable, major modifications in family relations elude serious consideration. In this way doctor-patient interaction helps reinforce not only current relations of economic production, but also the major supporting institution of the family.

The medical management of leisure and pleasure also occurs in this encounter. Planning for the summer vacation is the background for the doctor's questions about the patient's children (ll. 196–198). The doctor then asks if the patient will "get away this summer." She replies about a possible trip by car to visit her mother-in-law in St. Louis. Despite the patient's concern about finances, the doctor encourages her to fly. He inquires whether she will be spending some time at the beach and implies that this would be a good idea; the patient's husband, however, is "not a beach loller" (ll. 209–234). The doctor's purposes here are not quite clear. He may have some concern (as in Encounter A) about the physical effects of long periods of sitting for a patient with heart disease. On the other hand, he seems to imply that relaxing at the beach may be more pleasurable than a "long haul" by car to visit one's mother-in-law. Although the doctor remains nondirective, the partial medicalization of leisure and pleasure, within an otherwise technically oriented encounter, is striking.

This encounter contrasts markedly with the previous one. Here both doctor and patient maintain a strong orientation to the technical problems of the patient's physical illness. The doctor shares information openly, and the patient participates actively. They convey an impression of mutual respect and cooperation. Yet similar themes of ideology and social control arise, albeit to a lesser degree. A primary goal of the encounter is the client's ability to function in her economic role; by not examining the problematic features of this role, the doctor implicitly supports it. Difficulties in family life, when questioned are amenable to stress reduction and adjustment rather than structural change. Medical mediation also arises in the realm of leisure and personal pleasure. Aside from the positive communication that occurs, the encounter still reinforces things as they are.

The patient in Encounter C is a 39-year-old white Irish Catholic netmaker who has a high school education. He is about to be married. Wanting to know all the details of his medical problems, he reports satisfaction with the doctor's explanation. The doctor is a 47-year-old white male, who denies a religious preference and reports his ethnic background as Russian. He states his area of specialization as general internal medicine. Patient and doctor have known each other about nine months. The patient's diagnoses, according to the doctor, are "ethanolism [alcoholism] under control" and "excess cigarettes with asthmatic bronchitis." The interaction occurs in a private suburban practice.

Encounter C (code 10/101/01)

```
 1 Doctor: OK. Let me explain what this is. [laughs] OK?
 2 Patient: Yeah.
 3 D: And the reason is that they're doing a research
 4    project. This doctor represents a doctor from
 5    Massachusetts General who, uh, is working with
 6    somebody at Stanford University, and they're
 7    doing a research project on patients. When
 8    you leave I write a summary, and then you
 9    write, you evaluate what I tell you and all
10    of that. So, if you don't want to, I'll
11    turn this off, but if you don't mind then/
12 P: /No.
13 D: Great, then I'll identify you as _____ and then we'll
14    start talking. Now, you got the Hinton tests at the
15    hospital/
16 P:          /Right.
17 D:                   /So that that's all set. . . .
18    Your premarital slip is all signed.
19 P: Right.
20 D: I have to just examine you to make sure that you have no
21    infectious diseases, which I'm sure you have not. I'm
22    more interested in your liver. Now what has your
23    situation been?/
24 P:                  /I . . .
25 D: How've you been?/
26 P:                       /feel a little . . .
27 D: You look great/
28 P:                   /tired.
29 D: Why? How much've you been working?
30 P: Not bad at all, running around the past week,
31    fooling around, lobstering/
32 D:                              /What did you say?
33 P: Lobster pots.
34 D: What are lobster pots?
35 P: For catching lobsters.
36 D: What's that got to do with you?
37 P: I'm tired.
38 D: Why are you, what are you doing with lobster pots?
39 P: Catching lobsters.
40 D: Where?
41 P: I've got a trailer down in _____, and I got a
42    boat down there.
43 D: Are you allowed to uh
44 P: Oh, yeah/
45 D:          /catch lobsters?
46 P: You catch 'em, only allowed ten pots.
```

Apparently the purpose of this visit, from the patient's point of view, is to obtain a report of a blood test for syphilis, so that he can get a marriage license ("Hinton," 1. 14). At the outset, however, the doctor asserts that the blood test is not the only item on the agenda: "I have to just examine you to make sure that you have no infectious diseases, which I'm sure you have not. I'm more interested in your liver" (ll. 20–22) — and many other areas of the patient's life as well. What begins as a straightforward request for technical information required by the state becomes a wide-ranging inquiry into the patient's medical status, social relations, and personal habits. Eventually, a variety of moral judgments issue forth, all under the rubric of medical advice.

Aside from its content, the overall form of the encounter is noteworthy. The doctor dominates the interaction through a long series of questions. After the patient responds, apparently as honestly as possible, the doctor then asks more questions. Meanwhile, the patient receives very little information as such. Instead, the doctor provides brief comments, rarely technical, and frequently moralistic. The encounter takes on a staccato quality, largely because of the doctor's interrogatory behavior. The format of repetitive questioning, although to some extent required by medical history taking, establishes the doctor's dominance in the interaction. Studies of sociolinguistics, outside the field of medical interaction, have found that repetitive questioning is a verbal style that both reflects and achieves interpersonal dominance (17). This encounter is a rather extreme example of the interrogatory format.

This style distorts the lengthy parenthetical discussion about lobstering (ll. 30–79). The doctor apparently intends this conversation partly to be sociable, although he himself may want to do some lobstering in the future. The doctor asks question after question, which the patient answers courteously but laconically. It is unclear whether the patient has any interest in discussing this topic. The doctor, however, pursues the details of lobstering relentlessly. Meanwhile, the patient mentions the only symptom that he reports in the entire encounter: he is "tired." The doctor hears this compliant twice in the lobstering conversation (ll. 28, 37) but either ignores or discounts the concern. Instead, the inquiry about the equipment, legalities, timing, and location of lobstering continues. Even if the patient wished to exert himself about his fatigue, it would be difficult to interrupt the flow of interaction.

That the patient is tired, however, does not escape the doctor entirely. The doctor connects fatigue to two issues, both of which he considers later in the encounter: work and marriage. After a long interlude on alcohol (which itself warrants further attention below), the doctor asks, "How's uh your general energy and strength?" The patient answers, now for the third time, "I'm tired." Immediately the doctor does some reality testing about the patient's work life: "but are you able to put out and work . . . a regular day?" When the patient responds affirmatively, the doctor congratulates his client for occupational reliability; "Wonderful," he says and then moves on to other questions (ll. 172–178). The patient himself seems not too keen about his job. For instance, he later notes that his going for a liver test

47 D: You are allowed ten pots?
48 P: Right, ten dollars, ten pots.
49 D: How did you, how are you allowed to get 'em?
50 P: By traps.
51 D: No, I mean why are you allowed to and I'm not
52   allowed to/
53 P: /You're allowed to. You just have to
54   file the permit.
55 D: Anybody can get a lobster pot?
56 P: Oh, yeah.
57 D: Do you catch lobsters?
58 P: Yes.
59 D: How many do you catch?
60 P: . . . last year I had four in, and uh, . . . well, we eat
61   very good every weekend.
62 D: What, you got four?
63 P: Well, I had four pots out/
64 D: /Yeah
65 P: and uh/
66 D: /How many lobsters did you get?
67 P: I think we were figuring on a weekend . . . after August
68 D: /Yeah/
69 P: /About eleven on the weekend.
70 D: My Gosh! . . . My Gosh! I didn't realize that. Where
71   are your pots?
72 P: Down at _____.
73 D: Where's that?
74 P: Uh, right up, up, up, uh
75 D: _____?
76 P: _____. _____.
77 D: _____? Oh, I see. You have a boat?
78 P: Yes.
79 D: Oh! I didn't know that. . . . And how's _____?
80 P: Good. Now.
81 D: And how are your sisters?
82 P: They're just . . . well . . . I don't get along with them . . .
83 D: Maybe you don't, but . . .
84 P: After next week it's all over.
85 D: Why?
86 P: I get married.
87 D: And then?/
88 P: /Sunday/
89 D: /And then?
90 P: Well, I'll move.
91 D: Where?
92 P: Where? Where'm I going to live? _____, maybe.
93 D: And where do your sisters. . . ?
94 P: Oh, they live at home.

95 D: Why do you think they'll then get off your back?

96 P: I dunno . . . I think . . . I'll just do my work.

97 D: What about your father?

98 P: Well, he's . . . good, I guess.

99 D: Who's going to live with him?

100 P: No one.

101 D: Going to live alone.

102 P: Right.

103 D: OK, fine. So then . . . who's going to watch over him?

104 P: Well . . . well, I guess my sisters . . . probably. I imagine

105   I will . . . 'bout the usual.

106 D: You'll share it.

107 P: Yeah.

108 D: Instead of you doing it all.

109 P: Right.

110 D: OK, Uh, the 32-dollar question: How's your cigarettes?

111 P: Bad.

112 D: How bad?

113 P: . . . I haven't cut down. Well, I mean, I started cutting

114   down, but I went back up again.

115 D: Why?

116 P: I don't know. I have a cigarette in my mouth

117   [inaudible]

118 D: Whenever you find that happening, put the cigarette out.

119   And then the 64-dollar question, of course, is how's the

120   booze?

121 P: I'll tell you, I've had a few beers, that's all.

122 D: Now . . .

123 P: At the stag party/

124 D: /Now . . .

125 P: I swear/

126 D: /You're skating on thin ice/

127 P: /I went to that

128   stag party last night; I didn't have a drink.

129 D: Really? For you/

130 P: /Right/

131 D: /Terrific.

132 P: Right.

133 D: How many guys?

134 P: Um . . . I have no idea. . . . Biggest one I've seen. [chuckles]

135 D: Really. Where was it?

136 P: Oh, the Italian restaurant.

137 D: My God! You had a hall?

138 P: Yep.

139 D: How many people?

140 P: I think there were 150 people.

141 D: Good God. And everybody drank?

142 P: Um hm.

143 D: You didn't? You had how much?

144 P: [chuckles] Cold Duck and beer/

145 D: /and no beer?

146 P: No. I'll tell you I had a beer afterwards, though.

147   I went to _____'s house afterwards and I had one beer

148   and we split that. That's all.

149 D: Now, that's great. That is . . .

150 P: Now will that one beer bother me? I'll never go back

151   on booze again/

152 D: /Look. It won't bother you if you can

153   stay there, you know/

154 P: /I can stay there/

155 D: /The thing that

156   bugs me, you said that the last time/

157 P: /Yeah, well I'm . . .

158   I'm a little smarter this time/

159 D: /That's right/

160 P: /than I

161   was last time.

162 D: That's right. And you know what, _____? You're going

163   to be smarter next year than you are this year.

164   The total . . .

165 P: I'll go without it.

166 D: Huh?

167 P: I'll go without it. There won't even be beer in the

168   uh, refrigerator up there.

169 D: Just terrific! Just terrific! Just terrific! How's

170   your appetite?

171 P: Same.

172 D: How's uh your general energy and strength?

173 P: I'm tired but/

174 D: /but are you able to put out and work?/

175 P: /Oh, yeah/

176 D: /and work a regular day?

177 P: Oh, yeah.

178 D: Wonderful. No symptoms of stomach trouble or . . .

179   coughing . . . or headaches?

180 P: Just the regular. I have had headaches, but I

181   think it's from the sinuses.

182 D: And your cigarettes. . . . And you're tired. . . . You're getting

183   married next . . . Sunday?

184 P: Right, right.

185 D: Shew! Have you gone to any AA at all?

186 P: Uh, just in the last three months, I missed the last

187   three ones. I uh got reminded of your appointment

188   today, and I remembered that I missed the one last

189   week and, the last two weeks . . . and I wish I

will provide "a good excuse" to miss work (ll. 270–271). On the other hand, the doctor reinforces his client's economic role and appears to take his patient's fatigue less seriously than if it interfered with productive labor.

Throughout the encounter, marriage, fatigue, alcohol, liver disease, and smoking seem intertwined. The doctor juxtaposes marriage and fatigue before interrogating the patient about Alcoholics Anonymous: "And you're tired. . . . You're getting married next . . . Sunday?" At the encounter's beginning, the doctor indicates that he is more interested in the patient's liver than in the medical requirements of the marriage license (ll. 20–23). Just before the session ends, the doctor connects bronchitis, marriage, and the liver: "You're all loaded with junk and wheezes. You're doing great. I signed the slip. You're all set for your wedding. Uh your liver's down to normal. . . . We're starting anew, just anew" (ll. 252–256). Although the patient is "doing great," the doctor nonetheless wants another liver test and notes that, because of heavy smoking, "you've got your lungs shot. . . . I've never heard it this bad." On the other hand, apparently because of the patient's upcoming wedding, the doctor advises a reduction in smoking rather than a complete stop: "I know, I'm not saying stop smoking, 'cause I can't, uh, because right now you're in a tense situation, but, uh, cut it down please" (ll. 272–278). Such mixed messages, voiced with the authority of scientific medicine, strain even the common-sense imagination.

Consistent, rational explanation seems a less important goal in this encounter than control over the patient's behavior. Control extends not only to the physical impact of such activities as smoking and drinking, but also to their moral implications. The doctor attaches symbolic values to these two problems. Smoking is "the 32-dollar question." When the patient gives a therapeutically incorrect answer, the doctor advises a straightforward act of will: "Whenever you find that happening, put the cigarette out" (ll. 110–118). Alcohol is "the 64-dollar question" and draws greater emphasis. The patient also gives the wrong answer to this question. At his prenuptial stag party, the patient has broken the vow of abstinence required by Alcoholics Anonymous. AA claims that, for an alcoholic, any drink creates a risk of full-scale readdiction. The doctor reaffirms this principle by stat-

```
190      did go because I gotta [inaudible] registered
191      and I coulda got it done there.
192 D: Have you seen him at all?
193 P: Since the last time? Yes uh huh I went last Tuesday.
194 D: You think he was helpful to you?
195 P: I think he was a lot better last time. He made sense
196      the last time, you know. I went in [mumbles]
197 D: Oh, really?
198 P: Yeah, and uh he made some sense. I mean, he wasn't
199      telling me about all his drinking problems. At least
200      you could sit down and talk with him, you know.
```

201 D: Yes I'd like to give you some sort of uh alcoholic
202   base uh, that is, when things get bad, you know you can
203   always come here.
204 P: Right, right.
205 D: You know that. You know that _____ will kick your ass,
206   and you know that you can always depend on me, too.
207   And then you also know that you'll have the AA who are
208   used to dealing with people like you. So that I think
209   that it's very important, not that you'll ever use it,
210   but if you do/
211 P: /I would go to him. I'll tell you if I
212   goofed again. I . . .
213 D: But we need contigency plans, and this is for, uh, sit
214   up on here [long pause] and come on down here a minute,
215   and let's poke a little and see. Let me listen to your
216   heart first. . . . Deep breath. . . . You hear that? Boy, your
217   lungs are loaded with uh wheezes. . . . Boy, you're smoking
218   up a storm.
219 P: I did last night something awful. 'Cause everybody was
220   on my back about . . .
221 D: Yeah, well when people get on your back, you can't go
222   to booze or cigarettes or . . . or sex/
223 P: /Oh, no/
224 D: /you've got to
225   think of something where you can hang out by yourself
226   and control/
227 P: /What are you gonna do when you're sitting
228   up at the table and the guys go after you?
229 D: Then you have to . . . here, take a deep breath, a real
230   deep breath, now, does this hurt at all?
231 P: I don't think so. I don't know.
232 D: Well, if I hit you here versus here, is that the same?
233 P: I . . . I . . . well, it's not a real bad pain, I mean.
234 D: Uh huh, very good.
235 P: I know you're pushin' it sort of.
236 D: Yeah, take a deep breath . . . real good. Wow, this has
237   improved considerably. This is excellent. Excellent.
238   Very good. Any skin problems?
239 P: Uh not that I know of.
240 D: No itching?
241 P: Uh I get this uh a couple of pimples up here, and I
242   got a bump on this arm, and this one broke here on
243   Wednesday night.
244 D: What's this?
245 P: Uhhh, it's for picking out eyes.
246 D: It's a dangerous thing to carry around. I'll never
247   argue with you when you have that on . . . [patient laughs].

ing that, despite the patient's drinking only "a few beers," he is "skating on thin ice" (ll. 119–126). Again the interrogation begins. In minute detail, the doctor questions the patient about alcohol consumption before, during, and after the stag party. Although he remains skeptical about the patient's intentions—"the thing that bugs me, you said that the last time"—the doctor extracts a promise that in the future, "There won't even be beer in the uh refrigerator up there." According to the doctor, this renewed vow is, "Just terrific! Just terrific! Just terrific!" (ll. 127–169).

The patient's promise, however, is not enough. To prevent recurrent alcoholism, he also needs social supports. After mentioning again the patient's impending marriage, the doctor stresses the importance of continuing participation in AA. When the patient reveals his irregular attendance, the doctor argues against relying solely on the patient's personal discretion and commitment: "Yes, I'd like to give you some sort of uh alcoholic base . . . we need contingency plans. . . ." The doctor offers three such supports: himself, an alcohol counselor, and AA as an organization: "when things get bad, you know you can always come here. You know that. You know that ____ will kick your ass, and you know you can always depend on me, too. And then you also know that you'll have the AA who are used to dealing with people like you" (ll. 185–213).

Aside from these practicalities, there is also a moral element here. When temptation beckons, self-control is paramount. Although social supports are desirable, ultimately the individual must resist personal decline through the force of will, and alone. Final responsibility for a healthy life, physically and morally, rests with the individual. Medically phrased moralism occurs during the physical examination when the patient asks what to do when social pressures encourage his deterioration into bad habits. The doctor replies: "Yeah, well when people get on your back, you can't go to booze or cigarettes or . . . or sex . . . you've got to think of something where you can hang out . . . by yourself and control." Knowing that such rectitude is easier said than done, the patient pushes harder: "What are you gonna do when you're sitting up at the table and the guys go after you?" For reasons unclear, the doctor then retreats into the physical examination but gives a physical instruction which ironically answers the patient's question through a double meaning: "Then you have to . . . here, take a deep breath, a real deep breath . . ." (ll. 219–230). This perhaps unintentional remark conveys an image of a man alone, restraining himself by any means possible from sensuous diversion and moral turpitude.

The doctor's concern about these issues, of course, is understandable. The patient's habits apparently are turning him into a physical wreck. Yet while heavily laden with value judgments, this encounter is nearly devoid of technical content concerning the patient's physical condition. The doctor provides no details about alcohol's impact on the liver or smoking's effect on the lungs. The doctor's medical observations are brief and uninformative, such as, "You hear that? Boy, your lungs are loaded with uh wheezes. . . . Boy, you're smoking up a storm" (ll.

248   Open your mouth. Say ah.
249 P: Ah.
250 D: Good. Now don't smoke that much. You're/
251 P: /I won't.
252 D: You're all loaded with junk and wheezes. You're doing
253   great. I signed the slip. You're all set for your
254   wedding. Uh, your liver's down to normal.
255 P: Whew!
256 D: Yeah, heh heh. We're starting anew, just anew.
257   _____, if you do good, that's it. If you don't do
258   good, I want to see you.
259 P: I won't.
260 D: Now I want to just . . . when was the last time we did a
261   liver test on you?
262 P: Uh, I was gonna have it done when I went in this/
263 D: /Yeah/
264 P: /time to the guy in AA with the telephone. And I'll
265   do the whole thing. I'll call him.
266 D: Could you just get a liver test sometime?
267 P: Yeah, I can just call him tomorrow.
268 D: That's what I mean. Could you just get that done and
269   please have it mailed to me?
270 P: Yeah. It would be a good excuse to get off next week
271   for a day. [laughs]
272 D: Great. _____, please, the smoking, huh? Your lungs/
273 P: /Yeah, all right/
274 D: /are, you know, you've got your lungs
275   shot. It's, it's, I never heard it this bad. I
276   know, I'm not saying stop smoking, 'cause I can't, uh,
277   because right now you're in a tense situation, but, uh,
278   cut it down, please. Good luck. Best wishes.
279 P: Thank you, doctor.
280 D: Have a happy life/
281 P: /Uh huh/
282   /Give my best to _____.
283 P: Right, uh you want me to come back?
284 D: Uh, I want the blood test first/
285 P: /Right/
286 D: /and then maybe just as a routine
287   check, uh, let's see, what is the date?
288   Uh, June, July, uh sometime in August
289   or September.
290 P: All right then.
291 D: If anything between then/
292 P: /I hope not.
293 D: Oh, yeah. Bye bye, _____.
294 P: Bye.

216–218), or "you've got your lungs shot" (ll. 272–275). Beyond the theme of self-control, the doctor also monitors the patient's role in economic production, as noted earlier. Regarding family relations, the doctor inquires about the patient's sisters and father, particularly what changes will occur after the patient's marriage. The doctor states, in no uncertain terms, that the sisters should do more to "watch over" the father, instead of the patient's "doing it all" (ll. 81–109).

In this interaction, ideologic messages about the patient's actions and attempts to control behavior in socially safe ways overshadow the technical communications of scientific medicine. Yet the symbolic aura of medicine supports the doctor's dominance, ensures the patient's relative passivity, and gives credence to ideologic messages that aim to control major facets of the patient's life experience. There are no heroes or villains here; it is doubtful that these processes reach conscious awareness. They occur in a caring relationship, where the professional's concern for his client's well-being is beyond dispute.

MEDICAL MICROPOLITICS AND SOCIAL CHANGE

The doctor-patient relationship, then, manifests contradictions that arise despite the best intents of well-motivated participants. Medical encounters are embedded in a social context. Dealing with physical problems represents only part of the interaction's content, and often a small part at that. Doctors' sharing of technical information is quite variable, as are communications explicitly grounded in scientific medicine.

On the other hand, messages of ideology and social control in medical encounters are rife. Such communications carry certain distortions; although they tend to be nontechnical, these messages convey the symbolic trappings of scientific medicine and the impression of the professional's superior technical knowledge. This communicative pattern supports the professional's dominance within the encounter. More important, ideologic messages extend beyond the encounter, to reinforce current social arrangements in work, the family, leisure, pleasure, sexuality, and other facets of social life. A primary, though sometimes implicit, goal is the client's continued participation in economic production. For women, this goal extends to the maintenance of the husband's economic role through housework and other familial responsibilities. Doctors make decisions about the certification of medical disability and eligibility for welfare payments. They also manage anger, anxiety, unhappiness, loneliness, depression, and related emotions; in the process, the social origins of many of these emotions escape notice.

The medicalization of social problems aims toward individual adjustment and mutes potential resistance. These micro-level processes tend to reinforce macro-level patterns of domination and subordination in society. Messages of ideology and social control are more than the foibles of individual doctors. Instead, such messages usually reflect a humanistic concern for the totality of a patient's experience.

In their education doctors internalize this concern as a mark of good medical practice. All this reveals the ambiguous nature of caring professional behavior.

Ambiguities within the doctor-patient relationship both reflect and help reproduce broader social contradictions and structures of oppression. Such issues as uneven development, the social origins of physical disease, the private-public duality, the class characteristics of the medical profession, and the costly corporate penetration of medicine—considered in earlier chapters—are problems at different levels of analysis from face-to-face medical interaction. Yet it is troubling to note that intimate interpersonal encounters between professionals and clients may help maintain these oppressive contradictions and social structures. That is, the medical encounter is one arena where the dominant ideologies of society are promulgated and where individuals' acquiescence is sought. The subtle force of this phenomenon derives from the presumed objectivity and helpfulness that the symbolism of scientific medicine conveys.

This is not to say that medicine is the only, or even the major, social institution, that promotes society's current structural arrangements. The family, educational system, criminal justice system, and many other institutions achieve similar effects in service of the status quo, but these impacts have received wider recognition than those of medicine. Further, it is foolish to think that changing the doctor-patient relationship in itself would lead to wider social change. Although medical encounters may reinforce structural patterns of domination and oppression, the struggle toward nondominating, nonoppressive doctor-patient relationships will not create social revolution (notwithstanding ardent claims by alternative health movements of various persuasions). Basic change in doctor-patient relationships needs to accompany change in the larger contradictions that impede a decent and humane health-care system. Just as medical encounters are only part of the problem, their modification will be only part of the solution.

Two questions remain: Does social revolution resolve the ambiguities of medical interaction observed here? What kind of medical relationship is the eventual aim? Regarding the first question, it is clear that revolution does not remove these micro-level contradictions. Although few observations of medical encounters in socialist countries are available, some very similar problems have persisted or arisen anew in postrevolutionary settings (18). In the former Soviet Union, the medical encounter became a tension-ridden experience, since workers could obtain exemption from work only through medical certification. The doctor-patient relationship thus tended to reproduce the relations of economic production, even after the means of production had become socially owned. More recently, as noted in chapter 1, analogous issues have emerged in the psychiatric labeling of political dissidents. Observations of medical encounters in Eastern European socialist countries have revealed that impersonality, lack of continuity, bureaucratization, and requests for certified absence from work have negatively affected doctor-patient relationships. In China, the class position of medical professionals was a major focus of the Cultural Revolution. Political struggle extended to face-to-face medical encounters, where patients and advocates who accompanied then demanded full information and equal participation in decision making. Since Mao's death these developments have, in part, reversed. In Cuba, where improved health care has received high priority, dissatisfaction with doctor-patient relationships contributed to two national reorganizations (*Medicina en la Comunidad*, Medicine in the Community, starting in 1974, and *Medicina General Integral*, Integral General Medicine, starting in 1984) that ensured the continuity of doctors in local communities and supported research on medical interaction. In short, the contradictions of the doctor-patient relationship do not disappear with social revolution and require continuing critical attention.

It is difficult to envision the characteristics of a desirable doctor-patient relationship under capitalism. Although the qualities of a "good" relationship are the subject of endless speculation, little of the available commentary deals with the ambiguities of medical humanism. Sensitivity, compassion, nurturance—all these admirable traits may encourage a client's adjustment and acquiescence to oppressive features of social and personal life. The problem really is quite close to that considered in previous chapters: What actions at the interpersonal level are nonreformist? That is, what kind of relationship heightens political understanding and motivates structural change rather than encouraging limited improvements that only perpetuate current conditions?

The empirical study summarized here provided not a single example that met this criterion of a nonreformist relationship. Some brief, preliminary, and somewhat utopian thoughts about such a relationship, however, may be appropriate in conclusion. These comments also point ahead to the next part of this book, which focuses on strategies for change.

First, in a nonreformist relationship, both participants try to overcome the domination, mystification, and distorted communication that result from asymmetric technical knowledge. Professionals try to communicate thoroughly, honestly, and in comprehensible language both the content and the limitations of their knowledge about physical problems. When patients do not understand or disagree, they say so openly. Because differences of education, class, gender, ethnicity, and race make communication more difficult, doctors actively seek full discourse by encouraging patients' participation, skepticism, and disagreement.

Second, doctors and patients avoid the medicalization of nonmedical problems. This involves a conscious attempt to prevent medicine's symbolism from extending to nonmedical spheres. When such issues as work, family life, leisure, pleasure, sexuality, and aging enter the conversation, both participants recognize that the doctor has neither training nor authority to arbitrate these areas. Because these issues involve social problems, it is necessary to seek social solutions. Likewise, feelings like anger, anxiety, unhappiness, depression, and loneliness frequently have social roots. A doctor's attempt to ease such emotions, either technically through medications or supportively through psychotherapeutic discussion, inappropriately may deflect attention from these underlying causes. Under such circumstances, reducing socially caused pain generally should not be the sole direction, however humanistic it may seem.

Instead, as a third goal, it is important to analyze the social roots of personal suffering. A doctor's participation in this analysis may or may not be appropriate; the health professional, for example, might refer a patient to a labor union, women's organization, cultural center, community group, or other agency for assistance. After further investigation, the client may decide that a change of social role is desirable in work, the family, or another institutional setting. In this decision, the client's autonomy is essential, but so is the availability of a support system. From the start, decision making and control in such areas are outside the professional's expertise and authority.

Fourth, physical illness may demand technical intervention as therapy, but social problems require resistance and political organizing. This distinction, often blurred by the undeniable impact of social conditions on physical health, is nonetheless essential to maintain if therapy is to include both physical and social elements. A nonreformist relationship encourages activism. When occupational toxins or stress produces physical symptoms, for instance, labor organizing is the preferred therapy, in addition to whatever physical treatment may be appropriate. For the tension headaches of tedious housework, sexual politics aim directly at social causes. Regarding alcoholism and other addictions that seek oblivion from the agonies of social life, social revolution may be the only remedy that even begins to correct the problem, as Engels and Allende noted long ago. These rather facile examples oversimplify the clinical issues; the point, however, is that a nonreformist doctor-patient relationship must foster long-term organized activism. Otherwise, the medical encounter dulls the pain of today, without hoping to extinguish it in the future.

Part Three

Policy, Practice, and Social Change

7

Medicine and Social Change:
Lessons from Chile and Cuba

Thus far, this book has concerned itself with problems more than with potential solutions. Its goal has been to clarify the difficulties of medicine in capitalist society, especially those stemming from the interrelationships among medicine, societal contradictions, and oppressive social structures. These interrelationships lead to a skepticism about meaningful change in the medical sphere, if unaccompanied by change in the social order.

It is tempting to stop here. Having analyzed the problems, one might wish to leave solutions to others, especially when solutions seem not at all straightforward. If one clear-cut conclusion suggests itself from this book, it is that strategies to improve medicine ultimately must be components of a wide-ranging strategy of social reconstruction. The latter is clearly beyond this book's scope and, for the United States at least, may be inappropriate during the present complex period of history. Nevertheless, it is important to confront more limited questions of policy and strategy; evasion of these issues leaves the arena of activism open mainly to alternatives that do not challenge the status quo in any important way.

This chapter and the next consider policy and strategy. The general perspective is the same as previously: the society in which medicine is situated shapes the changes that occur in the medical sphere. Reformist reforms in medicine make small material improvements without challenging current patterns of political power and economic domination. Nonreformist reforms do create real changes in power and finance; they also heighten political consciousness by exposing social inequities. The purpose here is to examine current health-care policies and strategies, to discern which are reformist versus nonreformist (although the distinction is seldom simple), and to advocate directions of medical-political activism. The discussion gains humility from the realization that policy making and strategizing in medicine play themselves out on a large social stage. What follows, then, takes guidance from Gramsci's homily that encourages "pessimism of the mind, optimism of the will" (1).

Chile and Cuba took different roads toward socialism, and their histories have much to teach about policy, strategy, and the nature of reform. Changes in health-care systems paralleled transformations that were occurring throughout the societies. Until 1973, Chile had a forty-one-year history of civilian government with strong traditions of social democracy and liberal programs of health and welfare. In Cuba prior to 1959, a dictatorship controlled the country, stark patterns of class privilege manifested themselves, and public health and welfare systems were rudimentary at best. Both Latin American nations suffered from economic underdevelopment and dependency. After Chile and Cuba won political independence from Spanish and British imperialism, they witnessed the extraction of economic resources by North American corporations. In Chile, economic imperialism particularly drained mineral resources like copper; in Cuba, sugar and tourism provided rich sources of foreign profit. Poverty and imperialism constrained the effectiveness of health and welfare programs in both nations, if such reforms received attention in social policy. When the *Unidad Popular* (UP, or Popular Unity) government headed by Salvador Allende took office during 1970, it aimed toward the nonviolent, gradual emergence of socialism. The military coup d'etat of 1973 abruptly terminated Chile's so-called peaceful road. On the other hand, Cuba's revolution was rapid, violent, and thorough in consolidating state power.

Both countries showed with exquisite clarity the linkages between medicine and social change. These linkages need careful consideration in strategic planning, even in countries like the United States, whose economic and political conditions are quite different. The experiences of Chile and Cuba illustrate the limitations of major health-care reforms in the context of unresolved social contradictions and the advantages of health policies tied to broad, social structural change. In Chile, underlying contradictions impeded crucial reforms, both within and outside the health sector. Cuba's accomplishments—in reorganizing the health-care system, in adopting rationalized policies about medical technology, in restructuring community medicine, and in modifying doctor-patient relationships—grew organically from a wide-ranging social revolution. Because Chile and Cuba entered periods of revolutionary transition from positions of economic underdevelopment, their experiences do not always lead to straightforward conclusions about advanced capitalist countries. The comparative histories of Chile and Cuba, however, convey certain lessons that apply regardless of a society's level of development and that are unifying themes of this book: health care is inextricably linked to a nation's political and economic systems; problems within the health system emerge from and reinforce the larger contradictions in society; and incremental reforms in the health system have little impact without basic change in the social order. The Chilean and Cuban experiences also demonstrate the positive effects for health care of nonreformist political struggle, as arduous and protracted in time as this struggle may be.

PRESOCIALIST HEALTH-CARE SYSTEMS

By 1970 Chile already had a tradition of public health care for low-income people. Recognizing the problems that Chileans faced in obtaining decent health care, Allende—acting as senator in 1952—proposed legislation that established a national health service (*Servicio Nacional de Salud*, SNS). The SNS comprised a nationwide system of public hospitals and clinics that provided services to people who could not afford the fees of private practitioners. In theory, then, health care became a right for all Chilean citizens in 1952.

In practice, however, the SNS fell short of its goals (2). Physicians tended to use SNS facilities while devoting a large part of their time and energy to wealthier patients in private practice. Because they could join the SNS voluntarily and could work on a part-time basis, doctors gained access to SNS hospitals and clinics, where they maintained offices to see both SNS and private patients. Although private practitioners were expected to work a fixed proportion of time for the SNS, these hours were not enforced. By the time the UP government took power in 1970, approximately 90 percent of Chilean physicians belonged to the SNS on a full- or part-time basis. In no sense, however, did this statistic represent commitment to public health.

The SNS also developed other weaknesses. In particular, it became a complex and cumbersome bureaucracy, which was notorious for its size (40,656 administrative employees worked for the SNS in 1967, as compared to 6,487 medical professionals) and for severe inefficiencies in delivering needed services. Even more important than these bureaucratic problems was the persistent maldistribution of services. As in countries without a national health service, doctors and health facilities tended to be located in wealthier neighborhoods. Expenditures for both ambulatory and hospital care in Santiago, the capital, were over four times those in rural areas. Although Santiago contained only one-third of Chile's population, approximately 60 percent of all Chile's physicians and 50 percent of dentists practiced there (3). The failure of the SNS was so clear that the national legislature created separate health services for the armed forces, the railroad industry, and white-collar workers including teachers, lawyers, and bureaucratic officials. While recognizing health care as a right of citizenship, the SNS that the UP inherited had done little to achieve its formal purposes.

Chile's national health insurance (SERvicio MEdico NAcional de empleados, SERMENA) began in 1968, many years after the establishment of the SNS. Rather than consolidating the health care available for Chileans, SERMENA added still another health system to the SNS and private practice. SERMENA was a voluntary plan for health insurance similar to the Blue Cross–Blue Shield plans in the

United States. It provided both hospitalization and ambulatory benefits for patients who decided to pay annual insurance premiums. In addition, SERMENA received public subsidies from government funds. SERMENA paid doctors on a fee-for-service basis for seeing patients covered under the insurance plan.

A primary motivation for SERMENA was to give continued support for fee-for-service private practice. During the 1960s Chile, like many other countries, faced rapid increases in the costs of medical care. Chile's middle class, who generally had used private practitioners rather than the SNS, felt these increases acutely. The medical profession therefore became concerned that it would lose much of its private clientele. As a result, in 1968 the liberal Frei administration established SERMENA, which provided nationally administered health insurance for the majority of professionals, the owners of small businesses, and government employees. In this way, SERMENA directed even more of Chile's health resources into the private sector. Like the SNS, SERMENA provided important benefits to private practitioners while requiring no fundamental changes that would improve the health care available to low-income Chileans.

While they had created a public health system, pre-UP governments had not overcome the inequities of the private-public contradiction. Although most Chilean physicians worked part-time for the SNS, they also continued their own practices. Doctors received greater financial reward from their private patients and felt little motivation to devote energy to patients covered under public programs.

Although the majority of Chilean citizens were "public" patients, overall health spending was greater in the private sector than in the public sector. During the late 1960s, per capita health expenditures were far higher for the small proportion of Chileans who obtained care from private practitioners than for those covered by SERMENA and the SNS. It was estimated that during 1969 fee-for-service private practice consumed approximately $100 per capita per year to serve 8 percent of the Chilean population; SERMENA used approximately $50 per capita per year to serve 22 percent of the population; the SNS, serving 70 percent of Chile's population, received about $33 per capita per year (4). In short, the private sector created a drain on the financial resources and personnel available to serve people in the public sector. Public subsidization of the private sector emerged earlier in Chile than in some advanced capitalist countries like the United States, although the dynamics were similar.

With the enactment of SERMENA, then, Chile's medical care assumed the form of a three-class system. The upper class enjoyed access to private practitioners, paid on a fee-for-service basis. The middle class obtained insurance coverage through SERMENA, which also paid doctors on a fee-for-service basis but with government subsidies financed by taxes. Low-income Chileans had the theoretical right to health care provided by the SNS. However, in practice, Chile's problem of medical maldistribution prevented low-income people from receiving adequate care.

By the late 1960s, the inequities of this three-class system gained wide recognition. Members of the Socialist and other leftist parties argued for the adoption of a unified health service, or *Servicio Unico*. The *Servicio Unico* essentially would have abolished the private sector—either by banning the private practice of medicine or by taxing private practice heavily. If enacted, the *Servicio Unico* theoretically would have provided services efficiently to people from all class backgrounds.

The concept of *Servicio Unico* clearly threatened the Chilean medical profession. Because this measure remained controversial, the UP coalition did not formally include it in the platform for the 1970 election (5). The platform, which represented a compromise adopted jointly by several left-oriented parties, merely noted that health care was a basic right of all citizens.

The official planning documents that the UP administration published shortly after gaining office again stressed the inequities of the private-public contradiction and argued for a redistribution of resources in favor of the public sector (6). At no time, however, did the UP government explicitly adopt a policy suppressing private practice. Therefore, although the UP favored a more equitable distribution of resources, and although many UP planners personally supported the concept of *Servicio Unico,* the new government entered office without a clear policy directed toward eliminating that private-public duality.

Despite its problems, the health-care system that the UP government inherited in Chile was vastly superior to Cuba's prerevolutionary system. Cuba's medical services before 1959 were so limited that they require little discussion. The government operated a small number of clinics and public hospitals in Havana and a few other cities. These facilities were maldistributed and riddled by corruption. Private practitioners and clinics, located almost exclusively in the capital and large cities, served high-income Cubans on a fee-for-service basis. Insurance groups, or *mutualistas,* administered private insurance plans for descendants from specific geographic regions of Spain and also for selected categories of industrial workers. The province of Havana contained 32 percent of the country's hospital beds and the only blood bank. There was not one public dental clinic. Cuba's only medical school, in Havana, trained doctors for private practice; most graduates remained in Havana, settled in other cities, or emigrated.

Before the revolution, low-income Cubans living in both urban and rural areas faced enormous obstacles in obtaining needed services (7). It is estimated that more than 60 percent of the population had no regular access to medical care. Doctors, clinics, and hospitals in the private sector were unavailable because of high fees and geographical maldistribution. Public-sector medicine was rudimentary and usually inaccessible. Traditional healers (*curanderos*) and birth attendants (*comadronas*) provided services to Cuba's poor, but these practitioners could have little impact on the diseases of underdevelopment. The infant mortality rate ranked among the world's worst. Cuba's people also suffered from a high incidence of such infectious diseases as tuberculosis, polio, malaria, intestinal parasites, acute diarrhea, diphtheria, and tetanus. Malnutrition heightened the risk of infection, and epidemics were frequent. In short, a coordinated public health system was nonexistent, expensive fees and maldistribution left much of the population without access to services, and patterns of disease and early death that are characteristic of underdevelopment ravaged the poor.

CONTRASTS IN REVOLUTION, REFLECTIONS IN MEDICINE

Chile's Revolution in Process

The Chilean revolution ended far from completion. Allende and the UP sought socialism through peaceful means; elections, organizing in workplaces and local communities, and gradual shifts in the control of major social institutions were typical strategies of the UP, both before and after Allende won the presidency in 1970. Although the UP assumed power over the executive branch of government through electoral processes, vast sectors of Chilean society remained autonomous. In particular, the UP did not gain control over the legislature, judiciary, and military. During its three years in office, the UP encouraged politicization in the health-care system and many other sectors. However, the UP never came close to the consolidation of state power. This weakness made the UP vulnerable to the armed overthrow that Allende's devotion to nonviolent and constitutional processes could not prevent.

Even before the coup, the UP's opponents struggled to create a situation of economic chaos, in which political stability would become impossible. The shortages of products accompanying Chile's economic crises deeply affected the medical system. Because health care was linked to Chile's economic situation, the more general effects of imperialism and underdevelopment are pertinent.

The economic policies that fostered the UP's downfall originated mainly in the United States. Multinational corporations viewed with dismay the prospect of a socialist government. Corporations such as International Telephone and Telegraph (ITT) actively conspired to prevent Allende from assuming the presidency after his election in 1970 (8). When the UP took office, it moved to nationalize key industries dominated by North American interests. The most dramatic economic initiative occurred in 1971, when Chile nationalized its copper mines. The financial establishment of the United States responded swiftly with an economic blockade of Chile. The Nixon Administration chose to deny additional foreign aid, loans, or credit. United States representatives to international sources of credit (such as the International Monetary Fund, Export-Import Bank, World Bank, and Inter-American Development Bank), as well as large banks in the United States traditionally offering credits to foreign nations, withheld loans for nonmilitary purposes.

Because of the country's dependence on loans for the purchase of imports, Chile faced severe shortages of consumer goods. United States business officials, of ITT in this case, predicted the consequences of a hard-line economic policy: "A more realistic hope among those who want to block Allende is that a swiftly deteriorating economy . . . will touch off a wave of violence, resulting in a military coup" (9). As expected, the dissatisfaction of middle-class Chilean consumers plunged the UP government into an increasingly untenable political position. While denying economic support in all civilian sectors, the United States government continued to provide financial and technical assistance to the Chilean military (10).

International imperialism and economic dependency tempered Chile's ability to achieve lasting health-care reforms. Because medical underdevelopment and economic underdevelopment were intertwined, limited economic resources hindered the UP's efforts. As the Chilean journalist Valenzuela has remarked, if Chile and similar countries spent the same proportion of their wealth for health care as did a developed country like the United States, the effect necessarily would be restricted by the underdeveloped country's much lower level of wealth. Valenzuela concludes: "Consequently every health policy should be narrowly united with the general policy regarding development of the country" (11).

Poor nations are especially vulnerable to forces that drain the limited resources they do possess. Multinational corporations operating in the Third World generally remove many times more profit than they invest. Products like medical instruments and drugs have been imported or have been manufactured in Chile by profitable subsidiaries of North American corporations. During the sixty years prior to the UP government, for example, foreign companies took approximately $9.8 billion in profits from Chile (12). This wealth, if not removed from the country, could have gone toward health and welfare, as well as general economic development.

In the health sector itself, resources also move from the Third World to developed countries. Doctors trained in countries like Chile frequently migrate to developed nations like the United States; this pattern leads to a loss of human resources and capital for the poorer countries. Because of the flow of physicians to the United States, Latin America incurs an annual loss of more than $200 million, an amount roughly equivalent to the medical aid that the United States gives to Latin America for a decade (13). When human and natural resources leave the country in vast quantity, no Third World nation can expect a truly significant improvement in health care.

The class position of medical professionals also poses a problem. A majority of physicians have class interests that frequently conflict with progressive social change. Although 20 to 30 percent of Chile's doctors did support the UP at various times, the Chilean Medical Association consistently opposed it, for two main reasons. First, as members of the upper middle classes, physicians found shortages of consumer goods intolerable. Although shortages and inflation resulted largely from economic sanctions imposed by the United States, most Chilean physicians blamed the UP government and Allende personally for Chile's difficulties.

Second, Chilean doctors saw potential threats to their own professional dominance over the health system. The UP's support of consumer-worker councils in

neighborhoods and hospitals (which are discussed below) implied a future transformation of the health system in the direction of popular control. Although the
councils remained advisory, doctors feared that eventually the councils would
attain greater power. Since doctors were a minority within these councils, organized medicine generally opposed their formation and hindered their work.

Because the UP lacked state power, physicians realistically understood that they
could disrupt health services and that the government could do little in response.
Doctors united with other conservative groups in Chile to create the general instability that paved the way for military dictatorship. In a series of work stoppages
and strikes, the Chilean Medical Association periodically paralyzed the health system. During the truck owners' strike in October 1972, the majority of Chilean
physicians refused to see SNS patients except on an emergency basis (14). Meanwhile, doctors continued to see patients in their private practices. Lower-income
Chileans, who legally were entitled to services through the SNS, were unable to
find adequate medical care. In addition, the Chilean Medical Association resisted
other UP measures, including the training of paraprofessional health workers,
immigration by foreign doctors to Chile, and reduction in the length of medical
education (15). As members of the national bourgeoisie, physicians consistently
opposed the government's struggle toward a socialized health system and a more
equalitarian society.

Cuba's Consolidation of State Power

Although the roots of Cuba's revolution dated back through several decades of
organizing and popular uprisings, in contrast to Chile the revolution itself was
swift and dramatic. By military actions mainly in the eastern provinces during
1958 and 1959, insurgent forces led by Fidel Castro, Che Guevara, and Camilo
Cienfuegos won decisive victories that culminated in the fall of the Fulgencio
Batista dictatorship and the dictator's flight to the United States.

After its military victory, the revolutionary government moved quickly to consolidate state power. The new government controlled the armed forces and the
executive branch. The legislature and judiciary ceased to exist in their prerevolutionary forms. Mass political organizations emerged throughout the country (16).
Previously clandestine local groups reconstituted themselves as Committees for
the Defense of the Revolution (CDRs). Organized in local neighborhoods and
workplaces, the CDRs initially concerned themselves with security and vigilance
against counterrevolutionary activities. Later, the CDRs became the primary political structures for popular representation in policy decisions. Other major mass
organizations included the Federation of Cuban Women, the association of small
farmers, and the trade unions. All the mass organizations elected representatives
at the local, regional, provincial, and national levels. The Cuban Communist Party,
which came to hold ultimate responsibility for national policy decisions, assumed

formal power after the mass organizations had established themselves. Cooperative relationships linked the mass organizations and the party's leadership. A new judicial system emerged. Popularly elected people's courts generally decided disputes and made judgments about criminal actions at the local level. Regional, provincial, and national courts adjudicated weightier conflicts, for example, those that arose between labor unions and administrators of factories.

This brief summary reveals one key difference from the Chilean revolution, a distinction that is important for strategic planning. In Chile, the revolutionary process was only beginning with the election of a socialist government. In Cuba, a military victory permitted a rapid consolidation of state power, with broad-based support from mass organizations, even before Fidel Castro declared that the revolution aimed toward the establishment of socialism. This distinction carried profound implications for all sectors of the societies, including medicine.

After the Cuban revolution, the medical system needed almost total reconstruction (17). As in Chile, physicians occupied a privileged class position before the revolution; most maintained urban private practices that served high-income patients. The revolution's swiftness and largely military nature permitted little organized resistance by the medical profession. Also, because Cuba's public health system, hospitals, and clinics were already inadequate, strikes or other work stoppages by the profession could have had a much more limited impact than they did in Chile. In 1959 physicians found themselves in a radically different society whose future was unpredictable and difficult to control.

The revolutionary government took no measures to change the conditions of private medical practice. Doctors could continue their practices as before the revolution, with the same fee-for-service arrangement. In fact, the government offered financial incentives to physicians if they would work part-time in public hospitals and clinics. Doctors even received the option of office space and the use of technical facilities in public hospitals. Physicians and other citizens who owned homes and offices before the revolution retained their ownership rights. During the first years after the revolution, then, health professionals faced little objective change in their ability to work as they pleased.

Subjectively, however, many private practitioners perceived enormous threats. As one of its first priorities, the new government began planning for a reorganized public health system that would overcome previous inequities linked to poverty and geographic isolation. Physicians could take a role in policy making, but other groups, including government leaders, the mass organizations, and representatives of nonprofessional health workers, also would participate in health-care planning; doctors therefore could anticipate a gradual loss of professional dominance and autonomy. In addition, creation of a nationally organized system posed long-term financial dangers for private practitioners. The government proposed clinics and hospitals that would provide publically financed, high-quality services which patients generally would receive free of charge. Clearly the availability of free care would be attractive not only to the poor and to people without previous access to services; at least part of practitioners' private clientele predictably would turn to the public sector.

These anticipated long-term changes in medicine combined with a more general loss of class privilege. Although the new government permitted limited holdings in private property, it did restrict private investment in land and corporations. Also, the government sought a more even distribution of goods and services. Monitoring and rationing led to greater availability of products for people who previously faced hardship in obtaining the necessities of life. As legal and black-market prices outside the rationing system inflated rapidly, some products were harder to obtain for those accustomed to a degree of luxury.

Real or imagined, such threats proved intolerable for a large segment of the Cuban medical profession. By 1962, three years after the revolution, nearly half of Cuba's physicians emigrated, mostly to the United States; in some specialties not a single physician remained. At the country's sole medical school, in Havana, whole departments simply ceased to function. During this period, physicians who were sympathetic to the revolution came from other countries to provide direct services and other assistance. Although these supporters offered a stopgap, the Cuban government faced a momentous crisis in the health-care system.

Forces of imperialism deepened this crisis still further. Shortly after it recognized the socialist character of the Cuban revolution, the Kennedy administration participated in a series of interventions aimed at the overthrow of the new government. Primary among these ventures was the Bay of Pigs invasion of 1961. This unsuccessful military maneuver set the stage for an economic boycott which lasted throughout the 1990s. Cuba's prerevolutionary economy was heavily dependent on the United States. In the medical sector, the United States generally was the sole supplier for equipment and pharmaceuticals; as an underdeveloped and dependent country, Cuba—like Chile—had paid a high price for medical products. Nevertheless, the United States had provided a regular source of needed equipment, supplies, and drugs. The economic boycott abruptly ended Cuba's ability to buy these goods, and severe shortages arose rapidly. For major radiologic and laboratory equipment, replacement parts were unavailable. In the long run, Cuba faced major decisions about the purchase of foreign technology, as opposed to the creation of new industries to manufacture medical products. The impact of imperialism, together with the prior class position of professionals, thus led to a further breakdown of the health-care system, as personnel left the country and supplies were difficult to obtain.

Yet, in contrast to Chile, the fact that the Cuban government had consolidated state power created the potential for basic change in medicine. While Chile's incomplete revolution permitted policies that generally remained reformist in character, the nature of Cuba's revolution encouraged more dramatic improvements that moved beyond reformism toward a structurally different health-care system.

REFORM VERSUS STRUCTURAL CHANGE IN MEDICINE

Reformism in Chile

Immediately after it took office, the UP government started a number of public health programs designed to improve the distribution of resources throughout the country (18). The UP's innovations emphasized nutrition, environmental health, and preventive care. Allende's analysis of the social origins of illness and his view of needed sociomedical change set the pattern for the UP's reforms. The government provided one-half liter per day of free milk to all children and pregnant or nursing mothers. Educational campaigns promoted better nutrition. The SNS developed a system of emergency care, whose purpose was to offer free emergency services to all citizens. To help reduce Chile's high rates of infant and perinatal mortality, the government set up a network of maternity clinics in small towns. In environmental health, the UP tried to decrease the incidence of occupational diseases like silicosis by requiring technical innovations in copper mining and other industries. In addition, the government initiated programs to improve sanitation and housing, especially for low-income areas.

The SNS also focused attention on preventive health measures. For example, Chile had for many years faced a serious problem of widespread alcoholism. To promote popular consciousness, the government published comic books that dealt humorously with public health issues and started treatment centers specializing in alcoholism.

The UP attempted to correct the maldistribution of health services that it inherited from previous administrations. By constructing new hospitals and clinics and by giving financial incentives to practitioners willing to work in rural provinces, the government tried to increase both ambulatory services and inpatient care in underserved areas. The UP also promoted short-term campaigns to focus attention on rural health problems. For instance, a "health train" sponsored by the government gave medical care to approximately 30,000 people during a tour of the southern provinces.

These health reforms were highly visible and widely publicized. Although their impact on the population's health status was impossible to measure during the brief three-year period of the UP government, these initiatives excited enthusiasm throughout the country. Ultimately, however, the programs did little to change the overall organization of the Chilean health system and remained at the level of reformist reforms.

Because the UP lacked state power, it could not employ compulsory mechanisms to achieve a thorough structural transformation of health care. In the first place, it did not nationalize the health system. Likewise, the government did not require doctors to serve in areas of the country that lacked adequate personnel. Nor could it expand significantly the resources available for public health, since it was unable to impose any major restrictions on private practice. Regarding expensive medical technology, although the UP government made some initial efforts to regulate the sales of drugs and equipment, it failed to achieve a national formulary that limited private profitability. In short, broad social contradictions, including uneven development and the private-public duality, persisted as structural limitations to change (19).

The government did focus attention on private practitioners' exploitation of the SNS. There was increasing criticism of the use of SNS facilities to treat private patients. In addition, doctors who worked part-time for the SNS faced pressure to adhere to stricter schedules in their SNS duties. Yet part-time physicians remained the only health workers in SNS who did not submit regular accountings of time at work.

Massive maldistribution of health personnel and facilities persisted throughout the UP government. Chile's doctors remained concentrated in Santiago; higher-income areas of Santiago enjoyed approximately six times more health workers and financial resources for health care than did low-income areas of the city. After nearly three years of UP administration, it was estimated that private practitioners continued to receive 60 percent of Chile's total health expenditures to care for 20 percent of the people; meanwhile 40 percent of the health expenditures went to the SNS to serve 80 percent of the population (20). The enthusiasm of the UP's reformism masked the fact that fundamental structural change in the health system did not occur.

The UP also encouraged democratization and decentralization. Because these modifications promised important shifts in financing and power, they were nonreformist reforms, to which health professionals reacted with anger and opposition. Although the UP's actions were sometimes inconsistent, in general the government supported increased worker and consumer control. In the industrial sector, this policy led to workers' administration of a number of factories, especially after several companies (for example, textiles, automotive repair industries, and metallurgical enterprises) were nationalized. In the health-care system, consumer-worker control gradually emerged at two levels: the community and the hospital.

Even before the UP government took office, the Ministry of Health had divided Chile into geographical health "zones" and each zone into several health "areas." In Santiago, for instance, there were four major health areas, each served by one base hospital. The area comprised a number of smaller localities, each encompassing a population of 50 to 75 thousand and served by one neighborhood health center (NHC). Generally the NHCs were located in low-income residential communities (*poblaciones*). These NHCs were administratively dependent upon an area hospital for personnel, medical supplies, and financing.

Part of the UP program was to decentralize medical care by putting greater emphasis on the NHCs. The goal of decentralization, together with efforts to democratize the health system and to encourage greater community participation, led to the enactment of *Decreto 602*, a government decree providing a structure for active participation by health workers and community representatives. *Decreto*

602 created four different councils, two on the NHC level and two on the level of the area hospital. Figure 7.1 presents a simplified diagram of the relations among these advisory councils, the NHCs, and the area hospitals.

On the NHC level, local health councils (*consejos locales de salud,* hereafter referred to as LHCs) were formed by representatives of all organized groups in the community and by the labor unions of professional and nonprofessional health workers. The tasks of the LHC were to discuss the health problems of the community, to suggest solutions, to cooperate in the promotion of health campaigns, and to act as an advisory link between the SNS and the community. Still on the NHC level, a second council acted as an executive body (*paritario*). This group included representatives elected from the LHC in addition to the director of the NHC. The purpose of the *paritario* was to act upon the suggestions of the LHC, although ultimate decisions remained in the hands of the medical director. Analogously, at the area hospital level, parallel councils (*consejos locales del area*) and executive groups (*paritarios*) were established, with similar tasks and advisory functions. In addition, the area councils participated in comprehensive health planning and the coordination of services and facilities throughout the area.

As a supplement intended to broaden the provisions of *Decreto 602,* the UP initiated a Program of Sociocultural Development. The Program created an integrated health team to work with community members in identifying each locality's needs. Cooperating with local organizations, the health team offered health information and emphasized people's direct participation as knowledgeable LHC

Figure 7.1 Structure of Popular Participation in Health Care under the Unidad Popular Government in Chile

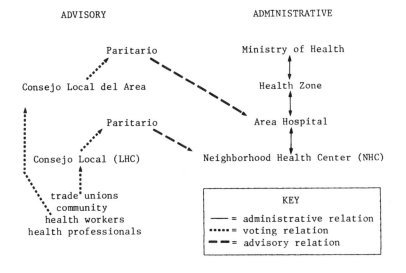

members. The health team encouraged patients' assertive behavior with doctors. This activity pointed toward greater personal autonomy in health care and reduced professional dominance within doctor-patient relationships. In general, the health team tried to raise the level of medical and political consciousness and to encourage activism.

As community participation grew stronger, many LHCs integrated themselves into other broad-based organizations concerned with food distribution, transportation, local security, and industrial production. When available health facilities appeared inadequate, LHC members took part in autonomous "committees to defend health." These groups became increasingly viable forms of popular power. They also provided a basis for the massive efforts needed to maintain health care during later strikes and boycotts by the medical profession.

Paralleling these changes on the neighborhood level, comparable democratization of decision making occurred in many hospitals, especially those affiliated with medical colleges. Within each specialty department, a governing council was formed; this council included elected representatives of professional and nonprofessional workers. The governing council made administrative and staffing decisions that formerly had fallen under the exclusive jurisdiction of high-ranking professionals. The influence of the departmental councils extended to the governance of the hospital as an institution. Departmental councils elected representatives — nonprofessional workers as well as physicians — to the council that made policy for the entire hospital. The restructuring of power relations in hospitals reflected the conscious thrust toward democratization that occurred also in other Chilean institutions such as industrial enterprises and the universities.

Decreto 602 provided a first step toward structural changes in the health system that involved nonreformist reforms. These measures promised a shift in existing power structures and encouraged community organization. On the other hand, the innovations contained important weaknesses, which many health workers and activists understood. As established, the councils and health teams did not produce a real change in power relations. Although they included a relatively low proportion of doctors (10 to 20 percent), the LHCs and *paritarios* remained basically advisory in nature. Actual decision-making power stayed in the hands of the medical directors of the NHCs. *Decreto 602* heightened consciousness about the contradictions that fostered problems of health care, including those of underdevelopment, professional dominance, and the private-public duality. But by 1973, when the military coup abruptly terminated these experiments in democratization and decentralization, the contradictions remained unresolved.

The coup's effects throughout society and particularly in the health system were devastating. Taking power six months after 44 percent of the Chilean people voted for the UP government in congressional elections, the military junta immediately needed to deal with its opponents; it chose mainly to execute the opposition. During the first three months of dictatorship, approximately 10,000 people died, in a total Chilean population of 8 million (21). The junta closed most NHCs that had operated in the *poblaciones* and rural areas. Decentralized medical services returned to the area hospitals, which members of the Chilean Medical Association again controlled. Community participation in health planning ended. The local and area councils that influenced health policy under the UP disbanded. Within hospitals, the consumer-worker councils on the departmental and hospital levels were abolished. Private practitioners, under military scrutiny, regained control of the health system. The dictatorship also discontinued most of the UP government's preventive health programs or, as in the case of free milk distribution to children, private entrepreneurs took control of these programs. Low-income Chileans experienced even more severe difficulties in obtaining medical care than they faced prior to the UP period.

The country's medical schools and the national school of public health were especially hard hit by the junta's policies. Medical students who expressed leftist political beliefs during the UP period were expelled. Faculty members in preventive medicine, social sciences, and public health were fired; entire departments in these disciplines were closed.

Throughout Chile, health workers suffered reprisals. For example, approximately two-thirds of the union of nonprofessional health workers were dismissed because of previous activities supporting the UP; one-third of the union of non-physician health professionals also were fired. Rates of unemployment for both professional and nonprofessional health workers rose as high as in any other single sector of the Chilean economy. Former directors of the NHCs were detained in the National Stadium with other political prisoners. At least thirty-five physicians were executed or died following torture. Medical school professors as well as general practitioners were imprisoned; torture was used routinely against doctors and other health workers. In addition, there were numerous reports that some military physicians cooperated in the administration of torture, particularly by supervising the use of drugs during torture sessions (22).

The Chilean experience has been deeply disturbing to those who uphold nonviolence and peaceful reform. Lacking state power and unwilling to arm the masses for military confrontation, the UP could not persuade the opposition to maintain legal and constitutional procedures. The brutality of Chile's dictatorship shows the harsh methods that are necessary to withstand a widely supported movement toward progressive change.

Structural Change in Cuba

The revolutionary transformation of Cuban society permitted a rapid reconstruction of its health-care system. Although Cuba's prerevolutionary medical services were rudimentary compared to Chile's, and although a large proportion of the country's physicians emigrated, the consolidation of state power allowed a remarkable series of nonreformist reforms and structural modifications. These changes fostered the creation of a health-care system which, to a variety of observers, appeared the most responsive and effective in all of Latin America (23).

Shortly after the revolution, the new government faced an immense crisis in health care. The government placed a high priority on recruitment into medicine and initiated a policy of open enrollment in medical school for qualified students; two additional medical colleges opened in provinces outside Havana. Medical education was free, and previous barriers of social class, race, and sex no longer affected the number or composition of the medical profession. Students from working-class and peasant families, blacks, and women quickly entered the study and practice of medicine. By the early 1970s, the ratio of doctors to population in Cuba resembled that of the United States and surpassed those of all other Latin American countries.

Government policies rectified geographical maldistribution. In exchange for free education, graduates have served a compulsory two-year period of practice in rural health centers and hospitals. Similar programs provided for a redistribution of nurses and allied health workers. In addition to personnel, the government sought to correct the severe maldistribution of health-care facilities; construction of hospitals and clinics in underserved areas received priority. Within a decade, each of Cuba's provinces contained a major regional hospital and an integrated system of clinics. More than half the new clinics were located in rural areas which previously had lacked such facilities altogether.

Despite these measures, the difficulties of rural practice led to a high turnover of physicians, who often returned to urban centers after compulsory service and undertook specialty training. To address the problem of continuity, in the mid-1970s the Ministry of Health began a program of "Medicine in the Community" (*Medicina en la Comunidad*). Among other initiatives, this program started teaching and research activities at decentralized clinics and required a rotation of professors between clinics and teaching hospitals. A second national reform, "General Integral Medicine" (*Medicina General Integral*), beginning in the mid-1980s, initiated family medicine training for all new physicians, as well as the requirement that at least one family practitioner live and work in each urban neighborhood and rural area throughout Cuba. Partly as a result of these policies, maldistribution and turnover have improved. A designated clinic and staff of health workers serve patients in every defined geographical location of the country.

The government also has sought to change prior patterns of class structure and racism that limited the accessibility of health care. Even when doctors were within traveling distance, the high fees of private practice had prevented low-income people from obtaining services. Racism compounded the problem, since the number of doctors and clients who were white was disproportionate to the ratio of whites to general population. In postrevolutionary Cuba, health care is free to the patient at the point of delivery. Public financing ensures that medical services, as well as most drugs and needed supplies, are available to patients, regardless of income. Patients receive preventive, ambulatory, and inpatient services without charge.

Blacks have entered the profession of medicine in proportion to population, and racism does not hinder patients from seeking and obtaining care.

While the consolidation of state power permitted effective planning to overcome maldistribution and inaccessibility, the mass organizations have taken an active role in preventive medicine. The Committees for the Defense of the Revolution have coordinated immunization campaigns in neighborhoods and workplaces; they also have assisted people in obtaining early attention for medical problems. The Federation of Cuban Women has helped coordinate prenatal, maternal, and infant care. Regarding occupational health, the association of small farmers and the trade unions have monitored workplace safety and have organized educational campaigns about work hazards. From time to time, when national goals of high productivity have interfered with safe working conditions, the trade unions have intervened to protect workers. In short, central planning and activism by the mass organizations have fostered prevention as well as accessible services.

These programs led to remarkable changes in morbidity and mortality, which demonstrate the impact of simple medical interventions in the context of prior underdevelopment. The incidence and prevalence of major infectious diseases fell drastically. Within fifteen years of the revolution, diphtheria, polio, tetanus, and malaria—cases of which still occurred in the United States—were eradicated in Cuba. Infant mortality fell from 52 to 27 per 1,000 within the same time period, and maternal mortality declined from 118 to 63 per 100,000. By the 1970s, Cuba resembled economically developed countries in illness and mortality patterns, as heart disease and cancer became the leading causes of death. In occupations like sugar production, the chronic lung disease of bagassosis would be a predictable consequence of high productivity standards; measures to reduce bagasse dust in cane processing and regular tests of workers' pulmonary function have helped prevent this and similar occupational diseases. Such accomplishments in rapidly modifying morbidity and mortality patterns would be hardly imaginable without the coordinated efforts of mass organizations and health workers.

After the early exodus of physicians, the private-public contradiction ceased to drain resources in any important way. Physicians who had engaged in private practice before 1959 could continue in the private sector on a full-time or part-time basis. New medical graduates, again in exchange for free education, vowed not to engage in private practice but to remain in the public sector. Since primary and specialty services were available in public clinics and hospitals, patients saw little reason to consult private practitioners, unless they had relationships from before the revolution. The private sector withered, as older practitioners died or retired.

Physicians' social class allegiance also has contributed to the successes of Cuban medicine. In contrast to Chile, where medical professionals consistently impeded the transition to socialism, Cuban physicians could do little in opposition other than to leave the country. After the crisis of the early 1960s, the class origins of the new Cuban medical profession changed quickly. A large proportion of new graduates came from working-class or peasant families. For them, the revolution has provided mobility into a satisfying and relatively prestigious field of work.

It might be expected that physicians trained after the revolution would enjoy certain privileges of higher class position. That is, a new class structure might emerge, based on differential expertise and responsibility. Even critical observers of the Cuban health-care system have found little evidence of such privilege. Doctors have greater access to publicly owned automobiles for work-related travel and receive somewhat higher salaries than do other medical workers (the differential between highest and lowest incomes in the health-care system is less than 20 percent of that in the United States), yet their housing and ability to buy consumer goods is approximately the same as other workers' (24). The commitment to public service, willingness to cooperate with the mass organizations, and tolerance for difficult conditions of practice all reflect, in large part, the medical profession's drastically different class origins and loyalties.

On the other hand, such characteristics of the profession do not imply that doctors lack power. The technical practice of medicine in Cuba follows traditional Western patterns. In general, doctors hold responsibility for day-to-day clinical decisions and lead the health-care teams in clinics and hospitals. Nurses and allied health workers take orders from physicians. Only in the mid-1990s did Cuba develop limited paraprofessional roles to permit practice by traditional healers or other workers who are less than fully trained. These policies came from a recognition by the country's leadership that the Cuban people were accustomed to the Western standard of medical professionalism. Physicians also have taken an active role in health-care planning on the national, regional, and local levels. Critics both within and outside Cuba have noted persisting professional dominance and the preservation of some hierarchical social relationships among health workers (25).

Although professional dominance remains a source of tension and ambiguity, it occurs within a framework of coordinated administration and democratic participation in decision making. During the early 1960s the Ministry of Public Health organized the health-care system so that planning and administration take place at the national, provincial, regional, and local levels. Figure 7.2 shows the structure of the system and the mechanisms for popular participation. At the local level, the family practitioners' offices, polyclinics, municipal hospitals, and rural hospitals provide direct medical services. The mass organizations elect representatives to the local people's commissions on health, which help implement such activities as immunization campaigns, control of infectious diseases, maternal and infant care, and occupational health monitoring. The local commissions also advise the administrative and clinical staffs about priorities and shortcomings. Since the reorganization of 1974, the municipal hospitals and polyclinics also are directly accountable to elected municipal assemblies. The assemblies, which are the formal structures of political representation known as "People's Power," have authority to request changes in the programs and personnel of the municipal hospitals and polyclinics when local needs warrant such changes or when dissatisfactions arise.

Figure 7.2   Structure of Popular Participation in Health Care in Cuba

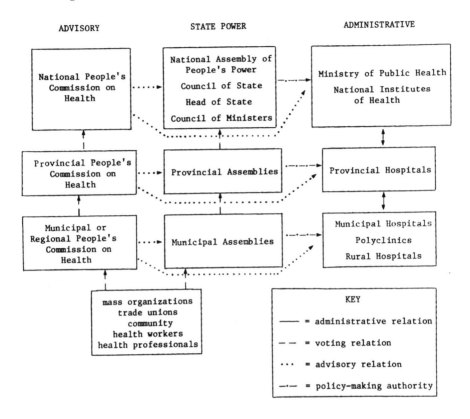

The municipal assemblies elect representatives to provincial assemblies, which contribute to policies of the provincial hospitals that serve as referral and teaching centers. At the national level, the Ministry of Public Health and the institutes of health in each medical specialty formulate health plans for the country as a whole. In policy decisions, the Ministry and institutes take guidance from the national assembly of People's Power.

This organizational structure permits centralized planning and priority making but also encourages decentralized implementation and flexibility. At each level of the system, medical professionals perform administrative and clinical tasks. To ensure responsiveness and accountability, however, the mass organizations, commissions on health, and assemblies take part in policy decisions. The principle of democratic centralism fosters participation by patients, community residents, and both professional and nonprofessional workers. Democratic participation balances central planning and coordination, so that bureaucratic rigidities are reduced.

The structure of the Cuban health-care system also helps control the proliferation of costly medical technology. At the national level, the Ministry of Public Health and the institutes of health evaluate the adoption of technical innovations, new equipment, and drugs. A national formulary of generic medications limits the drugs which physicians can prescribe. As in other industries, pharmaceutical production occurs within a nationalized and centrally planned enterprise (*empresa*), which manufactures about 75 percent of the drugs and medical equipment used throughout the country. In addition to cutting costs, the Cuban pharmaceutical and equipment industry has partly overcome the devastating effects of the economic boycott by the United States, which has caused shortages of drugs and supplies, as well as the loss of the Soviet Union as a major trading partner.

For costly innovations like coronary care units (CCUs), the Ministry of Public Health prepares an evaluation and plan that take into account the resources of the society as a whole. For example, the Ministry has recognized that CCUs are useful for some patients with complex cardiac problems and that supervised home care for patients in isolated areas is not always feasible. Most regional hospitals therefore have installed CCUs, although municipal and rural hospitals have cared for some heart attack patients without CCU facilities. Similar considerations have led to the adoption of renal dialysis, radiation therapy, and other expensive programs at the national and provincial levels but not at the local level. These policies have permitted the selective use of technologic advances without a wasteful drain of scarce resources.

In addition to major structural transformations, the Ministry of Public Health also has devoted attention to the nuances of the doctor-patient relationship. As noted previously, staff turnover and an orientation toward specialty medicine led to widespread dissatisfaction. As part of the programs of medicine in the community and family medicine, research and teaching efforts have emphasized the quality of professional-client interaction. Since the mid-1970s primary care teams, composed of doctors, nurses, and allied health workers, have assumed responsibility for a designated panel of patients. Participation by psychologists, sanitary workers, epidemiologists, and social workers on these teams supports an integrated approach to each patient and family.

The primary care team does not medicalize problems that have social or psychological roots. Instead, team members try to facilitate change in patients' living or working conditions that interfere with health and well-being. Educational campaigns in neighborhoods and workplaces encourage citizens to express discontent and to suggest improvements, either to the primary care team directly or through the mass organizations.

Many problems remain in the Cuban health-care system, as openly acknowledged within Cuba. In particular, the difficulties posed by underdevelopment and the United States' economic embargo limit further accomplishments; professional dominance and discontinuities of staffing in rural areas still require attention. Yet Cuba has transformed its rudimentary and crisis-ridden medical services into a rationalized and accessible system, whose accomplishments are startling even to the most skeptical observers. The rapidity and comprehensiveness of these advances depended on revolutionary social change that consolidated state power and that claimed wide popular support.

IMPLICATIONS OF THE CHILEAN AND CUBAN EXPERIENCES

As Allende liked to point out, the probability of peaceful evolution toward socialism was greater in Chile than in perhaps any other country. Elsewhere, since obstacles to change are greater and forces of reaction stronger and more sophisticated, the events in Chile become especially disheartening. Retrospectively, it is not difficult to find strategic errors by which the UP facilitated its own downfall, errors that arose in health policy as well as in other areas. The UP's mistakes, of course, occurred in the context of hostile economic maneuvering by multinational corporations and agencies of the United States government. The instability produced by the international economic boycott in part deflected the UP's attention away from crucial strategic opportunities. In Chile, social contradictions rooted in underdevelopment, imperialism, the private-public duality, and professional dominance did not reach resolution. Cuba needed to deal with similar social contradictions. However, Cuba's rapid and decisive revolution allowed a wide-ranging reconstruction of the health-care system, a reconstruction that went far beyond Chile's partial and ultimately unsuccessful reformism.

Mass Mobilization, State Power, and the Private Sector

The health councils established in Chile to increase consumer-worker influence eventually took part in broader mass mobilization. The councils allied with local groups concerning security, transportation, food supplies, and other urgent matters. Mass mobilization, however, seldom received direct support from the UP government. When mobilization occurred around health issues, it reflected a spontaneous movement by consumers and workers. The lack of explicit encouragement for mass political action was similar to the UP's hesitancy to promote mobilization in other areas of Chilean society. Critics of the UP have asked why the government—which apparently was well aware of a planned military coup many months in advance—failed to arm the workers. There are many tactical explanations for this failure, but the failure itself was consistent with the government's general stance toward mass mobilization.

In Cuba, mass mobilization was a key factor in the military success of the revolution. Previously clandestine groups in neighborhoods and workplaces transformed themselves into the Committees for the Defense of the Revolution. The CDRs became the primary organizations responsible for internal security but later took an active role in health-care activities. In addition to the CDRs, the Federation of Cuban Women, the association of small farmers, the trade unions, the commissions on health, and the assemblies of People's Power at the local, provincial, and national levels participated in policy making and implementation of health programs. Mass mobilization led to a variety of accomplishments, of which a transformed health-care system was only one.

For the duration of the UP regime in Chile, the private-public contradiction persisted. In the government's planning documents, officials drew attention to the large proportion of Chile's health expenditures devoted to the care of the rich by private practitioners, and to the relatively small amount of money spent by the SNS for the poor. The government stated its intention to make more resources available for the public sector and to expand services and facilities for low-income Chileans. Until the coup, however, little progress had occurred toward meeting this goal.

The persistence of the private-public contradiction in the health system reflected an overall failure to achieve state power. The UP government missed a possible chance to gain control of several key institutions—legislature, judiciary, and military—in 1971, when popular support, as shown by national elections, was at its height (26). Many observers believed that the time had come to consolidate state power and that the likelihood of a successful coup would be much greater if the UP did not take this opportunity. However, Allende apparently believed that attempts to control the military or other major institutions should proceed through standard administrative procedures. In short, 1971 passed with most institutions outside the executive branch still controlled by a national bourgeoisie that opposed progress toward socialism.

The situation was no different in the health system. The establishment of an effective socialized health system depended on the decline of the private sector. As long as physicians could work in both private practice and the SNS and could depend on private practice for high incomes from wealthy patients, Chileans would continue to suffer from multi-class medical care.

During this period the UP government did not make a serious effort to nationalize the health system. Public hospitals and clinics received somewhat more funding, and some new services became available, particularly in the field of maternal and infant care. At no time, however, was there a move to restrict or to abolish private practice. The basis of this passivity apparently was a political judgment that an effort to restrict private practice would result in enormous opposition from the medical profession. Ultimately the Chilean Medical Association did strike against the government, even though the UP had not explicitly attempted to suppress private practice. In Chile and many other countries, the private-public contradiction has remained a primary structural impediment to change.

Because the Cuban revolution resulted in a rapid consolidation of state power, the new government could move quickly to build a public health system. Although the limited medical services that existed before the revolution temporarily declined still further with the exodus of Cuban physicians, the Ministry of Public

Health was able to construct accessible facilities, to redistribute personnel, and to wage health campaigns in cooperation with the mass organizations. The government did not directly suppress private practice but recruited medical professionals committed to practice in the public sector. The availability of free public services of high quality implied that over time the private sector would wither, as in fact occurred. The private-public contradiction did not undermine the accomplishments of Cuban medicine, and the resolution of this contradiction depended largely on success in achieving state power.

Medicine and Social Change

The Chilean and Cuban experiences also show that incremental reforms in health care have little lasting effect without basic change in society. One reason that meaningful reform is so difficult when unaccompanied by broader social change is the impact of class structure. In the prerevolutionary context, health professionals — either by birth or by occupational mobility — are members of the upper or upper middle classes. As such, they hold class interests that often impede progress toward a more egalitarian distribution of goods and services. Doctors, like bankers and corporate managers, possess economic advantages and customary life-styles that they do not willingly sacrifice on behalf of the poor. Besides economic interests, health professionals hold dominant positions in the institutions where they work. Because of their technical expertise, physicians usually believe that professional dominance over health policies is justified; innovations that limit the profession's control over the conditions of practice are perceived as threatening.

The Chilean medical profession worked against the UP government's attempts to bring equity and democratization to the health system. Objects of the profession's opposition included the training of paraprofessionals, reducing the length of medical education, immigration by foreign doctors, and consumer and worker control over health policy. Physicians also were acutely sensitive to economic pressures that reduced available consumer goods. Thus, the UP government faced inherent and continuing conflict with the interests of the medical profession.

The Cuban revolution led to a transformation of class structure, including the class position of medical professionals. When half the medical profession left the country, the government mandated active recruitment of students into the study of medicine. Young people from working-class and peasant families entered medical schools in unprecedented numbers. Their free education fostered a commitment to public service. These graduates were less accustomed to the privileges of higher class position than were their predecessors and were more willing to cooperate in decentralized and democratically controlled programs. Professional dominance remained a problem in Cuba, but resistance from the profession did not impede reorganization of the health-care system.

The comparative histories of Chile and Cuba, moreover, reveal the vulnerability of incremental reforms. Allende viewed his presidency as a transitional period in which a series of reforms would culminate in a socialist restructuring of society. The government encouraged the establishment of local health councils, workers' organizations, and other new groupings whose eventual purpose was a thorough transformation of power relations in Chilean society. With occasional exceptions, however, these organizations did not achieve a redistribution of power. While such attempts at popular control contained a potential for nonreformist change, they disintegrated in the face of armed attack in the military coup. In Cuba, the mass organizations initially formed as part of the revolutionary process; they later became a basis for popular participation in health policy which endured and deepened over time.

The Chilean experience in particular demonstrates that dominant groups in society do not surrender power peacefully. In this light, it appears that societal transformation is a precondition for popular control and lasting reform of health services. In Chile, where the potential for a peaceful transition toward socialism and a democratized health system was great, Allende's hope that popular control would evolve by peaceful means proved a vain dream. More than ever before, it became clear that the struggle toward a humane health system cannot succeed without a concomitant struggle toward fundamental change in the social order.

If the attempt to achieve nonreformist reform and peaceful transition failed in Chile, what are its chances in advanced capitalist nations like the United States? Here the political power, economic resources, and military strength of those opposed to structural change are even more extensive. In contrast to many countries of the Third World, societal transformation within the advanced capitalist nations will be a long and difficult process whose contours are difficult to predict. Meanwhile, the tenuous character of reform cannot be wished away. Strategies in health care must be linked to more general political strategy. Otherwise, the outcomes will be no less transitory than those of Chile's sad example.

8

Conclusion: Health Praxis, Reform, and Political Struggle

$\mathbf{P}$raxis is the uniting of theory and practice, study and action. A recurring argument of this book is that understanding the problems of medicine and society is not enough; knowledge alone will not solve the difficulties that beset us. Research and analysis must be linked to political action. For meaningful improvements in the health-care systems of the United States and other advanced capitalist countries, it is important to understand the roots of illness and suffering that extend beyond the health sector, but it is also necessary to move beyond study to the practicalities of change. This concluding chapter suggests some directions of progressive health praxis.

REFORMIST VERSUS NONREFORMIST HEALTH POLICY

Health praxis includes a careful study of policy proposals and the advocacy of reforms that will have a progressive impact. To review Gorz's distinction again, reformist reforms leave intact current political and economic structures, while providing small material improvements that may reduce social discontent. Nonreformist reforms achieve true changes in power and finance and, by increasing political tension and activism, create the potential for wider political action. Although the distinction is not always straightforward, it is important to analyze which health reform proposals are reformist and which are nonreformist, and to take an advocacy role accordingly.

National Health Insurance (NHI)

NHI has received cyclic attention as a health policy for the United States since the 1930s. At times the likelihood of its enactment has seemed high and at other times remote; the prominence of NHI in public debate has reflected the prevailing political climate. Since NHI doubtless will continue to wax and wane in policy analysis, the reforms that it promises deserve scrutiny. The following paragraphs summarize the characteristics of many NHI proposals presented during the past two decades.

Because it would not change the overall structure of the health-care system in any basic way, NHI is a reformist reform. NHI would produce modifications in payment mechanisms rather than in the organization of the health-care system. Under NHI the federal government would insure payment for health services, though not necessarily all such services. The crucial point is that NHI is not a method of reorganizing the system; there is nothing in NHI to guarantee that doctors or other practitioners would work in different ways, in different areas, or in relation to different patients. The nature of private practice would remain intact, and the organization of hospitals and other medical institutions would not change in any basic way. Some NHI proposals may offer financial incentives to organize the system differently, but in general there is no requirement to do so. Potentially, NHI would tend to equalize patients' ability to pay, while not improving the accessibility or quality of services for much of the population.

Most plans for NHI would not lead to full payment for all medical services used by an individual or family. The key concept here involves copayments, which are deductible provisions requiring that a person pay out-of-pocket some fixed percentage of each dollar spent for health services. Except in instances of extreme poverty, an individual or family would pay the initial costs up to a specified amount before NHI takes over.

Copayments also must be seen in the context of the question: who will pay for NHI? NHI likely would be financed by new and compulsory taxation, for the most part by fixed payroll deductions. The financing arrangements for NHI therefore would be regressive; that is, low-income people would pay disproportionately for the benefits of NHI. Even the portion of premiums that comes from employers probably would be paid largely by employees, since employers keep wages low as health benefits increase. Although various tax mechanisms could relieve the burden of health insurance for low-income patients, legislators have devoted little attention to forms of taxation that would favor the poor. The combined effect of copayments and payroll deductions will not result in a progressive system of paying for NHI.

The administration of NHI also is important. In most NHI proposals receiving serious attention, private insurance companies would serve as the fiscal intermediaries of NHI. They would distribute NHI payments from the government to health providers, with compensation for doing so. If NHI allowed participation by the insurance industry, private companies would be able to siphon off profits from NHI. Since the government could administer NHI, there is little reason for continuing participation by the insurance industry, but NHI planning rarely has sought to eliminate the role of private insurers.

NHI would not modify the organizational structure of hospitals or private practice. Hospitals would be reimbursed for services delivered. Some incentives aim toward institutional efficiency, but these regulations generally remain vague. Individual practitioners would be paid through a fee schedule established by professional associations. Doctors would have an incentive, but no requirement, to form group practices. There would be some limited cost controls. Local comprehensive health planning agencies would approve the nature and quantity of services, but in general, these agencies have been politically weak in monitoring hospitals. Several features of NHI—especially the role of the private insurance industry and rate setting by health professionals—indicate that costs will continue to rise. These costs would be paid mainly by a regressive system of taxation.

Regarding accessibility, NHI proposals contain few provisions for improving geographical maldistribution of health professionals. Fee schedules might be higher in some proposals for doctors who practice in underserved areas, but such incentives cannot ensure that health workers will practice in these areas. Experience with universal health insurance in Canada, for example, shows that poor people continue to encounter access barriers due to both income and geography, despite the success of the Canadian system (1).

In summary, NHI may reduce the financial difficulties of some patients; it would help ensure payment for health professionals and hospitals. On the other hand, NHI would do very little to control profit for medical industries or to correct problems of maldistributed health facilities and personnel. Most plans also would preserve a major role for the private insurance industry. Planners have not devoted much attention to methods of taxation that would ease the financial problems of low-income patients. In short, although NHI raises hopes of fundamental improvements, its incremental approach and reliance on private market processes would protect the same economic and professional interests that currently dominate the health-care system.

Managed Care and Peer Review

Other examples of reformist reforms are managed care organizations (MCOs) and professional review organizations (PROs). Originally, MCOs were mostly nonprofit "health maintenance organizations," which sought to improve health outcomes and to control costs by managing primary care and preventive services. Since 1989, however, the majority of MCOs have adopted for-profit status, and no new nonprofit MCO has been initiated. Under managed care, a family or individual, or an employer on their behalf, pays a fixed "capitation fee" on a prepaid basis and then presumably receives all services that are needed during the year. Although a comprehensive account of managed care is beyond the scope of this chapter (2), a few key features are pertinent to the notion of managed care as a general health-care reform strategy.

Two assumptions underlie managed care. First, the group setting is said to provide administrative advantages. By coordinating staffs and equipment, managers can organize work processes more effectively. Managed care also is supposed to improve quality control. Administrators can monitor practitioners' behavior more closely. However, research on existing MCOs has found little evidence of improved quality. Regarding the presumed administrative advantages, critics have pointed out that administrative control can lead to increasing bureaucratization, wasteful procedures, and micromanagement of clinical decisions (3).

Another assumption is that MCOs reduce costs. The reason is that the organization's income is inversely related to costs, since the capitation fee is fixed. That is, the more cheaply doctors can practice, with a fixed prepaid payment, the higher the organization's income will be. This incentive for higher income supposedly reduces unnecessary visits, hospitalizations, and surgery. Studies of MCOs, however, reveal that the actual cost reduction in these plans is quite variable (4). Furthermore, the lower costs reported by MCOs usually overlook utilization that occurs outside the plan. An MCO may have low costs but also long waiting times for appointments, hurried visits, impersonal interactions, and bureaucratization. A survey by the California Carpenters Union, for instance, revealed a 30 to 40 percent utilization of services outside the Kaiser-Permanente system by Kaiser members. This survey indicated that many patients covered by Kaiser went elsewhere for part of their care because of dissatisfaction. The costs of these outside services did not enter into calculations that showed cost reduction.

Regarding the distribution of health care, federal legislation offers certain incentives to set up facilities in rural and ghetto areas. However, there is no requirement to do so. Otherwise, nothing leads one to believe that managed care will improve distribution. Very few MCOs ultimately have served areas where medical care previously was unavailable.

Professional review organizations have been established mainly to control costs through "peer review." The intent is to reduce unnecessary hospital admissions, surgical procedures, and so forth. In addition, quality is to be monitored by reviewing doctors' actual practice and seeing whether it conforms to currently accepted medical standards. Several problems, however, have become obvious.

PROs often are organized and controlled by local medical societies or other groupings of doctors. In general, consumers and other health workers have little or no role in the composition of PROs. The established norms of etiquette which Freidson and others have described for the professions indicate that PROs will do little to reduce professional dominance or improve actual standards (5).

In addition, PROs generally rely on written records for monitoring quality. Doctors' retrospective account of what happens in doctor-patient encounters can be shaped to conform to prevailing standards. It has been shown many times that such accounts differ markedly from others' observations of the same encounters. In PROs there is no attempt to monitor actual doctor-patient interaction. Quality is judged by technical criteria applied to the doctors' written records; it is not assessed by consumers' evaluation or by observations of the doctor-patient relationship. The limited research on the impact of PROs has shown very little effect on doctors' behavior.

Will PROs reduce costs? Available evidence reveals no appreciable cost reduction. Often organized on a for-profit basis, PROs receive even more funds to carry out a quality-assessment function. Finally, there is nothing in PROs that will improve maldistribution.

To summarize, managed care and PROs preserve professional and administrative dominance in health care. Historically, professionals have played the major role in development and policy making for these organizations. There have been few incentives to improve existing patterns of maldistributed services. Moreover, private corporations have entered this field rapidly, running for-profit MCOs and marketing technologic aids for peer review. Limited research has provided conflicting data about these organizations' long-term impact on the outcomes of medical practice. There is little evidence that professional etiquette permits upper-echelon health workers to criticize each other in a meaningful way. Again, in the face of these reforms, the broad structure of the current health system would remain nearly the same.

National Health Service (NHS)

An NHS would be radically different from any of the reform proposals discussed thus far. A fundamental principle of an NHS is that health care is a right of citizenship. Thus, an NHS strives toward equity in the availability of services, across geographical boundaries and income differentials. Essentially all postrevolutionary socialist countries have established an NHS as the basic organizational structure of the health-care system. Some nations, like Great Britain and Chile, have created NHSs in prerevolutionary contexts while retaining an economy based mainly in capitalist private enterprise.

Support for an NHS in the United States has been rare. For instance, in the national debate regarding NHI during the Clinton Administration, the NHS model was not seriously considered (6). Since the mid-1970s, planners have worked with members of Congress in drafting preliminary proposals for an NHS. Although these proposals have faced dim political prospects, they deserve careful consideration. Plans for an NHS contain many nonreformist elements, yet one needs to appraise them with a critical eye in view of current political realities. The following summary uses as a model the NHS legislation written and reintroduced during the 1990s by Congressman Ronald Dellums and his associates (7). While the Dellums proposal contains many features that remain highly controversial, it clearly depicts the contours of fundamental changes that go beyond the potentialities of more limited reforms.

The Dellums bill provides for comprehensive care, including diagnostic, therapeutic, preventive, rehabilitative, environmental and occupational health services, dental and eye care, emergency and routine transportation to medical facilities, child care, homemaking, social work, and counseling. These services would be free at the "point of delivery"; that is, the fee-for-service principle no longer would apply, either for direct payment from patients or for indirect payment from third parties. To improve geographical maldistribution of health professionals, the NHS would provide free education and training in return for required periods of service by medical graduates in underserved locations. Moreover, poor communities— those suffering from uneven development—would receive supplementary funding for facilities, equipment, special programs, and other needs.

Financing for the NHS would come from taxation of individual and corporate income, plus a tax on gifts and estates. The taxation would be progressive, in that individuals and corporations with higher incomes would pay taxes at a higher rate. The NHS would aim toward the elimination of private profit in the health-care system. A national commission would establish a uniform formulary of drugs, devices, equipment, and supplies. Regional branches of the NHS would purchase these goods in their cheapest generic form. Tax revenues for the NHS would be collected in a national trust fund, which would disburse payments to health facilities, salaries to workers, moneys for supplies, equipment, drugs, and construction, and funds for administration and policy-making groups. In short, insurance corporations and other companies could no longer profit by acting as financial intermediaries.

During a transition period, the NHS would purchase private hospitals and related facilities, which then would be subject to standardized budgeting procedures. Nationalization would permit regionalized coordination of hospital services and would reduce profiteering by professionals and corporations. An ongoing survey of local health needs, based in part on a census of the population, health statistics, and prior deficiencies, would determine the budget of each local service area. NHS planners argue, largely from the experience of other countries, that strict budgeting, nationalization, curtailing administrative waste, and reduction of private profit would stop the escalating pattern of health-care costs.

Politically, the proposed legislation calls for policy making through democratic processes in local communities. The NHS proposal designates elected boards at four tiers of organization: community, district, region, and nation. Each board is to be composed of two-thirds users of services and one-third health workers.

As drafted, the legislation matches services and decision-making structure to the size of the area served. The basis unit, governed by the community board, is a population area of some 25,000 to 50,000 people. Services to be offered at a neighborhood health center include primary care, preventive medicine, and monitoring of workplaces and the environment. The next larger unit, the district, would contain a general hospital directed by the district board and would provide inpatient and some consulting services for a number of communities.

The regional unit comprises several districts, served by a training institute and a specialty-oriented teaching hospital. The elected representatives on the regional board are responsible for the recruitment and selection of students for medicine, nursing, and other health-care occupations. Likewise, the regional board would license graduates and make assignments for their required service. Purchase and distribution of drugs and equipment for the regional and district hospitals and the community health centers also are responsibilities of the regional board and its staff.

The national board, whose representatives are elected from the regional boards, is responsible for nationwide planning and budgeting. To carry out this policy work the board would appoint six commissions, focusing on the following issues: (1) quality (including certification of facilities and personnel, general distribution, and priorities in research); (2) planning and education for the health-care labor force; (3) occupational safety and health; (4) pharmaceutical and medical supplies (including establishment of a national formulary and periodic evaluation of new drugs and equipment); (5) health rights; and (6) financial and budgetary planning.

On balance, an NHS is a nonreformist reform. If enacted, it would create major changes in current patterns of power and finance. An NHS would place stringent limitations on private profit in the health sector. Most large health institutions gradually would come under public ownership. The development of a national drug and medical equipment formulary promises to curtail monopoly capital in the health system. Financing by progressive taxation would benefit low-income patients, and periods of required practice in underserved areas would address the problem of inequities in accessibility. Centralized health planning would combine with policy input from local boards to foster responsiveness and accountability throughout the system

NHSs in some socialist countries have created remarkable achievements. Horrendous health problems that antedated socialist revolutions have rapidly declined. Social changes that foster economic security, adequate nutrition, and sanitation enhance the effectiveness of medical care per se in these countries (8). Although problems have been recognized in the health-care systems of all socialist countries, a few examples of positive accomplishments are appropriate. The former Soviet Union eliminated its chronic problem of epidemics and cut its infant mortality rate by more than half in one generation. Since the "triumph" of capitalism in the former Soviet Union during the early 1990s, health indicators have deteriorated rapidly as the prior health-care system crumbled and as economic insecurity prevailed (9). In China, devastating problems like schistosomiasis and syphilis came under control. Cuba eradicated polio and diptherhia and has reduced its infant mortality rate to the lowest of any Latin American country. Advances in medical care and health status also have followed socialist revolutions in Eastern Europe, Vietnam, Mozambique, Angola, and Tanzania.

In the context of advanced capitalism, however, it is a mistake to dwell on these accomplishments. Contrary to Marx's predictions, most countries undergoing socialist revolutions have been predominantly agrarian societies characterized by severe economic underdevelopment. Socialism in these countries has improved health not only by reorganizing health-care systems but also through fundamental social change ensuring adequate living conditions for a majority of the population. The transition from advanced capitalism to socialism doubtless would lead to improved health status for previously deprived classes and racial groups; but the impact on the overall health of the population predictably would be less dramatic than in countries moving to socialism from a position of general underdevelopment.

In those countries which have established an NHS in a prerevolutionary context while retaining an economy based mainly in private enterprise, the NHS has reduced financial and geographic inequities. However, problems have remained that derive in large part from unresolved social contradictions. An NHS within a capitalist society, under some circumstances, can contain elements of reformist reform. Despite the many accomplishments of the British NHS, for example, many analysts have pointed to its effects in reducing the militancy of labor during Britain's recurrent economic crises. There is even evidence that "buying off" labor was a major motivation for economic and professional elites who otherwise would have opposed the British NHS (10). A key question here is whether an NHS emerges as a top-down or bottom-up phenomenon. The Dellums proposal for democratic decision making and local control would be meaningful only if it accompanied widespread educational efforts, organizing, and politicization. Without activism at the community level, the formal democratic structure would remain an empty shell resembling other arenas of oligarchic politics.

Another issue concerns the private-public contradiction. In the quite different settings of Great Britain and Chile, for example, large private sectors and professional dominance persisted. The private-public contradiction allowed private practice, pharmaceutical and equipment companies, and other profit-making enterprises to drain public resources while maintaining prior patterns of economic and political power.

The private-public contradiction suggests an even more troubling problem. Is a strategy sound which argues for a single-sector reform within the broader context of class structure and the capitalist economy? Private practitioners comprise the majority of a powerful profession, who predictably would oppose an NHS unless they received considerable advantages. Between 1946 and 1948, the Labour Party in Britain split the medical profession by offering a lucrative financial incentive to private consultants under the new NHS (Minister of Health Aneurin Bevan said, in his now famous metaphor, that he "choked their mouths with gold"), thus overcoming the organized resistance of general practitioners (11). Private gain and professional dominance within the British NHS have remained major drawbacks. Unless an NHS emerges along with wider social change, similar compromises to win the profession's mere participation would seriously hinder the NHS's goals. The Dellums bill is vague on the abolition of private practice and seems to indicate that young graduates trained by the NHS will replace private practitioners through gradual attrition. Unless this question is resolved, the private sector would continue to undermine the public purposes of an NHS.

In addition to the medical profession, private corporations predictably would take action to weaken or exploit an NHS constructed according to the Dellums framework. Although the Dellums bill would create a national formulary of drugs and medical equipment, it would not seek to nationalize industries manufacturing these products. The NHS still would need to buy materials from corporations which the state would subsidize. Similar considerations apply to the construction and maintenance of facilities, transportation, use of utilities, and many other goods and services that an NHS would have to consume but could not itself produce. In short, unless nationalization of a variety of related industries accompanied the establishment of an NHS, corporations would continue to gain profits. Ironically, this profit-making activity would receive shelter within the institutional structure of an NHS explicitly committed to reduce profit in health care.

To summarize, an NHS faces dim political prospects under advanced capitalism. Even if enacted, an NHS could not succeed fully without other transformations of the medical profession and industries producing health-related goods and services. Nevertheless, an NHS envisioned in proposals like the Dellums bill provides a model of a nonexploitative health-care system whose structure would address most of the current system's problems. An NHS would create major shifts in power and finances. Establishing an NHS also would highlight persisting contradictions, including professional dominance and profits generated by a nonprofit organization. To address these contradictions, continuing activism would be necessary. This activism might well lead to other goals, such as the nationalization of industries whose products the NHS requires. It is foolish to downplay the difficulties that would precede and follow the enactment of an NHS. Despite these problems, an NHS is a nonformist reform that—along with other directions of activism discussed below—deserves advocacy as a key part of health praxis.

PROBLEMS AND PROSPECTS OF SOCIALIST HEALTH-CARE SYSTEMS

For strategic planning, the successes of socialist systems are perhaps less instructive than are their failures. Because of central planning and social ownership of the means of production, socialism does address the major social contradictions of profit versus safety, uneven development, and the exploitation of illness for private economic gain. On the other hand, some problems persisting or arising anew in socialist systems suggest strategic concerns that should guide activism, in behalf of an NHS and in other struggles.

The Problem of Bureaucracy Must Be Surmounted

An attempt to construct a coordinated NHS involves the formation of a bureaucracy organized from the national level. The dehumanizing and alienating manifestations of bureaucracy have appeared in several socialist countries which have tried to establish effective health-care systems; as a result, patients often face difficulties in receiving the services they seek. Bureaucratic obstacles to adequate health care arise primarily at two points: overcentralization of policy making and inefficient referral networks.

Centralized planning can produce a health-care system which is rational on paper but cumbersome in reality. Each region of a nation experiences unique problems that relate to such variables as the principal economic enterprise, terrain and transportation, and degree of urbanization. Rural areas organized around agriculture, for example, show an incidence of occupational diseases and difficulties of access to medical facilities markedly different from those of urban districts with predominantly industrial enterprise. Several Eastern European countries constructed health-care systems that, in practice, failed to take into account such local variations. Particularly in rural areas, patients encountered severe inconveniences in obtaining needed services despite national policies which made health care theoretically available to all citizens. Clearly, it is difficult for a centralized bureaucracy to plan adequately for the diverse needs of an entire population.

A second bureaucratic problem concerns the availability of general practitioners as opposed to specialists. General practitioners staff local health centers and must see a large number of patients each day. Specialists are available in provincial areas but spend most of their time at large regional hospitals; patients with nonacute conditions who require specialty attention often must wait long periods of time and travel great distances to obtain care at these hospitals. Because the separation of general versus specialty services is fairly rigid, difficulties arise at both the local and provincial levels. For patients whose conditions fall within the competence of general practitioners at local health centers, medical care tends to be brief and perfunctory. For problems requiring specialists, patients face inconvenient delay and geographic inaccessibility; their care at the provincial hospitals tends to be impersonal. In short, the balance of general and specialty services tends to be poorly matched to the specific health needs of local patient populations.

The problems of bureaucracy emerge in any attempt to formulate a framework for an NHS. The solution does not lie in a simple assertion that bureaucratic forms be minimized. Some mechanism must be designed through which planning—particularly for the allocation of resources and personnel—can occur on a national level. Such a mechanism inevitably would involve some degree of bureaucratic organization. It is a fallacy to believe, as many have argued, that bureaucracy itself necessarily leads to an alienating, cumbersome health-care system. Bureaucracy exerts its worst effects when it interferes with the day-to-day activities of specific localities. From this view, the problem of bureaucracy becomes an issue of central versus local control.

National Goals, Local Control

The role of a centralized bureaucracy in a progressive health system need not be complex. (Planning for the Dellums NHS bill has considered this role, but not in detail.) First, a nation must determine at the federal level the priority which health care is to receive within a spectrum of national goals. Budgetary implications follow directly from this decision. For example, the relatively small proportion of the national budget devoted to health activities in the United States, in comparison to continued support of the military and related industries, reflects policy preferences of the nation's political and economic elite.

Reordering of priorities at a national level is a vital precondition for reorganization in the health-care system. Obviously, in the United States and other advanced capitalist nations, this redirection is an awesome task that will require concerted political action over many years. It is difficult to be optimistic that such basic changes will occur in the near future. Nevertheless, it is important to recognize the potential outcomes of a shift in national goals to emphasize health and welfare needs. With this redirection, changes would ensue in central budgetary processes; resources now allocated to capital-intensive, defense-related industries could become available for health care, housing, nutrition, child care, and similar human services.

Following these major modifications in national priorities, the scope of central bureaucratic activities would be quite limited. The major task of the bureaucracy at the national level would pertain to the allocation of resources—the transfer of funds from a central collecting point to the clinics and hospitals which provide care. One reasonable suggestion is that funds distributed to specific health centers or hospitals be determined by the number of patients using those institutions; another is that communities with more immediate needs (i.e., higher rates of illness, lower average income, and so forth) receive greater initial funding. The crucial point is that the centralized bureaucracy would not play a major role in health policy; it also would not control the day-to-day activities of local and district health facilities. Major decisions would be made at the community level, thus circumventing the problem that a federal bureaucracy may set uniform procedures not appropriate to the diverse needs of groups and localities within the nation. Because they are best acquainted with local health needs and working conditions, health workers and community residents could unite to form boards responsible for the policies of health centers and hospitals.

As mandated by the Dellums NHS bill, for instance, board members would be elected through democratic procedures. The specific details of consumer-worker control need not be rigidly defined. Effective local governance would depend on flexibility in establishing decision-making structures appropriate for different localities. In communities with ethnic or racial minorities, arrangements would be made to encourage representation from these groups. Moreover, groupings such as women's organizations, migrant workers, and high-risk occupations could provide the basis for particular health facilities. In these cases, the composition of local health councils could be modified to take into account the unique needs of the clinics' clientele. Several local health-care projects in the United States have tried to follow such principles of community-worker control (12).

There are several problems inherent in this projected scheme. Perhaps the most serious is the expansionary tendency of bureaucracies. Although the initial intention might be a limited bureaucracy, encroachment by bureaucrats into the activities of local health boards would need to be prevented. Also, the widely recognized tendency toward oligarchy might affect local control. In many democratic organizations, the leadership often grows away from the constituency it represents. Furthermore, especially in relationships with the professional providers of medical services, local health boards can become objects of co-optation, providing legitimation for decisions which actually would continue to be made by a professional elite.

None of these comments about socialist systems implies that reforms in capitalist systems will be successful, for reasons already discussed. The contradictions of capitalism that impede the creation and functioning of an NHS also stand in the way of more refined goals, like the minimization of bureaucracy and achievement of community-worker control. Nevertheless, it is important to realize that the advent of socialism does not in itself solve these organizational problems. In the context of capitalism, advocacy of an NHS needs to convey forthrightly both the accomplishments and limitations of socialist systems.

HEALTH CARE AND POLITICAL ACTIVISM

Health workers concerned about social change face difficult dilemmas in their day-to-day work. Clients' problems often have roots in the social system. Examples abound: drug addicts and alcoholics who prefer numbness to the pain of unemployment and inadequate housing; persons with occupational diseases that require treatment but will worsen upon return to illness-generating work conditions; housewives harassed by responsibilities at home and lacking opportunities for fulfilling work experience; people with stress-related cardiovascular disease; elderly or disabled people who need periodic medical certification to obtain welfare benefits that are barely adequate; prisoners who develop illness because of prison conditions. Health workers usually feel obliged to respond to the expressed needs of these and many similar clients.

In doing so, however, health workers engage in patching. On the individual level, patching permits clients' continued functioning in a social system that is often the source of the problem. Patching also involves the sometimes unwitting communication of messages that exert social control and that reinforce society's dominant ideologies. At the societal level, the cumulative effect of these interchanges is the patching of a social system whose patterns of oppression frequently cause disease and personal unhappiness. The medical model that teaches practitioners to serve individual patients deflects attention from this difficult and frightening dilemma. Even health workers who are highly critical of our society devote much of their clinical work to patching the system's victims; frequently this work has the paradoxical effect of preserving the system's overall stability. These observations do not impugn the efforts of caring health workers but point out some of the unintended consequences of clinical work.

The contradictions of patching have no simple resolution. Clearly health workers cannot deny services to clients, even when these services permit clients' participation in illness-generating social structures and do not attack the deeper roots of their problems. On the other hand, it is important to draw this connection between social issues and personal troubles (13). Although the contradictions of patching are difficult for practitioners who want progressive social change, their recognition leads to certain conclusions about health praxis. The most basic conclusion is that health work in itself is not sufficient. Instead, health workers should try to link their clinical activities to efforts aimed directly at basic sociopolitical change.

Arguments against the current system do not reveal simple avenues for change. Although socialism has produced improvements in health-care systems and health status in some countries, difficulties remain, and the route to socialism in advanced capitalist countries like the United States is not clear in any case, even to the most optimistic and dogmatic proponents. On the other hand, political action focusing on health care should accompany activism that extends beyond the health-care system alone. The goal here is to encourage health praxis that points to progressive change in the social order.

Because problems of health care derive in large part from problems of society, strategies for change should deal with this linkage. As an overall strategy, activism should expose, highlight, and in some cases exacerbate the social contradictions which are sources of health problems. These efforts also should address the structures of oppression that the social organization of medicine both reflects and helps maintain. Social contradictions create points of weakness and vulnerability. In confronting these contradictions, especially during crises, activism can aim toward nonreformist goals and longer-term change in society. If specific issues in health care have social roots, these interrelationships should be a focus of organizing. Health workers need to consider the subtle ways that medical services can permit clients' functioning in a social system which is a source of their difficulties. By taking action to change the social origins of medical problems, health workers and other activists can begin to address the limitations of patching.

For those readers interested in political activism, it may be helpful to return full circle and to think about alternatives for action under the headings developed in the first part of this book. The overview that follows is not exhaustive, nor does it provide straightforward solutions to the problems raised here. Concerning the practicalities of political action, there is bound to be disagreement. Directions of activism also predictably will shift over time. The purpose is to convey the range of current nonreformist strategies that trace medical problems to underlying conditions of society and then to specify some priorities.

Class structure in the health-care system mirrors the more general contradictions of social class. Members of the corporate and upper middle classes dominate the policy-making bodies of North American health-care institutions. Coalitions of community residents and health workers are trying to gain greater control of medical centers, hospitals, and clinics (14). In communities resisting the expansion of private medical centers, local residents have demanded positions on the boards of these institutions. Through this participation, low-income community members have exerted pressure to limit expansion and to obtain needed services. While private medical centers have expanded, public hospitals have contracted; besides reducing services, public-sector cutbacks have led to layoffs and unemployment for many health workers. Community-worker coalitions have played a key role in resisting cutbacks in services and closures of public hospitals. Community organizing also has led to the formation of locally controlled clinics, whose clients elect representatives to make policy decisions. Workers at these clinics usually participate in policy making. The success of community-worker coalitions has varied in different localities. In many areas, activism by these coalitions has led to more accessible and responsive services as well as broader participation by community residents and workers in health policy.

Class structure also manifests itself in the stratification of workers within health-care institutions. Union organizing, which occurs in medical centers throughout the United States, can modify this stratification. In the past, different professional orientations have caused technicians, nurses, doctors, and other groups to start separate unions. These groups generally negotiate with the same administrators and governing boards, but often with a reduced power base because of professional divisions. In countering the divisive impact of professionalism, the unionization effort needs to overcome these divisions. Unionization in health care also should go beyond narrow economic goals. Although workers' economic interests are of great importance, unions should seek greater control over the work process and participation in policy making. Union organizing in health care is not an end in itself but can be a useful strategy when it aims toward wider shifts in political and economic power.

Racism heightens the impact of class structure in the health-care system. To address the combined effects of racism and social class, minority groups have organized to increase their recruitment into medicine and to obtain better medical care. Minority caucuses have formed at many health science schools. Chicano, Puerto Rican, black, and other minority organizations have created programs to improve services in local communities and to oppose racism in medicine. Affirmative action to combat racism has achieved only limited success. After increases in the admission of blacks to medical schools in the late 1960s and early 1970s, for example, enrollment subsequently declined again, and recruitment of minorities into the health professions has declined even further with legal rulings and legislative decisions which place limits on affirmative action. Similarly, although the utilization of medical services by minorities rose after the passage of Medicaid and Medicare legislation during the 1960s, problems like high infant mortality and racial differences in access to diagnostic procedures and treatments still affect minorities. These issues will continue to be a focus for activists concerned with racism in health care.

With the growth of *monopoly capital,* the economy remains volatile, with frequent and recurrent crises. Uneven development persists, as rural areas and low-income urban districts face a maldistribution of medical and other needed services. The private-public contradiction, by which public funds subsidize private medical centers and corporations while public facilities face cutbacks, worsens such inequities even further.

The expansion of private medical centers has been a major expression of monopoly capital in the health-care system. In many cities the growth of private hospitals and medical schools has threatened housing and the survival of low-income communities. Activists have organized against private medical expansion. Most often, health planning provisions, which are supposed to assess the need for expansion and to control costs, have had very little impact. Organizers in several cities, however, have been able to stop unnecessary expansion. In others, as discussed above, low-income residents have obtained positions on the governing boards of private medical centers. Organizing against private medical expansion also calls attention to the many forms of public subsidization of the public sector. These subsidizations include public payment for low-income patients, government grants and loans for new construction, and tax advantages because of private hospitals' nonprofit status. Such uses of public moneys weaken public-sector medicine, whose funding tends to decline as private medical centers expand. Meanwhile, private hospitals still try to transfer uninsured patients to public facilities after patients are stabilized as required by federal legislation; the "dumping" of indigent patients from the private to the public sector remains a target of organizing. Political activism that opposes private expansion and that aims toward a stronger public sector is a key part of health praxis.

Other work, based largely in medical schools and hospitals, deals with the profits of large corporations and advocates a reduction of private finance capital in reorganization of the health-care system. For example, in researching the financial operations of private medical centers, activists have uncovered major sources of profit for banks, trusts, and insurance companies. Despite their nonprofit status, many private hospitals accept loans and investments from financial institutions that later receive high rates of interest. Frequently, officers of the same financial institutions sit on the governing boards of the hospitals that obtain loans and investments. Local organizers have worked to publicize and to change these economic relationships. At the national level, activists also have called for a reduction of private finance capital in medicine. This work, for instance, has opposed the role of the private insurance industry in publicly funded insurance programs, managed care organizations, and peer review.

The "medical-industrial complex," especially the pharmaceutical and medical equipment industries, has drawn heavy criticism for promoting costly, ineffective technology and exploiting illness for private profit. Locally, organizers in hospitals and community clinics have insisted on the development of generic drug formularies and have opposed the promotion of drugs within their institutions by pharmaceutical companies. Similar actions by medical and nursing students have prevented the use of misleading educational materials from drug houses.

Another important local effort emphasizes expensive technology at private medical centers. Corporations develop and promote technologic innovations like coronary care units, fetal monitoring, and radiologic scanning devices. Although their effectiveness in improving morbidity and mortality is largely unverified, private medical centers buy these devices in an uncoordinated fashion. The proliferation of technology increases the costs of medical care and diverts attention from simpler services that are sorely needed. Organizers in several cities have rallied opposition against private hospitals' purchase of advanced technologies, especially when these institutions do not provide adequate medical care to low-income residents.

Policies of the state continue to protect the economic system based in private profit and monopoly capital. The state supports the private sector, for example, by public subsidization of expending medical centers and firms doing business in medical products. The state also helps legitimate the current social order by providing health and welfare services in the public sector. Especially during periods of recession, however, the contradictions of state expenditures lead to cutbacks of public services. These cutbacks can have devastating effects on needed medical care. The analysis and redirection of state policies are essential goals for activists concerned about the difficulties that the private-public duality creates.

The impact of *medical ideology* has motivated attempts to demystify current ideologic patterns and to develop alternatives. These efforts emphasize the complex etiology of many health problems, the frequent inappropriateness of technologic solutions, and the medicalization of social problems. Educational campaigns, often in community clinics or trade unions, focus on illness-generating conditions in the workplace and environment. Several groups have publicized and acted against the growing social control function of medicine in such areas as drug addiction, genetic screening, contraception and sterilization abuse, and psychosurgery. These efforts have heightened sensitivity to the messages of ideology and social control that health professionals transmit within the doctor-patient relationship. The women's and self-help movements have developed less esoteric medical care, which reduces professional dominance and fosters personal autonomy. Alternative health programs also have emerged that try to develop nonhierarchical and noncapitalist forms of practice; these ventures then would be available as models of progressive health work when future political change permits their wider acceptance.

Because of the powerful economic and political interests that dominate the health-care system, the alternative health movement cannot succeed unless it connects itself to broader political activism as well. Sometimes proponents of the alternative health movement retreat into their own activities. The assumption here seems to be that the development of more humane and holistic practice is an important end in itself. Alternative medicine is attractive to some parts of the population, especially to people who hold countercultural values. Components of alternative medicine ultimately may also be useful for people in low-income and minority communities. In these communities, uneven development and deprivations of class structure lead to maldistribution and inaccessibility of even the simplest kinds of services. Alternative visions will not in themselves correct these structural sources of oppression. With this qualification, the attempt to counteract the dominant ideologic patterns of medicine is an important part of nonreformist strategy.

The social contradictions that foster problems of health care extend beyond the national boundaries of the United States. Political activism should address these *international issues*. One concern is the foreign operation of the pharmaceutical and medical equipment industries. Multinational corporations have cultivated markets abroad for expensive technologies like coronary care units; often these technologies are inappropriate in the context of underdevelopment, when more basic needs cannot be met. Pharmaceutical companies have used people in Third World countries for testing of drugs whose safety is unknown; an example is that of oral contraceptives, which drug companies tested and sold in Latin America before their complications became apparent. Moreover, drug houses frequently sell medications in Third World countries when regulatory agencies disapprove their use in the United States because of risks and complications (15). The promotion of infant formula instead of breast milk in countries where formulas are dangerous because of unsanitary water supplies is another example of exploitative behavior by pharmaceutical companies. Several groups based in North American hospitals and medical schools have documented these activities of the pharmaceutical and equipment industries. This information has been useful both in the United States and abroad to restrict the dumping through export of products which otherwise could not be sold. North American corporations dealing in drugs and equipment benefit greatly from their activities in underdeveloped countries; these activities should be a target of political work in the United States.

In several countries with totalitarian governments aided by the United States, health workers have suffered imprisonment and torture. Medical professionals supporting dictatorships, on the other hand, have taken part in torture and related activities that have jeopardized their colleagues' safety (16). Several international groups have formed to assist persecuted health workers and to speak out against medical complicity in torture. Publicizing detrimental effects on health and safety, these groups have called for an end to military and economic assistance for such regimes.

Another phase of international work involves support for countries that have undergone progressive change linking medicine and society. Health workers from the United States have traveled to such countries as Cuba, Vietnam, Tanzania,

Mozambique, Angola, Zimbabwe, and Nicaragua. These visits, sometimes involving extended stays, generally serve two purposes. In the first place, health workers can provide direct services. Especially during the early years after a revolution, when professionals tend to leave a country because of their threatened class position, visiting health workers can fill a critical need. Second, visitors on their return can spread information about the impact of imperialism and about health care in postrevolutionary societies. Health brigades organized in the United States and Western Europe have sent money and medical supplies to countries with severe shortages. The educational work that accompanies these actions fosters further organizing within dominant nations that have been responsible for many damaging effects of imperialism and underdevelopment.

Illness-generating social conditions have extremely important implications for political action. Proof that some occupations are associated with specific disease and mortality patterns has led to interventions in workplaces and unions. Organizations of medical and science workers have taken part in occupational safety and health projects. The purposes of these efforts are to publicize the problems, to inform unions and local communities about hazards and possible solutions, and to exert pressure on companies and government regulatory agencies for stricter enforcement.

Activists in unions and the women's movement have focused on work- and stress-related illness. They also have recognized the illness-generating potential of economic cycles; this finding has formed one basis of requests for cost-of-living clauses in contracts and job security provisions that would dampen the effects of these cycles. Organizing against sexism has included demands for improved work conditions that recognize differential risks for men and women but that rectify discriminatory wage patterns.

Such efforts in occupational and environmental health seek to enhance workers' control over the conditions of work and communities' ability to eliminate environmental hazards. Confronting the contradiction between profit and safety is necessary to modify the social origins of illness. This problem becomes ever more critical, as illness-generating conditions of the workplace and environment threaten humanity's survival (17).

What are the priorities? The range of nonreformist activism shows many areas in which change is needed; several problems are particularly urgent. Strategies to address these problems deserve high priority.

First, the recurrent fiscal crisis of advanced capitalism presents both dangers and opportunities. Stagnation and cutbacks in health care and other public services have heightened tensions throughout the society. The ultra-right has emerged as a well-financed and politically powerful interest group. Some elements of the ultra-right have developed a striking public presence and leadership style. Such organizations reveal an authoritarian fervor that, as many observers have noted, is reminiscent of fascism. At the same time, openly racist groups have grown in size and public visibility; under conditions of economic and political instability, polarization along class and racial lines is likely to deepen. Antiracist activism has become a crucial priority in workplace and community organizing. In the health-care system, as community-worker coalitions, unions, and similar organizations go about their work, they should view race and class as interrelated structures of oppression.

International work, especially in opposition to militarism, is a second priority. Medicine, capitalism, and imperialism historically have been intertwined. Medical and public health professionals, as noted earlier, have played an important role on behalf of imperialist expansion. Dominant nations frequently have tried to maintain their power through direct military intervention, as in Indochina. At other times these efforts are subtler, as in the economic destablization of new governments or covert military support for dictatorships. The availability of nuclear weapons (including the notion that such weapons can be used in a limited way within specific geographic areas) vastly increases the stakes of political action against militarism. Warfare, if unchecked, will lead to devastating effects on health and well-being throughout the world.

Third, there is the inescapable problem of illness-generating conditions in the workplace and environment. During the past two centuries, the world has become a dumping ground for toxic wastes. Environmental exploitation has emerged as a damaging effect of capitalist development, but similar problems also have arisen in socialist countries. Epidemics of cancer and other chronic diseases have appeared among workers in a variety of industries. The hazards of nuclear power and stockpiled weapons threaten humanity because of potential accidents as much as the intentional use of these technologies. In capitalist societies, the structure of private profit consistently impedes efforts to deal systematically with occupational and environmental health problems; these medical consequences emerge from the very fabric of our society as currently organized. Changing the social roots of illness-generating conditions must be a major goal if we are to have a future at all.

A common criticism of the Marxist position is that it presents many problems with few solutions. Some useful directions of political strategy, however, are clear. Social contradictions lie behind many medical problems; the social organization of medicine both reflects and fosters structures of oppression. These contradictions and oppressive structures are important targets of political activism. The urgency of such problems justifies impatience, but patience is needed. Because of the resistance it will encounter, the struggle for change will be a protracted one and will involve action on many fronts. The present holds little room for complaisance or misguided optimism. Our future health-care system, as well as the social order of which it will be a part, depends largely on the praxis we choose now.

Notes

PREFACE TO THE SECOND EDITION

1. John Reed's vision of the Russian Revolution's global importance might apply to the Soviet Union's unfolding: J. Reed, *Ten Days That Shook the World* (New York: Modern Library, 1935).

2. M. Gorbachev, *Perestroika: New Thinking for Our Country and the World* (New York: Harper & Row, 1987), pp. 3–45.

3. E. K. Ligachev, *Inside Gorbachev's Kremlin: The Memoirs of Yegor Ligachev* (New York: Pantheon, 1993).

4. D. A. Barr and M. G. Field, "The Current State of Health Care in the Former Soviet Union: Implications for Health Care Policy and Reform," *Am. J. Public Health* 86 (1996): 307–312.

5. K. Marx and F. Engels, *The Communist Manifesto* (New York: Appleton-Century-Crofts, 1955), p. 12.

CHAPTER 1. HEALTH CARE, SOCIAL CONTRADICTIONS, AND THE DILEMMAS OF REFORM

1. The following discussion is based on many sources. Useful theoretical analyses include: K. Marx, *A Contribution to the Critique of Political Economy* (New York: International, 1970 [1859]), especially pp. 19–23; Mao Tse-Tung, *On Contradiction* (New York: International, 1953); G. Lukacs, *History and Class Consciousness: Studies in Marxist Dialectics* (Cambridge: MIT Press, 1971), pp. 1–26, 223–255; E. Balibar, "The Basic Concepts of Historical Materialism," in L. Althusser and E. Balibar, eds., *Reading Capital* (London: New Left Books, 1970), pp. 199–308; M. Godelier, "Structure and Contradiction in Capital," in R. Blackburn (ed.), *Ideology and Social Science* (New York: Pantheon, 1972); R. Heilbroner, *Marxism: For and Against* (New York: Norton, 1980), pp. 61–89; P. M. Sweezy, *Four Lectures on Marxism* (New York: Monthly Review Press, 1981).

2. Cf. E. W. Smith and A. Smith, *Minamata* (New York: Holt, Rinehart and Winston, 1975).

3. Ibid., pp. 140–143.

4. K. Marx and F. Engels, *The Communist Manifesto* (New York: Monthly Review Press, 1964 [1858]), pp. 13–16, 29–31.

5. J. Powles, "On the Limitations of Modern Medicine," *Sci. Med. Man* 1 (1973): 1–30.

6. A. L. Cochrane, *Effectiveness and Efficiency: Random Reflections on Health Care* (London: Nuffield Hospitals Trust, 1972); R. J. Haggerty, "The Boundaries of Health Care," *Pharos* 35 (1972): 106–111; T. McKeown, *The Role of Medicine: Dream, Mirage, or Nemesis?* (Princeton: Princeton University Press, 1979); T. McKeown, *The Modern Rise of Population* (New York: Academic Press, 1977); E. H. Kass, "Infectious Diseases and Social Change," *J. Inf. Dis.* 123 (1971): 110–114.

7. Kass, "Infectious Diseases."

8. T. McKeown, *Role of Medicine*, p. 85. The impact of social class on health outcomes continues as a central focus of social epidemiology. For instance, see P. M. Lantz, J. S. House, J. M. Lepkowski, D. R. Williams, R. P. Mero, and J. Chen, "Socioeconomic Factors, Health Behaviors, and Mortality: Results from a Prospective Study of U.S. Adults," *JAMA* 279 (1998): 1703–1708; G. Pappas, W. C. Hadden, L. J. Kozak, and G. F. Fisher, "Potentially Avoidable Hospitalizations: Inequalities in Rates between U.S. Socioeconomic Groups," *Am. J. Public Health* 87 (1997): 811–816; L. E. Montgomery, J. L. Kiely, and G. Pappas, "The Effects of Poverty, Race, and Family Structure on U.S. Children's Health," *Am. J. Public Health* 86 (1996): 1401–1405; N. Krieger and S. Sidney, "Racial Discrimination and Blood Pressure: The CARDIA Study of Young Black and White Adults," *Am. J. Public Health* 86 (1996): 1370–1378; R. A. Hahn, E. Eaker, N. D. Barker, S. M. Teutsch, W. Sosniak, and N. Krieger, "Poverty and Death in the United States — 1973 and 1991," *Epidemiology* 6 (1995): 490–497; G. Pappas, S. Queen, W. Hadden, and G. Fisher, "The Increasing Disparity in Mortality between Socioeconomic Groups in the United States, 1960 and 1986," *N. Engl. J. Med.* 329 (1993): 103–109.

9. J. Habermas, "Technology and Science As 'Ideology,'" in *Toward a Rational Society*, ed. Jürgen Habermas (Boston: Beacon, 1970), p. 82.

10. F. Moseley, *The Falling Rate of Profit in the Postwar United States Economy* (New York: St. Martin's Press, 1991); F. Verdera, "Adam Smith on the Falling Rate of Profit," *Scot J. Pol. Econ.* 39 (1992): 100–110.

11. McKeown, *Role of Medicine*, pp. 190–198.

12. Major discussions of these themes include D. Noble, *American by Design* (New York: Knopf, 1977), pp. 33–65; M. S. Larson, *The Rise of Professionalism* (Berkeley: University of California Press, 1977), pp. 19–39, 136–158; and E. R. Brown, *Rockefeller Medicine Men* (Berkeley: University of California Press, 1979), pp. 98–191.

13. For Marx's early views, see K. Marx, "Estranged Labor," in *The Economic and Philosophic Manuscripts of 1844* (New York: International, 1964). The major analysis of deskilling is H. Braverman, *Labor and Monopoly Capital* (New York: Monthly Review Press, 1974).

14. I. K. Zola, "Medicine As an Institution of Social Control," *Sociol. Rev* 20 (1972): 487–504; B. Ehrenreich and J. Ehrenreich, "Health Care and Social Control," *Soc. Policy* (May–June 1974): 26–40; H. Waitzkin, "Latent Functions of the Sick Role in Various Institutional Settings," *Soc. Sci. Med.* 5 (1971): 45–75.

15. H. Waitzkin and B. Waterman, *The Exploitation of Illness in Capitalist Society* (Indianapolis: Bobbs-Merrill, 1974), pp. 45–46.

16. F. F. Piven and R. A. Cloward, *Regulating the Poor* (New York: Vintage, 1971), pp. 3–79.

17. A. Gorz, *Socialism and Revolution* (Garden City, N.Y.: Anchor, 1973), pp. 135–177.

CHAPTER 2. SOCIAL STRUCTURES OF MEDICAL OPPRESSION

1. F. Engels, *The Condition of the Working Class in England in 1844* (Moscow: Progress Publishers, 1973 [1845]).

2. K. Marx and F. Engels, *The Communist Manifesto* (New York: Monthly Review Press, 1964 [1848]).

3. R. Virchow, *Gesammelte Abhandlunge aus dem Begiet der oeffentlichen Medicin und der Seuchenlehre* (Berlin: Hirschwald, 1879), v. 1, pp. 305, 321–334.

4. R. Virchow, *Ueber den Hungertyphus und einige verwandte Krankheitsformen* (Berlin: Hirschwald, 1868); H. Berliner, "Notes on the Historical Precursors of Materialist Epidemiology," *Health Movement Organziation* 1 (1976): 5–7.

5. E. H. Ackerknecht, *Rudolf Virchow* (Madison: University of Wisconsin Press, 1953), pp. 159–181; R. Virchow, *Briefe an seine Eltern* (Leipzig: Engelmann, 1907), pp. 121–164.

6. T. McKeown, *The Role of Medicine* (Princeton: Princeton University Press, 1979), pp. 12–116.

7. A. Flexner, *Medical Education in the United States and Canada* (New York: Carnegie Foundation, 1910).

8. E. R. Brown, *Rockefeller Medicine Men: Medicine and Capitalism in the Progressive Era* (Berkeley: University of California Press, 1979), pp. 135–191; H. Berliner, "A Larger Perspective on the Flexner Report," *Int. J. Health Serv.* 5 (1975): 573–592; S. J. Kunitz, "Professionalism and Social Control in the Progressive Era: The Case of the Flexner Report," *Soc. Problems* 22 (1974): 16–27.

9. V. Navarro, *Social Security and Medicine in the USSR: A Marxist Critique* (Lexington, Mass.: Heath, 1977); S. Allende, *La Realidad Medico-Social Chilena* (Santiago: Ministero de Salubridad, Prevision y Asistencia Social, 1939); N. Bethune, "A Plea for Early Decompression in Pulmonary Tuberculosis," *Can. Med. Assoc. J.* 27 (1932): 36–42; N. Bethune, "Wounds," in *"Away with All Pests. . .": An English Surgeon in People's China,* edited by J. S. Horn (New York: Monthly Review Press, 1969); T. Allan and S. Gordon, *The Scalpel, the Sword: The Story of Doctor Norman Bethune* (Toronto: McClelland and Stewart, 1952); E. Guevara, " On Revolutionary Medicine," in *Venceremos,* edited by J. Gerassi (New York: Simon & Schuster, 1969); G. Harper, "Ernesto Guevara, M.D.: Physician—Revolutionary Physician—Revolutionary," *N. Engl. J. Med.* 281 (1969):1285–1289.

10. For classic discussions, see K. Marx, *A Contribution to the Critique of Political Economy* (New York: International, 1971 [1859]), pp. 27–63, and K. Marx, *Capital,* Vol. 1 (Moscow: Progress Publishers, 1963 [1890]), Parts III–V.

11. The data that follow are adapted from U.S. Bureau of Labor Statistics, 1998–1999, *Occupational Outlook Handbook,* http://stats.bls.gov.

12. V. Navarro, "A Historical Review (1965–1997) of Studies on Class, Health, and Quality of Life," *Int. J. Health Services* 28 (1998): 389–406; V. Navarro, *Medicine Under Capitalism,* p. 155.

13. *Navarro, Medicine Under Capitalism,* pp. 139–141; U.S. Bureau of Labor Statistics, 1998–1999.

14. H. Waitzkin and B. Waterman, *The Exploitation of Illness in Capitalist Society* (Indianapolis: Bobbs-Merrill, 1974), pp. 65–75; J. C. Cantor, E. L. Miles, L. C. Baker, and D. C. Barker, "Physician Service to the Underserved: Implications for Affirmative Action in

Medical Education," *Inquiry* 33 (1996): 167–180; S. Fisher, *Nursing Wounds* (New Brunswick, NJ: Rutgers University Press, 1995).

15. G. Ziem, "Medical Education since Flexner," *Health/PAC Bull.* 76 (1977): 8–14, 23; M. A. Simpson, *Medical Education: A Critical Approach* (London: Butterworths, 1972); K. T. Leicht and M. L. Fennell, "The Changing Organizational Context of Professional Work," *Ann. Rev. Sociol.* 23 (1997): 215–231. In comparison to research on gender and racial differences, remarkably few studies deal with social class differences in mobility into medical careers.

16. Brown, *Rockefeller Medicine Men.*

17. *Fortune,* April 28, 1997, pp. F-54–55.

18. T. Bodenheimer and K. Grumbach, *Understanding Health Policy: A Clinical Approach* (Norwalk, CT: Appleton and Lange, 1998); J. Canham-Clyne, S. Woolhandler, D. Himmelstein, *The Rational Option for a National Health Program* (Stony Creek, CT: Pamphleteer's Press, 1995); H. Waitzkin, "The Strange Career of Managed Competition: Military Failure to Medical Success? *Am. J. Public Health* 84 (1994): 482–489; V. Navarro, *The Politics of Health Policy: The U.S. Reforms, 1980–1994* (Cambridge, MA: Blackwell, 1994).

19. B. Ehrenreich and J. Ehrenreich (eds.), *The American Health Empire* (New York: Vintage, 1970); D. Kotelchuck (ed.), *Prognosis Negative* (New York: Vintage, 1976); M. Silverman, M. Lydecker, and P. R. Lee, *Bad Medicine: The Prescription Drug Industry in the Third World* (Stanford: Stanford University Press, 1992); P. Davis (ed.), *Contested Ground: Public Purpose and Private Interest in the Regulation of Prescription Drugs* (Oxford: Oxford University Press, 1996); J. P. Weiner, A. M. Stoline, E. Gorovitz, and A. S. Relman, *The New Medical Marketplace: A Physician's Guide to Health Care in the 1990s* (Baltimore: Johns Hopkins University Press, 1993); R. Kuttner, "The American Health Care System—Wall Street and Health Care," *N. Engl. J. Med.* 340 (1999): 664–668.

20. For classic analyses, see Marx and Engels, *The Communist Manifesto,* p. 5, and V. I. Lenin, *The State and Revolution* (New York: International, 1932 [1917]), pp. 7–20; C. Offe, *Modernity and the State: East, West* (Cambridge, MA: MIT Press, 1996); J. O'Connor, *The Fiscal Crisis of the State* (New York: St. Martin's, 1973).

21. Waitzkin and Waterman, *Exploitation of Illness,* pp. 8–16; H. Waitzkin and H. Modell, "Medicine, Socialism, and Totalitarianism: Lessons from Chile," *N. Engl. J. Med.* 291 (1974): 171–177; H. Modell and H. Waitzkin, "Medicine and Socialism in Chile," *Berkeley J. Sociol.* 19 (1974): 1–35; J. K. Iglehart, "The American Health Care System: Medicare," and "The American Health Care System: Medicaid," *N. Engl. J. Med.* 320 (1999): 327–332, 403–408; K. Stocker, H. Waitzkin, and C. Iriart, "The Exportation of Managed Care to Latin America," *N. Engl. J. Med.* 320 (1999): 1131–1136.

22. Bodenheimer and Grumbach, *Understanding Health Policy.*

23. H. Waitzkin, B. V. Akin, L. M. de la Maza, F. A. Hubbell, H. Meshkinpour, L. Rucker, and J. S. Tobis, "Deciding against Corporate Management of a State-Supported Academic Medical Center," *N. Engl. J. Med.* 315 (1986): 1299–1304; A. B. Bindman, D. Keane, and N. Lurie, "A Public Hospital Closes: Impact on Patients' Access to Care and Health Status," *JAMA* 264 (1990): 2899–2904. Chapter 5 analyzes this problem in more depth.

24. Discussions on health services include V. Navarro, "Social Class, Political Power, and the State and Their Implications in Medicine," *Soc. Sci. Med.* 10 (1976): 437–457;

V. Navarro, "A Historical Review (1965–1997) of Studies on Class, Health, and Quality of Life." For a sociohistorical analysis of public welfare, see F. F. Piven and R. A. Cloward, *Regulating the Poor* (New York: Vintage, 1971).

25. See, for example, Committee on Government Operations, United States Senate, *Confidence and Concern: Citizens View American Government: A Survey of Public Attitudes* (Washington: Government Printing Office, 1973).

26. For more extensive discussion of these themes, see Offe, *Modernity and the State*; Navarro, "Social Class, Political Power, and the State."

27. Classic analyses of these issues in Marxism include Marx, *A Contribution to the Critique of Political Economy*, pp. 19–23; F. Engels, *The Origin of the Family, Private Property and the State* (New York: International, 1972 [1891]), pp. 94–146. Major reinterpretations are A. Gramsci, *Selections from The Prison Notebooks* (New York: International, 1971), pp. 12–14, 257–264, 364–377; L. Althusser, *Lenin and Philosophy and Other Essays* (New York: Monthly Review Press, 1971), pp. 127–186. Chapter 6 examines these issues in more detail.

28. Brown, *Rockefeller Medicine Men*, pp. 112–134; H. Waitzkin, "The Strange Career of Managed Competition"; "Is Our Work Dangerous? Should It Be?" (presentation on receipt of Leo G. Reeder Career Recognition Award, American Sociological Association, August 1997). *J. Health Soc. Beh.* 39 (1998): 7–17.

29. Watizkin and Waterman, *Exploitation of Illness,* pp. 36–65; H. Waitzkin, *The Politics of Medical Encounters: How Patients and Doctors Deal with Social Problems* (New Haven: Yale University Press, 1991); I. K. Zola, *Socio-Medical Inquiries* (Philadelphia: Temple University Press, 1983), pp. 241–296.

30. G. Markowitz and D. Rosner, "Doctors in Crisis: A Study of the Use of Medical Education Reform to Establish Modern Professional Elitism in Medicine," *Am. Q.* 25 (1973): 83–107; H. R. Holman, "The 'Excellence' Deception in Medicine," *Hosp. Pract.* 11 (April 1976): 11–21.

31. V. Navarro, "The Underdevelopment of Health or the Health of Underdevelopment: An Analysis of the Distribution of Human Health Resources in Latin America," *Politics Soc.* 4 (1974): 267–293.

32. Brown, *Rockefeller Medicine Men*.

33. Silverman, *Drugging of the Americas;* Silverman, Lydecker, and Lee, *Bad Medicine*.

34. Regarding these issues in the former Soviet Union, Cuba, and Chile, see Navarro, *Social Security and Medicine in the USSR;* V. Navarro, "Health Services in Cuba: An Initial Appraisal," *N. Engl. J. Med.* 287 (1972): 954–959; D. A. Barr and M. G. Field, "The Current State of Health Care in the Former Soviet Union: Implications for Health Care Policy and Reform," *Am. J. Public Health* 86 (1996): 307–312; T. H. Tulchinsky and E. A. Varavikova, "Addressing the Epidemiologic Transition in the Former Soviet Union: Strategies for Health System and Public Health Reform in Russia," *Am. J. Public Health* 6 (1996): 313–320; H. Waitzkin, K. Wald, R. Kee, R. Danielson, and L. Robinson, "Primary Care in Cuba: Low- and High-Technology Developments Pertinent to Family Medicine," *J. Fam. Pract.* 45 (1997): 250–258; V. Navarro, "Health, Health Services, and Health Planning in Cuba," *Int. J. Health Serv.* 2 (1972): 397–432; Waitzkin and Modell, "Medicine, Socialism, and Totalitarianism"; Modell and Waitzkin, "Medicine and Socialism in Chile."

35. Cf. B. S. Levy and V. W. Sidel, eds., *War and Public Health* (New York: Oxford University Press, 1996).

36. Waitzkin, Wald, Kee, Danielson, and Robinson, "Primary Care in Cuba"; W. C. Hsiao, "The Chinese Health Care System: Lessons for Other Nations," *Soc. Sci. Med.* 41 (1995): 1047–1055; C. M. Grogan, "Urban Economic Reform and Access to Health Care Coverage in the People's Republic of China," *Soc. Sci. Med.* 41 (1995): 1073–1084; Barr and Field, "The Current State of Health Care in the Former Soviet Union"; Tulchinsky and Varavikova, "Addressing the Epidemiologic Transition in the Former Soviet Union."

37. See sources on Chile in footnote 34 and discussion in chapter 7.

38. M. Turshen, "The Impact of Colonialism on Health and Health Services in Tanzenia," *Int. J. Health Serv.* 7 (1977): 7–35; O. Gish, *Planning the Health Sector: The Tanzanian Experience* (New York: Holmes and Meier, 1976); M. Turshen, ed., *Women and Health in Africa* (Trenton, N.J.: Africa World Press, 1991); M. Turshen, *Privatizing Health Services in Africa* (New Brunswick, NJ: Rutgers University Press, 1999).

39. D. W. Light, "Managed Care in a New Key: Britain's Strategies for the 1990s," *Int. J. Health Serv.* 28 (1998): 427–444; "From Managed Competition to Managed Cooperation: Theory and Lessons from the British Experience," *Millbank Q.* 75 (1997): 297–341.

40. A. Jacobs, "Seeing the Difference: Market Health Reform in Europe," *J. Health Polit. Policy Law* 2 (1998): 1–33; P. Garpenby, "Health Reform in Sweden in the 1990s: Local Pluralism versus National Coordination," *J. Health Polit. Policy Law* 20 (1995): 695–717; M. Whitehead, R. A. Gustafsson, and F. Diderichsen, "Why Is Sweden Rethinking Its NHS Style Reforms?" *Br. Med. J.* 315 (1997): 935–939.

41. H. Brenner, *Mental Illness and the Economy* (Cambridge: Harvard University Press, 1973); H. Brenner, "Mortality and the National Economy," *Lancet* (September 15, 1979): 568–573; R. A. Catalano and W. A. Satariano, "Unemployment and the Likelihood of Detecting Early-Stage Breast Cancer," *Am. J. Public Health* 88 (1998): 586–589; D. Dooley, R. Catalano, and G. Wilson, "Depression and Unemployment: Panel Findings from the Epidemiologic Catchment Area Study," *Am. J. of Community Psychology* 22 (1994): 745–765; R. Catalano and S. Serxner, "The Effect of Ambient Threats to Employment on Low Birthweight," *J. Health Soc. Behav.* 33 (1992): 363–377; R. Catalano and S. Serxner, "Neonatal Mortality and the Economy Revisited," *Int. J. Health Serv.* 22 (1992): 275–286.

42. J. Eyer and P. Sterling, "Stress-Related Mortality and Social Organization," *Rev. Rad. Pol. Econ.* 8 (Spring 1977): 1–44; J. Eyer, "Hypertension As a Disease of Modern Society," *Int. J. Health Serv.* 5 (1975): 530–558; Krieger and Sidney, "Racial Discrimination and Blood Pressure"; P. S. Schnall, C. Pieper, J. E. Schwartz, R. A. Karasek, Y. Schlussel, R. B. Devereux, A. Ganau, M. Alderman, and K. Warren, "The Relationship between 'Job Strain,' Workplace Diastolic Blood Pressure, and Left Ventricular Mass Index," *JAMA* 263 (1990): 1929–1935.

43. N. Krieger and S. Sidney, "Racial Discrimination and Blood Pressure"; N. Krieger, S. K. van den Eeden, D. Zava, and A. Okamoto, "Race/Ethnicity, Social Class, and Prevalence of Breast Cancer Prognostic Biomarkers: A Study of White, Black, and Asian Women in the San Francisco Bay Area," *Ethnicity & Disease* 7 (1997): 137–149; T. Theorell and R. A. Karasek, "Current Issues Relating to Psychosocial Job Strain and Cardiovascular Disease Research," *J. Occup. Health Psychology* 1 (1996): 9–26; P. L. Schnall, P. A. Landsbergis, and D. Baker, "Job Strain and Cardiovascular Disease," *Annu. Rev. Public Health* 15 (1994): 381–411; R. Karasek and T. Theorell, *Healthy Work: Stress, Productivity and the Reconstruction of Working Life* (New York: Basic Books; 1990).

44. K. J. Greenlund and R. H. Elling, "Capital Sectors and Workers' Health and Safety in the United States," *Int. J. Health Serv.* 25 (1995): 101–116; *Struggle for Workers'*

Health: A Study of Six Industrialized Countries (Farmingdale, NY: Baywood, 1986); A. W. McCoy, *The Politics of Heroin: CIA Complicity in the Global Drug Trade* (Brooklyn, NY: Lawrence Hill, 1991); A. W. McCoy and A. A. Block, eds., *War on Drugs: Studies in the Failure of U.S. Narcotics Policy* (Boulder, CO: Westview, 1992).

45. M. Witt, "Production with Safety?" *Cubatimes* 1, 4 (Winter 1981): 3–5; For a more pessimistic view concerning the Soviet Union, see Komarov, *The Destruction of Nature* (White Plains, N.Y.: M. E. Sharpe, 1981).

46. K. Rothenberg, B. Fuller, M. Rothstein, T. Duster, M. J. Ellis Kahn, R. Cunningham, B. Fine, K. Hudson, M. C. King, P. Murphy, G. Swergold, and F. Collins, "Genetic Information and the Workplace: Legislative Approaches and Policy Changes," *Science* 275 (1997): 1755–1757; T. Duster, *Backdoor to Eugenics* (New York: Routledge, 1990); J. M. Stellman, "Women's Health Perspectives from the ILO Encyclopedia of Occupational Health Safety," *Epidemiologia e Prevenzione* 20 (1996): 191–193; J. M. Stellman and S. D. Stellman, "Cancer and the Workplace," *Ca: A Cancer Journal for Clinicians* 46 (1996): 70–92; J. M. Stellman and S. D. Stellman, "Social Factors: Women and Cancer," *Seminars in Oncology Nursing* 11 (1995): 103–108.

CHAPTER 3. THE SOCIAL ORIGINS OF ILLNESS: A NEGLECTED HISTORY

1. Early works that considered the social origins of illness, but with a different analytic perspective, include: G. Rosen, "What Is Social Medicine?" *Bull. Hist. Med.* 21 (1947): 674–733; G. Rosen, *A History of Public Health* (New York: MD Publications, 1958), especially pp. 192–293; R. Sand, *The Advance to Social Medicine* (London: Staples Press, 1952), especially pp. 295–343, 507–589; H. E. Sigerist, *Civilization and Disease* (Ithaca: Cornell University Press, 1944), pp. 6–64.

2. F. Engles, *The Condition of the Working Class in England in 1844* (Moscow: Progress Publishers, 1973 [1845]).

3. For a sympathetic critique, see S. Marcus, *Engels, Manchester, and the Working Class* (New York: Vintage, 1974).

4. Engels, *Condition*, p. 135.

5. E. Chadwick, *Report on the Sanitary Condition of the Labouring Population of Great Britain* (Edinburgh: Edinburgh University Press, 1965 [1842]), especially pp. 80–254.

6. Engels, *Condition*, pp. 141–142.

7. Ibid., pp. 142–143.

8. Ibid., pp. 190–193.

9. Ibid., p. 230.

10. Ibid., p. 200.

11. Ibid., pp. 279–284.

12. F. Engels, *Herr Eugen Dühring's Revolution in Science [Anti-Dühring]* (New York: International, 1966 [1878]); F. Engels, *Dialectics of Nature* (New York: International, 1940).

13. R. Virchow, *Cellular Pathology* (New York: De Witt, 1860).

14. R. Virchow, *Disease, Life, and Man.* Translated by L. J. Rather (Stanford: Stanford

University Press, 1958), pp. 27–29. Unless otherwise noted, I have prepared the translations from German and Spanish.

15. E. H. Ackerknecht, *Rudolf Virchow: Doctor, Statesman, Anthropologist* (Madison: University of Wisconsin Press, 1953), p. 52.

16. Virchow, *Disease, Life, and Man*, pp. 142–150.

17. R. Virchow, *Werk and Wirkung*, (Berlin: Rütten & Loenig, 1957), pp. 94–96.

18. R. Virchow, *Gesammelte Abhandlungen aus dem Gebiet der Öffentlichen Medicin und der Seuchenlehre* (Berlin: Hirschwald, 1879), v. 1, pp. 305, 321–334.

19. Virchow, *Werk und Wirkung*, pp. 42, 104.

20. Virchow, *Gesammelte Abhandlungen*, v. 1, pp. 121–122; Ackernecht, *Rudolf Virchow*, pp. 125–129.

21. Virchow, *Werk und Wirkung*, p. 110.

22. Ibid., p. 55; Ackerknecht, *Rudolf Virchow*, pp. 131–138.

23. Virchow, *Werk und Wirkung*, pp. 127, 108.

24. Ibid., p. 106.

25. Ibid., p. 117; Virchow, *Disease, Life, and Man*, p. 106.

26. S. Allende, *La Realidad Medico-Social Chilena* (Santiago: Ministerio de Salubridad, Prevision y Asistencia Social, 1939).

27. Ibid., pp. 6, 8.

28. Ibid., p. 75.

29. Ibid., p. 86.

30. Ibid., p. 105.

31. Ibid., p. 119.

32. Ibid., p. 124.

33. Ibid., pp. 189–190.

34. Ibid., p. 191.

35. Ibid., p. 198.

CHAPTER 4. TECHNOLOGY, HEALTH COSTS, AND THE STRUCTURE OF PRIVATE PROFIT

1. H. W. Day, "An Intensive Coronary Care Area," *Dis. Chest* 44 (1963): 423–427.

2. D. T. Campbell and J. C. Stanley, *Experimental and Quasi-Experimental Designs for Research* (Chicago: Rand McNally, 1963), pp. 6–13.

3. B. Lown, A. M. Fakhro, W. B. Hood, et al., "The Coronary Care Unit: New Perspectives and Directions," *JAMA* 199 (1967): 188–198.

4. United States Department of Health, Education, and Welfare, Heart Disease Control Program, *Proceedings of the National Conference on Coronary Care Units*. DHEW Publication No. 1764 (Washington: Government Printing Office, 1968).

5. United States Department of Health, Education, and Welfare, Heart Disease and Stroke Control Program, *Guidelines for Coronary Care Units*. DHEW Publication No. 1824 (Washington: Government Printing Office, 1968).

6. Metropolitan Life Insurance Company, "Geographical Distribution of Coronary Care Units in the United States," Statistical Bulletin 58 (July–August, 1977): 7–9.

7. O. L. Peterson, "Myocardial Infarction: Unit Care or Home Care?" *Ann. Intern.*

Med. 88 (1978): 259–261; Editorial, "Antidysrhythmic Treatment in Acute Myocardial Infarction," *Lancet* 1 (1979): 193–194; Editorial, "Coronary-Care Units—Where Now?" *Lancet* 1 (1979): 649–650; H. Waitzkin, "How Capitalism Cares for Our Coronaries: A Preliminary Exercise in Political Economy," in *The Doctor-Patient Relationship in the Changing Health Scene,* edited by E. B. Gallagher. DHEW Publication No. [NIH] 78–183 (Washington: Government Printing Office, 1978); S. P. Martin, M. C. Donaldson, C. D. London, et al., "Inputs into Coronary Care during 30 Years: A Cost Effectiveness Study," *Ann. Intern. Med.* 81 (1974): 289–293.

8. S. Hofvendahl, "Influence of Treatment in a CCU on Prognosis in Acute Myocardial Infarction," *Acta Med. Scand. (Suppl.)* 519 (1971): 1–78; I. Christiansen, K. Iversen, A. P. Skouby, "Benefits Obtained by the Introduction of a Coronary-Care Unit: A Comparative Study," *Acta Med. Scand.* 189 (1971): 285–291; J. C. Hill, G. Holdstock, J. R. Hampton, "Comparison of Mortality of Patients with Heart Attacks Admitted to a Coronary Care Unit and an Ordinary Medical Ward," *Br. Med. J.* 2 (1977): 81–83; K. Astvad, N. Fabricius-Bjerre, J. Kjaerulff, et al., "Mortality from Acute Myocardial Infarction before and after Establishment of a Coronary Care Unit," *Br. Med. J.* 1 (1974): 567–569.

9. H. G. Mather, D. C. Morgan, N. G. Pearson, et al., "Myocardial Infarction: A Comparison between Home and Hospital Care for Patients," *Br. Med. J.* 1 (1976): 925–929; H. G. Mather, M. G. Pearson, K. L. Q. Read, et al., "Acute Myocardial Infarction: Home and Hospital Treatment," *Br. Med. J.* 3 (1971): 334–338; J. C. Hill, J. R. Hampton, J. R. A. Mitchell, "A Randomised Trial of Home-versus-Hospital Management for Patients with Suspected Myocardial Infarction," *Lancet* 1 (1978): 837–841; A. Colling, A. W. Dellipiani, R. J. Donaldson, "Teesside Coronary Survey: An Epidemiological Study of Acute Attacks of Myocardial Infarction," *Br. Med. J.* 2 (1976): 1169–1172; A. W. Dellipiani, W. A. Colling, R. J. Donaldson, et al., "Teesside Coronary Survey—Fatality and Comparative Severity of Patients Treated at Home, in the Hospital Ward, and in the Coronary Care Unit after Myocardial Infarction," *Br. Heart J.* 39 (1977): 1172–1178.

10. E. Mandel, *An Introduction to Marxist Economic Thought* (New York: Pathfinder, 1970), p. 52.

11. R. J. DeSalvo, "Medical Marketing Mixture—Update," *Med. Marketing & Media* 13 (September 1978): 21–35.

12. Warner-Lambert Pharmaceutical Company, *Annual Report* (Morris Plains, NJ, 1969), p. 8.

13. American Optical Company, *Annual Report* (Southbridge, MA, 1966), p. 9.

14. Warner-Lambert, *Annual Report* (1967), p. 7.

15. Warner-Lambert, *Annual Report* (1968), p. 25.

16. Warner-Lambert, *Annual Report* (1969), pp. 18–19.

17. Warner-Lambert, *Annual Report* (1970), p. 19.

18. Warner-Lambert, *Annual Report* (1975), p. 5.

19. Warner-Lambert, *Annual Report* (1970), p. 16.

20. *People & Taxes,* November 1978, p. 4.

21. Hewlett-Packard Company, *Annual Report* (Palo Alto, California, 1966), p. 11.

22. Hewlett-Packard, *Annual Report* (1969), p. 11.

23. Hewlett-Packard, *Annual Report* (1966), p. 4.

24. Hewlett-Packard, *Annual Report* (1969), p. 15.

25. Hewlett-Packard, *Annual Report* (1974), p. 2.

26. Hewlett-Packard, *Annual Report* (1971), p. 5.

27. Hewlett-Packard, *Annual Report* (1973), pp. 18–19.

28. Lown, Fakhro, Hood, et al., "Coronary Care Unit."

29. A. A. Scitovsky and N. McCall, *Changes in the Costs of Treatment of Selected Illnesses, 1951–1964–1971.* DHEW Publication No. [HRA] 77-3161 (Washington: Government Printing Office, 1977).

30. American Heart Association, *Annual Report* (New York: 1967), p. 11.

31. Day, "Intensive Coronary Care Area."

32. American Heart Association, *Annual Report* (New York, 1968), pp. 2, 13–14.

33. John A. Hartford Foundation, *Annual Report* (New York, 1963), p. 58.

34. W. R. Hewlett Foundation, *Annual Report to the Internal Revenue Service* (Palo Alto, California, 1967, 1971).

35. Day, "Intensive Coronary Care Area."

36. B. S. Bloom and O. Peterson, "End Results, Cost, and Productivity of Coronary-Care Units," *N. Engl. J. Med.* 288 (1973): 72–78.

37. J. O'Connor, *The Fiscal Crisis of the State* (New York: St. Martin's Press, 1973), pp. 64–72, 92–174.

38. United States Department of Commerce, Domestic and International Business Administration, *Global Market Survey: Biomedical Equipment.* USDC Publication, unnumbered (Washington: Government Printing Office, 1973).

39. H. Braverman, *Labor and Monopoly Capital* (New York: Monthly Review Press, 1974), especially pp. 85–152.

40. E. F. Rosinski, "Impact of Technology and Evolving Health Care Systems on the Training of Allied Health Personnel," *Milit. Med.* 134 (1969): 390–393.

41. F. J. Moore, "Information Technologies and Health Care: The Need for New Technologies to Offset the Shortage of Physicians," *Arch. Intern. Med.* 125 (1970): 351–355.

42. F. L. Foster, G. G. Casten, and T. J. Reeves, "Nonmedical Personnel and Continuous ECG Monitoring," *Arch. Intern. Med.* 124 (1969): 110–112; P. J. Sanazaro, "Physician Support Personnel in the 1970's," *JAMA* 214 (1970): 98–100; G. O. Barnett and A. Robbins, "Information Technology and Manpower Productivity," *JAMA* 209 (1969): 546–548.

43. B. Waterman, "The Coronary Care Labor Force," unpublished data.

44. C. J. Hitch and R. N. McKean, *The Economics of Defense in the Nuclear Age* (New York: Atheneum, 1967).

45. A. C. Enthoven, "Consumer-Choice Health Plan," *N. Engl. J. Med.* 298 (1978): 650–658, 709–720.

CHAPTER 5. SOCIAL MEDICINE AND THE COMMUNITY

1. W. J. Bicknell and D. C. Walsh, "Certificate-of-Need: The Massachusetts Experience," *N. Engl. J. Med.* 292 (1975): 1054–1061; E. Rothenberg, *Regulation and Expansion of Health Facilities: The Certificate of Need Experience in New York State* (New York: Praeger, 1976).

2. H. Waitzkin, J. Wallen, and J. Sharratt, "Homes or Hospitals? Contradictions of the Urban Crisis," *Int. J. Health Serv.* 9 (1979): 397–416.

3. For more details about the struggle in Boston and comparisons with other cities, see H. Waitzkin, "Expansion of Medical Institutions into Urban Residential Areas," *N. Engl. J. Med.* 282 (1970): 1003–1007; H. Waitzkin and J. Sharratt, "Controlling Medical Expan-

sion," *Society* 14 (January–February 1977): 30–35; H. Waitzkin, "What to Do When Your Local Medical Center Tries to Tear Down Your Home," *Sci. for the People* 9 (March–April 1977): 22–23, 28–39; J. Grady, C. Ploss, and H. Waitzkin, "Dilemmas of Community Organizing: Mission Hill in Boston," *Soc. Policy* 9 (May–June 1978): 43–52.

4. M. Fried, *The World of the Urban Working Class* (Cambridge: Harvard University Press, 1973), p. 143–177, 270–290.

5. Health/PAC West, *The Profit in Non-Profit Hospitals* (San Francisco: Health Policy Advisory Center, n.d.).

6. D. Harvey, *Social Justice in the City* (Baltimore: Johns Hopkins University Press, 1973), especially pp. 120–194; D. Harvey, *Justice, Nature and the Geography of Difference* (Cambridge, MA: Blackwell, 1996); A. Merrifield and E. Swyngedouw, *The Urbanization of Injustice* (London: Lawrence & Wishart, 1996).

7. J. O'Connor, *The Fiscal Crisis of the State* (New York: St. Martin's, 1973), pp. 1–12, 64–70, 97–178.

8. Regarding the history of public hospitals, see B. G. Rosenkrantz, *Public Health and the State: Changing Views in Massachusetts,* 1842–1936 (Cambridge: Harvard University Press, 1972), pp. 97–127; M. J. Vogel, "The Transformation of the American Hospital," in *Health Care in America,* edited by S. Reverby and D. Rosner (Philadelphia: Temple University Press, 1979).

9. J. Colombotos, "Physicians and Medicare: A Before-After Study of the Effects of Legislation on Attitudes," *Am. Sociol. Rev.* 34 (1969): 318–335.

10. M. I. Roemer and J. A. Mera, "'Patient Dumping' and Other Voluntary Agency Contributions to Public Agency Problems," *Med. Care* 11 (1973): 30–39.

11. D. U. Himmelstein, S. Woolhandler, M. Harnly, M. B. Bader, R. Silber, H. D. Backer, and A. A. Jones, "Patient Transfers: Medical Practice As Social Triage," *Am. J. Public Health* 74 (1984): 494–497.

12. M. B. Bader and M. Harnly, "Emergency Room Transfers in Alameda County," testimony to the Alameda County, California, Board of Supervisors, 1981.

13. R. L. Schiff, D. A. Ansell, J. E. Schlosser, A. H. Idris, A. Morrison, and S. Whitman, "Transfers to a Public Hospital: A Prospective Study of 467 Patients," *N. Engl. J. Med.* 314 (1986): 552–557.

14. W. Shonick, "The Public Hospital and Its Local Ecology in the United States," *Int. J. Health Serv.* 9 (1979): 359–396; A. B. Bindman, D. Keane, and N. Lurie, "A Public Hospital Closes: Impact on Patients' Access to Care and Health Status," *JAMA* 264 (1990): 2899–2904.

15. H. Waitzkin, B. V. Akin, L. M. de la Maza, F. A. Hubbell, H. Meshkinpour, L. Rucker, and J. S. Tobis, "Deciding against Corporate Management of a State-Supported Academic Medical Center," *N. Engl. J. Med.* 315 (1986): 1299–1304.

16. Bindman, Keane, and Lurie, "A Public Hospital Closes."

17. For more details about the history of community clinics, see J. D. Stoeckle and L. M. Candib, "The Neighborhood Health Center—Reform Ideas of Yesterday and Today," *N. Engl. J. Med.* 280 (1969): 1385–1391; R. M. Hollister, B. Kramer, and S. S. Bellin, *Neighborhood Health Centers* (Lexington, MA: Lexington, 1974).

18. I am indebted to Leslie Cohen and Jack Geiger for clarification of these issues.

19. R. W. Chamberlin and J. F. Radebaugh, "Delivery of Primary Health Care—Union Style," *N. Engl. J. Med.* 294 (1976): 641–645; P. Rudd, "The United Farm Workers Clinic Delano, California: A Study of the Rural Poor," *Public Health Rep.* 90 (1975): 331–339.

CHAPTER 6. THE MICROPOLITICS
OF THE DOCTOR-PATIENT RELATIONSHIP

1. K. Marx, *Capital* (Moscow: Progress Publishers, 1971 [1894]), v. 3, pp. 370–390, 790–794.

2. For an early and incompletely developed analysis, see K. Marx and F. Engels, *The German Ideology* (New York: International, 1939 [1846]), pp. 3–78.

3. Economic determinacy and ideology are among the most difficult problems in Marxist theory. For example, although Marx mainly used the term "ideology" to refer to the false consciousness engendered by the capitalist class, later Marxist theorists have broadened the usage of the term. The relative impact of economic versus nonmaterial forces also has been a central focus of debate within Marxism. Although the complexities of the debate are beyond my purposes here, pertinent discussions include: R. Lichtman, "Marx's Theory of Ideology," *Socialist Rev.* 5, 1 (Nov. 1975): 45–76; R. L. Heilbroner, *Marxism: For and Against* (New York: Norton, 1980), especially pp. 61–89; Žižek, "The Spectre of Ideology" and "How Did Marx Invent the Symptom," in S. Žižek, ed., *Mapping Ideology* (London: Verso, 1994).

4. A. Gramsci, *Prison Notebooks* (New York: International, 1971), pp. 123–202, 375–377, 406–407.

5. L. Althusser, "Ideology and Ideological State Apparatuses" in *Lenin and Philosophy and Other Essays* (New York: Monthly Review Press, 1971).

6. Ibid., pp. 132–133.

7. J. Habermas, "Science and Technology As 'Ideology,'" in *Toward a Rational Society* (Boston: Beacon, 1971), pp. 81–122; J. Habermas, *Knowledge and Human Interests* (Boston: Beacon, 1971), especially pp. 214–273, 301–317; J. Habermas, *Theory and Practice* (Boston: Beacon, 1974), pp. 1–40, 195–282; J. Habermas, *Legitimation Crisis* (Boston: Beacon, 1975), especially pp. 33–96; J. Habermas, *Communication and the Evolution of Society* (Boston: Beacon, 1979), pp. 1–68, 130–177; M. Kelly, ed., *Critique and Power: Recasting the Foucault/Habermas Debate* (Cambridge, MA: MIT Press, 1994).

8. Habermas, "Science and Technology," pp. 83–84.

9. Ibid., p. 111.

10. Ibid., p. 113.

11. Habermas, *Communication,* pp. 119–120.

12. Regarding medical social control of economic production, see E. R. Brown, "Public Health in Imperalism: Early Rockefeller Programs at Home and Abroad," *Am. J. Public Health* 66 (1976): 897–903; E. R. Brown, *Rockefeller Medicine Men* (Berkeley: University of California Press, 1979), pp. 112–134. For differing views of the family: T. Parsons, *The Social System* (Glencoe: Free Press, 1951), pp. 297–321, 428–454; C. Lasch, *Haven in a Heartless World* (New York: Basic Books, 1977), pp. 97–110, 167–189; J. Denizot, *The Policing of Families* (New York: Pantheon, 1979), pp. 169–198; M. Poster, *Critical Theory of the Family* (New York: Seabury, 1978); For an account of the sick role in repressive institutions: H. Waitzkin, "Latent Functions of the Sick Role in Various Institutional Settings," *Soc. Sci. Med.* 5 (1971): 45–75. Major general accounts of medicalization include I. Illich, *Medical Nemesis* (New York: Pantheon, 1976). Concerning social control and professional dominance, see E. Freidson, *Profession of Medicine,* (Chicago: University of Chicago Press, 1988); E. Freidson, *Profes-*

sionalism Reborn: Theory, Prophecy, and Policy (Chicago: University of Chicago Press, 1994).

13. Empirical studies of doctor-patient interaction (few of which refer to the interaction's social and historical context) are reviewed critically in H. Waitzkin, *The Politics of Medical Encounters* (New Haven: Yale University Press, 1991); D. L. Roter and J. A. Hall, *Doctors Talking with Patients: Improving Communications in Medical Visits* (Westport, CT: Auburn House, 1993); R. C. Smith, *The Patient's Story: Integrated Patient-Doctor Interviewing* (Boston: Little, Brown, 1996); M. Lipkin, Jr., S. M. Putnam, and A. Lazare, eds., *The Medical Interview: Clinical Care, Education, and Research* (New York: Springer, 1995); B. Korsch and C. Harding, *Intelligent Patients' Guide to the Doctor-Patient Relationship* (New York: Oxford University Press, 1997).

14. H. Waitzkin, "Information Giving in Medical Care," *J. Health Soc. Behav.* 26 (1985): 81–101; Waitzkin, *The Politics of Medical Encounters.*

15. Waitzkin, "Information Giving in Medical Care."

16. J. G. Hardman and L. E. Limbird, eds., *Goodman & Gilman's The Pharmacological Basis of Therapeutics* (New York: McGraw-Hill, 1996).

17. E. G. Mishler, "Studies in Dialogue and Discourse: II. Types of Discourse Initiated by and Sustained through Questioning," *J. Psycholing. Res.* 4 (1975): 99–121.

18. J. S. Horn, *"Away with All Pests . . .": An English Surgeon in People's China* (New York: Monthly Review Press, 1969), pp. 53–66, 175–183; V. W. Sidel and R. Sidel, *Serve the People: Observations on Medicine in the People's Republic of China* (Boston: Beacon, 1973), pp. 99–110; S. Conover, S. Donovan, and E. Susser, "Reflections on Health Care," *Cubatimes* 1, 4 (Winter 1981): 20–25; H. Waitzkin, K. Wald, R. Kee, R. Danielson, and L. Robinson, "Primary Care in Cuba: Low- and High-Technology Developments Pertinent to Family Medicine," *J. Fam. Pract.* 45 (1997): 250–258.

CHAPTER 7. MEDICINE AND SOCIAL CHANGE: LESSONS FROM CHILE AND CUBA

1. A. Gramsci, *Selections from the Prison Notebooks* (New York: International, 1971), p. 175.

2. Oficina de Planificación Nacional, *Antecedentes sobre el Desarrollo Chileno, 1960–1970* (Santiago, 1971), ch. 3 ("La Salud Pública"); V. Navarro, "What Does Chile Mean?" *Milbank Mem. Fund Q.* 52 (1974): 93–130; E. Santa Cruz, "Cáracter Clasista de la Medicina Chilena," *Punto Final* (Santiago), June 19, 1973, pp. 11–13. The analysis of Chile and Cuba that follows derives largely from my own personal observations and those of Hilary Modell, whose important contribution to our work on the Chilean health system I gratefully acknowledge.

3. D. J. Morris, *We Must Make Haste—Slowly: The Process of Revolution in Chile* (New York: Vintage, 1973), pp. 125, 143–145, 157–175, 195, 217, 240–242, 297; T. L. Hall and P. S. Diaz, "Social Security and Health Care Patterns in Chile," *Int. J. Health Serv.* 1 (1971): 362–377.

4. *An Analysis of Cost Expenditures in Latin America for the Period 1965–1970* (Baltimore: Johns Hopkins University, School of Hygiene and Public Health, unpublished manuscript, 1974).

5. S. Allende, *English and Spanish Texts of His Political Platform, the Program of the Popular Front, and His Biography* (Washington: Editorial Ardilla, n.d.), pp. 2–6, 39.

6. Oficina de Planificación Nacional, *Antecedentes.*

7. M. Gilpin and H. Rodriguez-Trias, "Looking at Health in a Healthy Way," *Cuba Rev.* 8 (March 1978): 3–15. For a detailed account of prerevolutionary medicine, see R. Danielson, *Cuban Medicine* (New Brunswick, NJ: Transaction Books, 1979), pp. 21–125; V. Navarro, "Health Services in Cuba," *N. Engl. J. Med.* 287 (1972): 954–959; V. Navarro, "Health, Health Services, and Health Planning in Cuba," *Int. J. Health Serv.* 2 (1972): 397–432.

8. Fidel Castro, "On Chilean Fascism and Revolution," in *The Chilean Road to Socialism,* edited by D. L. Johnson (Garden City: Anchor, 1973), pp. 337–359; D. L. Johnson, ed., *The Chilean Road to Socialism* (Garden City: Anchor, 1973), pp. 35, 47–51, 120, 125–129; North American Congress on Latin America, "Secret Memos from ITT" (released by Jack Anderson), *NACLA Latin America and Empire Report,* April 1972; International Telephone and Telegraph, "Memorandum," dated September 17, 1970, cited in *New York Times,* March 24, 1972.

9. International Telephone and Telegraph, "Memorandum."

10. See also R. M. Nixon, "Policy Statement: Economic Assistance and Investment Security in Developing Nations," press release, January 19, 1972; F. Bonilla and R. Girling, eds., *Structures of Dependency* (Stanford: Stanford University Press, 1973).

11. J. Valenzuela Feijoo, "Apostoles y Mercaderes de la Salud," *Punto Final* (Santiago), June 19, 1973, pp. 2–11.

12. North American Congress on Latin America, *New Chile* (Berkeley: Waller Press, 1972), pp. 81–117, 150–167.

13. O. Ozlak and D. Caputo, "The Migration of Medical Personnel from Latin America to the United States: Toward an Alternative Interpretation," presented at the Pan American Conference on Health Manpower Planning, Ottawa, Canada, September 10–14, 1973; R. Stevens and T. Vermuelen, *Foreign Trained Physicians and American Medicine,* DHEW Publication No. [NIH] 73-325 (Washington: Government Printing Office, 1973); V. Navarro, "The Underdevelopment of Health or the Health of Underdevelopment: An Analysis of the Distribution of Health Resources in Latin America," *Politics Soc.* 4 (1974): 267–293.

14. Morris, *We Must Make Haste.*

15. Santa Cruz, "Cáracter Clasista"; Valenzuela, "Apostoles y Mercaderes"; Navarro, "What Does Chile Mean?"

16. For accounts of the Cuban mass organizations, see R. R. Fagen, *The Transformation of Political Culture in Cuba* (Stanford: Stanford University Press, 1969), especially pp. 69–103; "New Forms of Democracy," *Cuba Rev.* 6 (September 1976): 1–36.

17. Gilpin and Rodriguez-Trias, "Looking at Health"; Danielson, *Cuban Medicine,* pp. 127–161.

18. R. Debray, *The Chilean Revolution—Conversations with Allende* (New York: Vintage, 1971), pp. 63–66, 84; North American Congress on Latin America, *New Chile,* pp. 16, 17, 21, 23, 52–58; R. E. Feinberg, *The Triumph of Allende: Chile's Legal Revolution* (New York: Mentor, 1972), pp. 81, 187, 240; Morris, *We Must Make Haste;* P. B. Cornely, R. Belmar, L. A. Falk, et al. "Report of the APHA Task Force of Chile," *Am. J. Public Health* 67 (1977): 31–36, 71–73.

19. E. Santa Cruz, "Ejemplo de Lucha por el Derecho a la Salud," *Punto Final* (Santi-

ago), June 19, 1973, pp. 14–16; A. Zimbalist and B. Stallings, "Showdown in Chile," *Monthly Rev.* 25 (October 1973): 1–24; K. Steenland, "Two Years of 'Popular Unity' in Chile: A Balance Sheet," *New Left Rev.* 78 (March–April 1973): 1–25; P. M. Sweezy, "Chile: The Question of Power," *Monthly Rev.* 25 (December 1973): 1–11; anonymous contributors, "Worker Control: (1) Its Structure under Allende; (2) At the Side of the Workers," *Sci. for the People* 5 (November 1973): 25–32.

20. Santa Cruz, "Ejemplo de Lucha."

21. J. Barnes, "Slaughterhouse in Santiago," *Newsweek,* October 8, 1973; L. R. Birns, ed., *The End of Chilean Democracy* (New York: Seabury, 1974), pp. 29–74; R. Rojas Sanford, *The Murder of Allende* (New York: Harper & Row, 1976), pp. 190–220; International Commission of Jurists, *Preliminary Report of the ICJ Mission to Chile* (Geneva, 1974).

22. The Chicago Commission of Inquiry into the Status of Human Rights in Chile, "Terror in Chile. I. The Chicago Commission Report," *New York Review of Books* 21 (May 20, 1974): 38–41; R. Styron, "Terror in Chile. II. The Amnesty Report," *New York Review of Books* 21 (May 30, 1974): 42–44; A. Argus, "Medicine and Politics in Chile," *World Medicine,* April 10, 1974, pp. 15–24; Chilean Medical Doctors in Exile, "An Appeal," Lima, Peru, March 8, 1974; A. Schester Cortes (military physician), "Policy to Be Followed with Members of the Popular Unity (UP)," Santiago, October 11, 1973.

23. For example, see Pan American Health Organization, *Health Conditions in the Americas,* vol. 2 (Washington, DC: The Organization [Scientific Publication No. 549], 1994).

24. For discussions of professional dominance in Cuba, see S. Conover, S. Donovan, and E. Susser, "Reflections on Health Care," *Cubatimes* 1 (Winter 1981): 20–25; J. M. Feinsilver, *Healing the Masses: Cuban Health Politics at Home and Abroad* (Berkeley: University of California Press, 1993).

25. Ibid.; Navarro, "Health, Health Services, and Health Planning in Cuba"; A. Cordova and J. Galigarcia, "Place of Social Science in the Medical Curriculum: An Integrated Study Plan for the Teaching of Medicine in the University of Havanna," *Soc. Sci. Med.* 11 (1977): 129–133.

26. Zimbalist and Stallings, "Showdown in Chile"; Sweezy, "Question of Power."

CHAPTER 8. CONCLUSION: HEALTH PRAXIS, REFORM, AND POLITICAL STRUGGLE

1. Pertinent work which deals with the many successes and limited failings of the Canadian national health program includes: T. Bodenheimer and K. Grumbach, *Understanding Health Policy: A Clinical Approach* (Norwalk, CT: Appleton and Lange, 1998); D. L. Williamson and J. E. Fast, "Poverty and Medical Treatment: When Public Policy Compromises Accessibility," *Can. J. Public Health* 89 (1998): 120–124; C. M. Bell, M. Crystal, A. S. Detsky, and D. A. Redelmeier, "Shopping around for Hospital Services: A Comparison of the United States and Canada," *JAMA* 279 (1998): 1015–1017; S. J. Katz, C. Charles, J. Lomas, and H. G. Welch, "Physician Relations in Canada: Shooting Inward As the Circle Closes," *J. Health Polit. Policy Law* 22 (1997): 1413–1431; S. J. Katz, T. P. Hofer, and W. G. Manning, "Hospital Utilization in Ontario and the United States: The Impact of Socioeconomic Status and Health Status," *Can. J. Public Health* 87 (1996): 253–256.

2. For critical overviews of the history of managed care, its limitations as the basis for a national health program, its impact on patient-doctor relationships, and pressures to expand its markets to Third World countries, see H. Waitzkin, "The Strange Career of Managed Competition: Military Failure to Medical Success?" *Am. J. Public Health* 84 (1994): 482–489; H. Waitzkin, "Is Our Work Dangerous? Should it Be?" (presentation on receipt of Leo G. Reeder Career Recognition Award, American Sociological Association, August 1997) *J. Health Soc. Behav.* 39 (1998): 7–17; H. Waitzkin and J. Fishman, "The Patient-Doctor Relationship in the Era of Managed Care," in J. Wilkerson, K. Devers, and R. Given, eds., *Competitive Managed Care: The Emerging Health Care System* (San Francisco: Jossey-Bass, 1997); K. Stocker, H. Waitzkin, and C. Iriart, "The Exportation of Managed Care to Latin America," *N. Engl. J. Med.* 320 (1999): 1131–1136.

3. Waitzkin and Fishman, "The Patient-Doctor Relationship in the Era of Managed Care."

4. R. Kuttner, "Must Good HMOs Go Bad?" *N. Engl. J. Med.* 338 (1998): 1558–1563, 1635–1639.

5. E. Friedson, *Profession of Medicine* (Chicago: University of Chicago Press, 1988).

6. The two models for NIH that were considered seriously during the first years of the Clinton Administration were those based on "managed competition" and on a "single-payer" system along the lines of the Canadian national health program. I personally devoted extensive efforts to supporting the latter approach, due to the rapidly growing barriers to health-care access, while recognizing that neither approach would have changed in a fundamental way the underlying relations of power and finance in the U.S. health-care system. The single-payer approach proved more palatable, since it would have eliminated parallel private insurance, thus decreasing the role of the private insurance industry. However, it would have preserved the overall structure of private practice, private ownership of hospitals, professional dominance, and a prominent position for for-profit managed care organizations. Regarding managed competition, see A. C. Enthoven and R. Kronick, "A Consumer-Choice Health Plan for the 1990s," *N. Engl. J. Med.* 320 (1989): 29–37, 94–101; P. Ellwood, A. Enthoven, and L. Etheredge, "The Jackson Hole Initiatives for a Twenty-first Century American Health Care System," *Health Econ.* 1 (1992): 149–168; P. Starr and W. A. Zelman, "A Bridge to Compromise: Competition under a Budget" *Health Aff (Millwood)* 12 (1993 Suppl): 7–23. On the single-payer approach, see D. U. Himmelstein, S. Woolhandler, and the Writing Committee of the Working Group on Program Design, Physicians for a National Health Program, "A National Health Program for the United States: A Physicians' Proposal," *N. Engl. J. Med.* 320 (1989): 102–108; J. Canham-Clyne, S. Woolhandler, and D. Himmelstein, *The Rational Option for a National Health Program* (Stony Creek, CT: Pamphleteer's Press, 1995).

7. R. V. Dellums et al., *Josephine Butler United States Health Service Act* (H.R. 1374) (Washington, D.C.: Government Printing Office, 1997).

8. See section on "International Comparisons" in chapter 2.

9. D. A. Barr and M. G. Field, "The Current State of Health Care in the Former Soviet Union: Implications for Health Care Policy and Reform," *Am. J. Public Health* 86 (1996): 307–312; T. H. Tulchinsky and E. A. Varavikova, "Addressing the Epidemiologic Transition in the Former Soviet Union: Strategies for Health System and Public Health Reform in Russia," *Am. J. Public Health* 6 (1996): 313–320.

10. V. W. Sidel and R. Sidel, *A Healthy State* (New York: Pantheon, 1977), pp. 129–157; V. Navarro, *Class Struggle, the State and Medicine: An Historical and Contem-*

porary Analysis of the Medical Sector in Great Britain (New York: Prodist, 1978), pp. 38–39.

11. J. Tudor Hart, "Bevan and the Doctors," *Lancet* 2 (1973): 1196.

12. See discussion and references on community health centers in chapter 5.

13. C. W. Mills, *The Sociological Imagination* (New York: Grove, 1959), pp. 8–11.

14. Examples of community-worker coalitions appear in Chapter 5.

15. M. Silverman, *The Drugging of the Americas* (Berkeley: University of California Press, 1976), pp. 106–134; M. Silverman, M. Lydecker, and P. R. Lee, *Bad Medicine: The Prescription Drug Industry in the Third World* (Stanford: Stanford University Press, 1992); P. Davis, ed., *Contested Ground: Public Purpose and Private Interest in the Regulation of Prescription Drugs* (Oxford: Oxford University Press, 1996).

16. For instance, see chapter 7 on Chile.

17. The most devastating social threat to humanity's survival, of course, is nuclear war. Although the complexities of this problem are beyond my scope here, the medical consequences of nuclear war remain important as nuclear weapons proliferate in Third World countries. See J. Schell, *The Gift of Time: The Case for Abolishing Nuclear Weapons Now* (New York: Metropolitan Books, 1998); B. S. Levy and V. W. Sidel, eds., *War and Public Health* (New York: Oxford University Press, 1996).

Selected Bibliography

Ackernecht, E. H. *Rudolpf Virchow: Doctor, Statesman, Anthropologist.* Madison: University of Wisconsin Press, 1953.

Allan, T., and Gordon, S. *The Scalpel, the Sword: The Story of Doctor Norman Bethune.* Toronto: McClelland and Stewart, 1952.

Allende, S. *La Realidad Medico-Social Chilena.* Santiago: Ministerio de Salubridad, Prevision y Asistencia Social, 1939.

Althusser, L. *Lenin and Philosophy and Other Essays.* New York: Monthly Review Press, 1971.

Amin S. *Unequal Development.* New York: Monthly Review Press, 1976.

Balibar, E. The basic concepts of historical materialism. In L. Althusser and E. Balibar, eds., *Reading Capital.* London: New Left Books, 1970.

Bennett A. E., ed. *Communication between Doctors and Patients.* London: Nuffield Hospitals Trust, 1976.

Belmar, R., and Sidel, V. W. An international perspective on strikes and strike threats by physicians: The case of Chile. *Int. J. Health Serv.* 5 (1975): 53–64.

Bethune, N. A plea for early decompression in pulmonary tuberculosis. *Can. Med. Assoc. J.* 27 (1932): 36–42.

———. Wounds. In J. S. Horn, ed., *"Away with All Pests . . .": An English Surgeon in People's China.* New York: Monthly Review Press, 1969.

Bettelheim, C., and Burton, N. *China since Mao.* New York: Monthly Review Press, 1978.

Bodenheimer, T., and Grumbach K. *Understanding Health Policy: A Clinical Approach.* Norwalk, CT: Appleton and Lange, 1998.

Boenheim, F. Einleitung. In R. Virchow, ed., *Werk und Wirkung.* Berlin: Rütten & Loenig, 1967.

Braverman, H. *Labor and Monopoly Capital.* New York: Monthly Review Press, 1974.

Brenner, H. *Mental Illness and the Economy.* Cambridge: Harvard University Press, 1974.

Brown, E. R. Public health in imperialism: Early Rockefeller programs at home and abroad. *Am. J. Public Health* 66 (1976): 897–903.

———. *Rockefeller Medicine Men: Medicine and Capitalism in the Progressive Era.* Berkeley, University of California Press, 1979.

Byrne, P. S., and Long, B. E. *Doctors Talking to Patients.* London: Her Majesty's Stationery Office, 1976.

Canham-Clyne, J., Woolhandler, S., and Himmelstein, D. *The Rational Option for a National Health Program.* Stony Creek, CT: Pamphleteer's Press, 1995.

Castells, M. *The Urban Question.* Cambridge: MIT Press, 1977.

Chadwick, E. *Report on the Sanitary Condition of the Labouring Population of Great Britain.* Edinburgh: Edinburgh University Press, 1965 (1842).

Chile Departamento de Planificación. *Biografía del Presidente Allende.* Santiago: Departamento de Impresos, 1972.

Cochrane, A. L. *Effectiveness and Efficiency: Random Reflections on Health Care.* London: Nuffield Hospitals Trust, 1972.

Colling, A., Dellipiani, A. W., and Donaldson, R. J. Teesside coronary survey: An epidemiological study of acute attacks of myocardial infarction. *Br. Med. J.* 2 (1976): 1169–1172.

Danielson, R. *Cuban Medicine.* New Brunswick, N.J.: Transaction Books, 1978.

Davis, P., ed. *Contested Ground: Public Purpose and Private Interest in the Regulation of Prescription Drugs.* Oxford: Oxford University Press, 1996.

Dellipiani, A. W. et al., Teesside coronary survey—Fatality and comparative severity of patients treated at home, in the hospital ward, and in the coronary care unit after myocardial infarction. *Br. Heart J.* 39 (1977): 1172–1178.

Dellums, R. V. et al., *Josephine Butler United States Health Service Act* (H.R. 1374). Washington, D.C.: Government Printing Office, 1997.

Denizot, J. *The Policing of Families,* New York: Pantheon, 1979.

Deppe, H. U. Rudolf Virchows Kampf um die Preussische Verfassung. *Blätter für deutsche und internationale Politik* 13 (1968): 961–974.

———, and Regus, M. *Seminar: Medizin, Gesellschaft, Geschichte.* Frankfurt am Main: Suhrkamp Verlag, 1975.

Ehrenreich, B., and Ehrenreich, J., eds. *The American Health Empire.* New York: Vintage, 1970.

———. Hospital workers: A case study of the new working class. *Monthly Rev.* 24 (January 1973): 12–27.

———. Health care and social control. *Soc. Policy* 5 (May–June 1974): 26–40.

Ehrenreich, B., and English, D. *Complaints and Disorders: The Sexual Politics of Sickness.* Old Westbury, N.Y.: Feminist Press, 1973.

———. *For Her Own Good.* New York: Anchor/Doubleday, 1978.

Ehrenreich, J., ed. *The Cultural Crisis of Medicine.* New York: Monthly Review Press, 1978.

Elling, R. H. Industrialization and occupational health in underdeveloped countries. *Int. J. Health Serv.* 7 (1977): 209–235.

Engels, F. *Dialectics of Nature.* New York: International, 1940.

———. *The Origin of the Family, Private Property and the State.* New York: International, 1942 (1891).

———. Briefe aus dem Wuppertal. In K. Marx and F. Engels, *Werke.* Berlin: Dietz Verlag, 1961.

———. *Herr Eugen Dühring's Revolution in Science* [*Anti-Dühring*]. New York: International, 1966 (1878).

———. *The Condition of the Working Class in England.* Moscow: Progress Publishers, 1973 (1845).

Eyer, J. Hypertension as a disease of modern society. *Int. J. Health Serv.* 5 (1975): 530–558.

———. Prosperity as a cause of death. *Int. J. Health Serv.* 7 (1977): 125–150.

————, and Sterling, P. Stress-related mortality and social organization. *Rev. Rad. Pol. Econ.* 8 (Spring 1977): 1–44.

Feinsilver, J. M. *Healing the Masses: Cuban Health Politics at Home and Abroad.* Berkeley: University of California Press, 1993.

Fletcher, C. M. *Communication in Medicine.* London: Nuffield Hospitals Trust, 1973.

Flexner, A. *Medical Education in the United States and Canada.* New York: Carnegie Foundation, 1910.

Frank, A. G. *Dependent Accumulation and Underdevelopment.* New York: Monthly Review Press, 1979.

Freidson, E. *Profession of Medicine.* Chicago: University of Chicago Press, 1988.

Fuchs, V. R. *Who Shall Live? Health, Economics, and Social Choice.* New York: Basic Books, 1974.

Gish, O. *Planning the Health Sector: The Tanzanian Experience.* New York: Holmes and Meier, 1976.

Gorbachev, M. *Perestroika: New Thinking for Our Country and the World.* New York: Harper & Row, 1987.

Gordon, L. *Woman's Body, Woman's Right: A Social History of Birth Control in America.* New York: Viking, 1976.

Gorz, A. Technical intelligence and the capitalist division of labor. *Telos* 12 (Summer 1972): 27–41.

————. *Socialism and Revolution.* Garden City, N.Y.: Anchor, 1973.

Gramsci, A. *Selections from the Prison Notebooks.* New York: International, 1971.

Guevara, E. On revolutionary medicine. In J. Gerassi, ed., *Venceremos.* New York: Simon and Schuster, 1969.

Habermas, J. Science and technology as "ideology." In *Toward a Rational Society.* Boston: Beacon, 1970.

————. *Knowledge and Human Interests.* Boston: Beacon, 1971.

————. *Theory and Practice.* Boston: Beacon, 1974.

————. *Legitimation Crisis.* Boston: Beacon, 1975.

————. *Communication and the Evolution of Society.* Boston: Beacon, 1979.

Harvey, D. *Justice, Nature and the Geography of Difference.* Cambridge, MA: Blackwell, 1996.

Heilbroner, R. *Marxism: For and Against.* New York: Norton, 1980.

Hill, J. C., Hampton, J. R., and Mitchell, J. R. A. A randomised trial of home-versus-hospital management for patients with suspected myocardial infarction. *Lancet* 1 (1978): 837–841.

Holman, H. R. The "excellence" deception in medicine. *Hosp. Pract.* 11 (April 1976): 11–21.

Horn, J. S. *"Away With All Pests . . .": An English Surgeon in People's China.* New York: Monthly Review Press, 1969.

Illich, I. *Medical Nemesis.* London: Calder & Boyars, 1975.

Kass, E. H. Infectious diseases and social change. *J. Inf. Dis.* 123 (1971): 110–114.

Kelman, S. Towards a political economy of health care. *Inquiry* 8 (1971): 30–38.

Kotelchuck, D., ed. *Prognosis Negative.* New York: Vintage, 1976.

Krause, E. *Power and Illness: The Political Sociology of Health and Medical Care.* New York: Elsevier, 1977.

————. *Death of the Guilds: Professions, States, and the Advance of Capitalism* (New Haven: Yale University Press, 1996).

Lall, S. Medicines and multinationals. *Monthly Rev.* 28 (March 1977): 19–30.

Lalonde, M. A. *New Perspective on the Health of Canadians.* Ottawa: Information Canada, 1974.

Larson, M. S. *The Rise of Professionalism.* Berkeley: University of California Press, 1977.

Lasch, C. *Haven in a Heartless World.* New York: Basic Books, 1977.

Law, S. *Blue Cross: What Went Wrong?* New Haven, Yale University Press, 1976.

Lenin, V. I. *The State and Revolution.* Peking: Foreign Languages Press, 1973 (1917).

Levy, B. S., and Sidel, V. W., eds. *War and Public Health.* New York: Oxford University Press, 1996.

Ley, P., and Spelman, M. S. *Communicating with the Patient.* London: Staples Press, 1967.

Lichtman, R. The political economy of medical care. In H. P. Dreitzel, ed., *The Social Organization of Health.* New York: Macmillan, 1971.

Lukacs, G. *History and Class Consciousness: Studies in Marxist Dialectics.* Cambridge: MIT Press, 1971.

Mandel, E. *An Introduction to Marxist Economic Thought.* New York: Pathfinder, 1970.

Mao Tse-Tung. *On Contradiction.* New York: International, 1953.

Marcus, S. *Engels, Manchester, and the Working Class.* New York: Vintage, 1974.

Markowitz, G., and Rosner, D. Doctors in crisis: A study of the use of medical educational reform to establish modern professional elitism in medicine. *Am. Q.* 25 (1973): 83–107.

Marx, K. *Capital.* Moscow: Progress Publsihers, 1963 (1890).

————. *The Eighteenth Brumaire of Louis Bonaparte.* New York: International, 1963 (1852).

————. *The Economic and Philsoophic Manuscripts of 1844.* New York: International, 1964.

————. *A Contribution to the Critique of Political Economy.* New York: International, 1971 (1859).

————, and Engels, F. *Gesamtausgabe.* Berlin: Marx-Engels-Verlag, 1931.

————. *The German Ideology.* New York: International, 1939 (1846).

————. *The Communist Manifesto.* New York: Appleton-Century-Crofts, 1955 (1848).

Mather, H. G., Morgan, D. C., et al. Myocardial infarction: A comparison between home and hospital care for patients. *Br. Med. J.* 1 (1976): 925–929.

Mather, H. G., Pearson, M. G., et al. Acute myocardial infarction: Home and hospital treatment. *Br. Med. J.* 3 (1971): 334–338.

McCoy, A. W. *The Politics of Heroin in Southeast Asia.* New York: Harper & Row, 1972.

McKeown, T. *The Modern Rise of Population.* New York: Academic Press, 1977.

————. *The Role of Medicine: Dream, Mirage, or Nemesis?* Princeton: Princeton University Press, 1979.

McKinlay, J. B. On the professional regulation of change. *Sociol. Rev. (Monogr.)* 20 (1973): 61–84.

————. The changing political and economic context of the patient-physician encounter. In E. G. Gallagher, ed., *The Doctor-Patient Relationship in the Changing Health Scene.* DHEW Publication No. [NIH] 78-183. Washington: Government Printing Office, 1978.

Merton, R. K. *Social Theory and Social Structure.* New York: Free Press, 1968.

Modell, H., and Waitzkin, H. Medicine and socialism in Chile. *Berkeley J. Sociol.* 19 (1974): 1–35.

Navarro, V. Health, health services, and health planning in Cuba. *Int. J. Health Serv.* 2 (1972): 397–432.

———. Health services in Cuba: An initial appraisal. *N. Engl. J. Med.* 287 (1972): 954–959.

———. What does Chile mean? An analysis of events in the health sector before, during, and after Allende's administration. *Milbank Mem. Fund Q.* 52 (1974): 93–130.

———. Social policy issues: An explanation of the composition, nature, and functions of the present health sector of the United States. *Bull. N.Y. Acad. Med.* 51 (1975): 199–234.

———. *Medicine under Capitalism.* New York: Prodist, 1976.

———. *The Politics of Health Policy: The U.S. Reforms, 1980–1994.* Cambridge, MA: Blackwell, 1994.

Noble, D. *America by Design.* New York: Knopf, 1977.

O'Connor J. *The Fiscal Crisis of the State.* New York: St. Martin's, 1973.

Offe, C. Advanced capitalism and the welfare state. *Politics Soc.* 2 (1972): 479–488.

———. The theory of the capitalist state and the problem of policy formation. In L. N. Lindberg et al., eds., *Stress and Contradiction in Modern Capitalism.* Lexington, MA.: Lexington Books, 1975.

Parsons, T. *The Social System.* Glencoe, IL: Free Press, 1951.

Piven, F. F., and Cloward, R. A. *Regulating the Poor.* New York: Vintage, 1971.

Powles, J. On the limitations of modern medicine. *Sci. Med. Man* 1 (1973): 1–30.

Reed, J. *Ten Days That Shook the World.* New York: Modern Library, 1935.

Renaud, M. On the structural constraints to state intervention in health. *Int. J. Health Serv.* 5 (1975): 559–571.

Roemer, M. I., and Mera, J. A. "Patient dumping" and other voluntary agency contributions to public agency problems. *Med. Care* 11 (1973): 30–39.

Rosen, G. What is social medicine? *Bull. Hist. Med.* 21 (1947): 674–733.

———. *A History of Public Health.* New York: MD Publications, 1958.

———. *From Medical Police to Social Medicine: Essays on the History of Health Care.* New York: Science History Publications, 1974.

Roter, D. L., and Hall, J. A. *Doctors Talking with Patients: Improving Communications in Medical Visits.* Westport, CT: Auburn House, 1993.

Sand, R. *The Advance to Social Medicine.* London: Staples Press, 1952.

Scitovsky, A. A., and McCall, N. *Changes in the Costs of Treatment of Selected Illnesses, 1951–1964–1971.* DHEW Publication No. [HRA] 77-3161. Washington: Government Printing Office, 1977.

Schell, J. *The Gift of Time: The Case for Abolishing Nuclear Weapons Now.* New York: Metropolitan Books, 1998.

Segall, M. Health and national liberation in the People's Republic of Mozambique. *Int. J. Health Serv.* 7 (1977): 319–325.

Shonick, W. The public hospital and its local ecology in the United States. *Int. J. Health Serv.* 9 (1979): 359–396.

Sidel, V. W., and Sidel, R. *Serve the People: Observations of Medicine in the People's Republic of China.* Boston: Beacon, 1973.

Sigerist, H. *Civilization and Disease.* Ithaca, NY: Cornell University Press, 1944.

Silverman, M. *The Drugging of the Americas.* Berkeley: University of California Press, 1976.

Silverman, M., Lydecker, M., and Lee, P. R. *Bad Medicine: The Prescription Drug Industry in the Third World.* Stanford: Stanford University Press, 1992.

Smith, E. W., and Smith, A. *Minamata.* New York: Holt, Rinehart, and Winston, 1975.

Smith, R. C. *The Patient's Story: Integrated Patient-Doctor Interviewing.* Boston: Little, Brown, 1996.

Stimson, G., and Webb, B. *Going to See the Doctor.* London: Routledge & Kegan Paul, 1975.

Stocker, K., Waitzkin, H., and Iriart., C. The exportation of managed care to Latin America. *N. Engl. J. Med.* 320 (1999): 1131–1136.

Strong, P. M. *The Ceremonial Order of the Clinic.* London: Routledge & Kegan Paul, 1979.

Turshen, M. *Privatizing Health Services in Africa.* New Brunswick, NJ: Rutgers University Press, 1999.

Virchow, R. *Cellular Pathology.* New York: De Witt, 1860.

―――. *Ueber den Hungertyphus und Einige Verwandte Krankheitsformen.* Berlin: Hirschwald, 1868.

―――. *Gesammelte Abhandlungen aus dem Gebiet der oeffentlichen Medicin und der Seuchenlehre,* vol. 1. Berlin: Hirschwald, 1879.

―――. *Briefe an seine Eltern.* Leipzig: Engelmann, 1907.

―――. *Werk und Wirkung.* Berlin: Rütten & Loenig, 1957.

―――. *Disease, Life, and Man.* Translated by L. J. Rather. Stanford: Stanford University Press, 1958.

Waitzkin, H. Latent functions of the sick role in various institutional settings. *Soc. Sci. Med.* 5 (1971): 45–75.

―――. *The Politics of Medical Encounters: How Patients and Doctors Deal with Social Problems.* New Haven: Yale University Press, 1991.

Waitzkin, H., and Fishman, J. The patient-doctor relationship in the era of managed care. In J. Wilkerson, K. Devers, and R. Given, eds. *Competitive Managed Care: The Emerging Health Care System.* San Francisco: Jossey-Bass, 1997.

Waitzkin, H., and Modell, H. Medicine, socialism, and totalitarianism: Lessons from Chile. *N. Engl. J. Med.* 291 (1974): 171–177.

Waitzkin, H., Wallen, J., and Sharratt, J. Homes or hospitals? Contradictions of the urban crisis. *Int J. Health Serv.* 9 (1979): 397–416.

Waitzkin, H., and Waterman, B. *The Exploitation of Illness in Capitalist Society.* Indianapolis: Bobbs-Merrill, 1974.

Waldron, I. Why do women live longer than men? I. *J. Hum. Stress* 2 (March 1976): 2–13.

―――, and Johnson, S. Why do women live longer than men? II. *J. Hum. Stress* 2 (June 1976): 19–31.

Wallen, J., Waitzkin, H., and Stoeckle, J. D. Physician stereotypes about female health and illness: A study of patient's sex and the informative process during medical interviews. *Women & Health* 4 (1979): 135–146.

Weber, M. Bureaucracy. In H. H. Gerth and C. W. Mills, eds., *From Max Weber.* New York: Galaxy, 1958.

Witt, M. Production with safety? *Cubatimes* 1, 4 (Winter 1981): 3–5.

Žižek, S., ed., *Mapping Ideology.* London: Verso, 1994.

Zola, I. K. *Socio-Medical Inquiries.* Philadelphia: Temple University Press, 1983.

Index

Abortion, 66
Academic medical center, 88–90
Accidents, 58, 67, 207
Activism, 35–36, 63–64, 69, 71–73, 162, 189,
  197, 200–207
Affirmative action, 202
Alameda County, California, 29–31, 107,
  112–15
Alameda Health Consortium, 113–15
Alcoholism, 57, 67, 149–59, 162, 175
Alienation, 33
Allende, Salvador, 39, 55–73, 166–67, 170–71,
  185–86
Allied health personnel, 92–94
Althusser, Louis, 120–22
American Heart Association, 90–91
American Optical Company, 80, 84–94
Angiosarcoma of liver, 9–10
Asbestos (asbestosis), 11–12

Back disease among farmworkers, 12–14
Bacon, Francis, 60
Batista, Fulgencio, 172
Bethune, Norman, 39
Black Panther Party, 110, 116
Blue Cross and Blue Shield, 45, 104, 167
Brain disease from mercury poisoning, 14–16
Braverman, Harry, 34
Brown, E. Richard, 123
Bureaucracy, 5, 24, 123, 167, 183, 192, 197–
  200
Burn-out of workers, 115, 116

Canada, 191
Cancer, 9–12, 30, 46, 181, 207; liver, 9–10;
  lung, 11–12
Capitalist class, 5, 40–41, 44
Capitation fee, 191–92

Castro, Fidel, 172–73
Centralization of health policy, 197–200
Certificate-of-need laws, 98
Chadwick, E., 56
Change. See Social change
Chile, 44, 51–52, 64–73, 85, 165–88, 193–96
China, 39, 49, 51–52, 160–61, 195
Chisso Corporation, 14–16
Cienfuegos, Camilo, 172
Civil rights, 93–110
Class, 5, 27, 31, 39–42, 48, 50–51, 53, 56–60,
  62–63, 64–69, 70–73, 100–01, 120–23,
  125, 168–69, 171, 173–74, 181–82,
  186–87, 201–02, 205–6; capitalist, 5,
  40–41, 44, 51, 57, 120; conflict, 6, 51–52;
  mortality rates and, 57–58, 62; social, 5,
  26–27, 31, 39–42, 48, 50–51, 53, 56–60,
  70–73, 120–23, 125, 168, 171, 173–74,
  181, 285–88, 201–2, 205; working, 5,
  41–42, 56–60, 62–63, 64–69, 100–101
Clinics, community, 109–17, 173–85, 194, 232
Closure of public hospitals, 107–8, 202
Co-insurance, 190
Commerce, U.S. Department of, 92
Committees for the Defense of the Revolution,
  Cuba, 172, 186
Communication, 119–62, 200; distorted, 122,
  125, 135–36; doctor-patient, 119–62
Communist Manifesto, 37, 44, 71
Community, 97–116; clinics, 109–17, 176–85,
  194, 202; development, 116–17; organizing
  against expanding medical centers,
  100–101; worker coalitions, 116–17, 202,
  207; worker control, 116–17, 176–85, 187,
  199, 202
Condition of the Working Class in England, 56–
  61, 69, 71
Conflict. See Class

Consumer-worker control, 175–79, 187–88, 229, 202,
Contraction, public medical, 104–9
Contradiction. *See* Social contradictions; Patching; Reform
Control over health institutions, 40–41, 198–200; social, 34–35, 48–49, 119–62, 200, 204
Coronary care unit, 27, 43, 77–96, 184, 204–5; political economy of, 83–94
Corporations, 7, 12, 14–16, 21–23, 29–31, 33, 43, 46, 50, 83–88, 93–98, 108, 119, 166, 170–71, 185, 193, 196, 203–4
Cost-effectiveness research, 77, 95
Costs, 24–31, 77–96, 103, 191–93, 194; containment of, 94–96, 191, 194
Countercultural movement, 110–13
Coup d'état, Chile, 178, 209–10, 212
Critical theory, 140–41
Cuba, 47, 53, 60–61, 181–82, 187–213, 224, 236
Cutbacks, 45, 95, 104–9, 115–17, 202, 203–4, 206
Cycles, economic, 54

Day, H. W., 91–92, 104
DBCP, 3
Decreto 602 (Decree 602), Chile, 176–78
Dellums, Ronald, 193–97, 198–200; proposal for national health service, 192–97
Democratization, 176–79, 182, 183, 187–88, 194–95, 199–200
Dependency, economic, 166, 170, 174
Depreciation, 104
Deskilling of labor, 34, 93–94
Development: and underdevelopment, 5, 20–24, 50–52, 55, 65–73, 166, 169–71, 174, 178, 184–85, 195–96, 205–6; uneven, 20–24, 27, 97–98, 113, 176, 194, 197, 203, 205
Dialectic materialism, 5–7, 60–61
Diminishing returns of medicine, 24–32
Disability, certification of, 127–29, 135
Distorted communication, 122, 125, 135
Doctor-patient relationship, 35, 49, 119–62, 184, 192, 204; empirical studies of, 108–9
Drug companies, 43, 47, 50–53, 68, 83–93, 95, 171, 174, 225, 203–6
Dumping of patients, 45, 104, 106–7, 203

Economic surplus, 83
Education, professional, 21, 97, 105
Effectiveness of medicine, 24–32, 78–83, 94, 119,

Encounters, doctor-patient, 119–62, 192
Engels, Friedrich, 23, 37–38, 53, 55–73
Engineering approach in medicine, 33–34
Environmental illness, 4, 6–16, 47–48, 55–73, 175, 205–7
Epidemics, 38–39, 61–63, 105–6, 195
Epidemiology, historical materialist, 53–55
Equality, 22–24, 70; and freedom, 22–24, 97–98
Equipment, medical, 42–42, 47, 50–53, 95, 174, 196, 203–5
Expansion, private medical, 98–104, 203
Expenditures, health, 24–32
Expertise, 6, 49, 181–82, 187
Exploitation of illness, 7–8, 29, 43, 88, 95, 197, 204

Family, 124, 135, 147–49, 159
Finance capital, 42, 203
Flexner Report, 39, 42
Frankfurt School, 121
Freidson, Eliot, 123, 192
Fried, Marc, 101

General practitioners, 198
Glomerulonephritis, 19
Gorz, André, 35–36, 189
Gramsci, Antonio, 120–21, 166
Great Britain, 44, 52, 56–60, 193–96
Guevara, Che, 39

Habermas, Juergen, 28, 121–23
Harrison, Donald, 89–90
Hartford, John A., Foundation, 78–80, 91
Health, Education, and Welfare, U.S. Department of, 80, 92, 111, 113
Health maintenance organizations, 191–93
Health policy, 71–73, 95–96, 111, 116–17, 165–207
Health praxis, 189–207
Heart disease, 30, 136–49, 181; congenital, 20; coronary care units, 27, 43, 77–96, 184
Hegel, G. W., 60–61
Hegemony, ideologic, 121
Hewlett, William, 89, 91
Hewlett, W. R., Foundation, 91
Hewlett-Packard Company, 83–93
Heyns, R. W., 91
Hill, J. C., 82
Hill-Burton Program, 22, 30, 103
Historical materialism, 5–7, 60–61
Historical materialist epidemiology, 53–55
Hospitals. *See* Public hospitals

Housing, 65–69, 175, 203; destruction by expanding medical centers, 99–104
Humanistic decline and technologic progress, 32–35, 93–94, 119–20, 161

Ideologic hegemony, 121–24
Ideologic state apparatuses, 121–22
Ideology, 22–24, 27–28, 47–57 97–98, 119–62, 200, 204–5; in doctor-patient relationship 119–62. *See also* Medical idelogy; Scientific ideology
Illich, Ivan, 123,
Illness, social origins of, 53–73
Illness-generating social conditions, 53–73, 200–201, 204, 206–7
Immunization, 26, 181, 182
Imperialism, 6, 49–51, 55, 64–73, 166, 171, 174, 185, 206, 207
Indochina War, 51, 92, 95
Industrialization, 8–9, 190–91
Infant mortality, 3–7, 24–28, 57, 62, 65–66, 169, 175, 181, 195
Infectious diseases, 25–26, 38–39, 56, 62–63, 64–67, 105–6, 109, 151, 169, 181–82
Institutions, health: control over, 40; stratification within, 40–41
Insurance companies, 42, 190, 194
Intensive care unit, 4, 27, 77–96
Interaction, doctor-patient, 119–62, 192
International comparisons, 49–53, 165–88, 205–6
International Telephone and Telegraph, 170

Kaiser-Permanente system, 192
Kass, Edward, 26

La Clínica de la Raza, 113–15
La Realidad Medico-Social Chilena, 64–69, 69, 72
Labor force, health care, 93–94
Lead Poisoning, 59
Legitimacy, 45, 92, 95, 101–2, 119, 120–24, 204; crisis, 46
Leisure, 133–35, 149, 159
Lenin, V. I., 39, 44
Life expectancy, 24–25
Local control, national goals, 198–99
Local health councils, Chile, 176–79, 188
Lown, Bernard, 80, 84–85, 88–89, 91
Lung disease, occupational, 11–12, 59, 181

Maldistribution, 16–24, 26, 45, 49–53, 57, 97–98, 167–68, 175–76, 179–80, 191–95, 202–3, 205
Mandel, Ernest, 83
Marx, Karl, 7, 23, 37, 61, 120, 195
Marxist analysis, 4–7, 28, 37–54, 55, 83, 120–23, 207; historical development in health care, 37–39
Mass mobilization, 185–87
Mass political organizations, 172, 180–88
Materialism, 5–7, 60–61
Mather, H. G., 82
McCall, N., 89
McKeown, Thomas, 26, 33
Medicaid, 19, 31, 44–45, 99, 103–9, 112, 202
Medi-Cal, 3, 107
Medical centers, 7, 21, 42, 88–90, 97–109, 203; academic, 88–90
Medical equipment, 43, 47, 50–53, 95, 174, 197, 204–5
Medical ideology, 47–49, 119–62
Medical-industrial complex, 43, 203
Medicalization of social problems, 34–35, 48–49, 119–63, 204
Medicare, 19, 31, 44–45, 103–9, 112, 202
Medicina en la Comunidad (Medicine in the Community), Cuba, 161, 180, 184
Mercury poisoning, 14–16
Mesothelioma, 11
Micro-level processes and macro-level contradictions, 119, 159–60
Mid-level practitioners, 111
Militarism, 207
Minamata Disease, 14–16
Minorities, 97–98, 106–8, 110–12, 116–17, 195, 199, 202, 206
Mobility, occupational, 41–42
Monopoly capital, 21, 33, 42–43, 68, 88, 97, 119, 195, 202–4
Mortality rates and social class, 57, 62
Multifactorial etiology, 61–62, 70–71
Myocardial infarction, 78–83, 89

National goals, local control, 198–99
National health insurance, 23, 42–47, 52–53, 167–68, 189–93, 195–96
National health service, 23, 52–53, 95, 167–68, 198–203, 175–79, 193–97, 204, 198–200
National Health Service Corps, 111, 113
Native Americans, 16, 110
Navarro, Vicente, 40–41
Negative selection, 47
Neighborhood health center, 176–79, 194

Nonprofit status of hospitals, 104
Nonreformist reforms, 35–36, 115–17, 161–62, 165–67, 175–177, 189–97, 201, 205, 206
Nuclear power, 206–7
Nuclear weapons, 206–7
Nutrition, 57, 66, 169, 175, 195

Occupational illness, 4, 6–7, 8–16, 47, 50, 53–54, 55–73, 175, 180, 182, 205–7
Occupational mobility, 41–42
Occupational Safety and Health Administration, U.S., 10
Oppression, medical, 37–54, 63, 77, 110, 119–20, 159–60, 165–66, 200–202, 207
Organizing, 162; against expanding medical centers, 99–100, 203; in community clinics, 115–17; in support of public hospitals, 108

Packard, David, 86
Parsons, Talcott, 123
Patching, contradictions of, 200–201
Patient-doctor relationship, 35, 49, 119–62, 184, 204
empirical studies of, 108–9
Patient dumping, 45, 104, 106–7, 203
Peer review, 191–93
People's Power, Cuba, 182–83
Peter Bent Brigham Hospital, 80, 88
Pharmaceutical industry, 43, 47, 50–53, 68, 83–93, 95, 171, 174, 196, 204–6
Philanthropies, 90–91, 95, 110–11, 114
Planning, health, 194–200, 203
Plastic, 9–10
Plus factor, 104
Political economy of coronary care, 83–94
Policy. *See* Health policy
Polvinyl chloride, 9–10
Popular Unity government in Chile, 165–207
Positive selection, 47, 92
Powles, John, 24
Praxis, health, 189–207
Prenatal care, 27–28
Prepaid group practice, 191–93
Prevention, 63, 175, 181
Private medical expansion, 98–104, 202, 203; public subsidization of, 104
Private-public contradiction, 35–36, 52–54, 61–62, 112, 125, 130–31, 190–91, 199, 202, 205, 209–11, 225, 233
Privatization of public hospitals, 107–08

Production, 6, 8–9, 69–70, 83–84, 120–24, 127, 133, 143–47, 155, 159–62, 197
Professional education, 21–22, 97, 105
Professional Standards Review Organizations, 191–93
Professionals, 6–7, 31, 119, 173–74, 176, 178, 181–82, 187–88, 191–93, 196–97, 202, 205; dominance, 123, 182, 185, 187, 192, 196–97
Profits, 5–16, 77–96, 166, 171, 190, 193–94, 196–97, 203, 204, 206–7; declining rate of, 29; and safety, 5, 7–16, 54, 55–60, 70, 197, 206
Public health service, 63, 69
Public Health Service, U.S., 80, 91
Public hospitals, 44–45, 104–9, 116, 201–2; closure of, 107–8, 202; privatization of, 107–8
Public medical contraction, 104–9, 201
Public-private contradiction, 29–30, 43–45, 52–53, 98, 109, 113–14, 167–68, 175–76, 178, 181, 185–87, 196, 203
Public subsidization of private medicine, 98, 104, 119, 168–69, 203–4

Quality of medical care, 191–93

Racial minorities, 4, 16, 64, 97–98, 106–7, 110–11, 116–17, 195, 199, 202, 206
Racism, 16, 64, 97–98, 110–11, 116, 180, 202, 206
Random controlled trial, 27, 78–79
Reductionism, 48,
Referral networks, 197–98
Reform, 3–36, 43, 52–53, 64–69, 71–73, 97, 115–17, 161–62, 165–66, 175–85, 187–88, 189–97, 201–2, 204–5, 206–7; contradictions of, 35–36, 52–53, 64–69; nonreformist, 35–36, 52–53, 97, 115–17, 161–62, 165–66, 175–76, 179, 187–88, 189–97, 201–2, 204–5, 206–7; reformist, 35–36, 52–53, 165–66, 175–76, 187–88, 189–97
Reformist reforms, 35–36, 52–53, 165–66, 175–76, 187–88, 189–97
Regional Medical Programs, 22
Repressive state apparatuses, 121–22
Reproductions of relations of production, 121–23, 125, 133, 143–47, 160
Revolution, 160–63, 166–67, 170–74, 179–80, 185, 187–88, 193, 205–6

Rhythm, heart, 78–79, 136–49
Rockefeller, David, 86
Ruge, Arnold, 60–61

Safety and profit, 6, 8–16, 54, 55–60, 70, 197, 206
Scientific ideology, 27–28, 48–49, 122–23
Scitovsky, A. A., 89
Selection, negative and positive, 47, 92
Self sufficiency, financial, 113–15
SERMENA, national health insurance in Chile, 167–68,
Servicio Nacional de Salud (National Health Service), Chile, 167–69, 175–79, 186
Servicio Único (Unified Health Service), Chile, 169
Sexism, 54, 110, 143, 205
Sick role, 123
Social change, 27, 35–36, 60, 62, 64, 68–69, 115–17, 147–49, 159–62, 165–207
Social class, 5, 26–27, 31, 39–42, 48, 50–51, 53, 56–60, 70–73, 120–23, 125, 168, 171, 173–74, 181, 285–88, 201–2, 205; mortality rates and, 57, 62
Social contradiction, 3–36, 52–53, 55–56, 62, 64, 68–73, 77, 83–84, 97–98, 109, 113–14, 119–20, 125, 159–61, 165–69, 176, 178–79, 185–87, 196–97, 199–201, 203–7
Social control, 34–35, 48–49, 119–62, 200, 204
Social medicine, 55, 60, 64, 73, 97–116, 119
Social origins of illness, 55–73, 175, 200–202, 206–27
Socialism, 5–6, 8–9, 16, 24, 34–35, 51–52, 72–73, 95–96, 160–61, 166–67, 173, 205, 185–87, 193–200, 206–7; transition to, 51–52, 72–73, 195
Soviet Union, 9, 35, 49–51, 160, 195
Specialists, 197–98
Stalinist period in Soviet Union, 34
Stanford University Medical Center, 89–90
State, 29–30, 43–47, 63, 95, 102, 119–23, 170, 172, 175, 180–87, 204; and coronary care, 92–93; definition, 43; general functions within health system, 45–46; ideological state apparatuses, 120–21; limits and mechanisms of state intervention, 46–47; power of, 170, 172, 175, 180–87; private-public contradiction, 43–47; repressive state apparatuses, 120–21
Strategy, political, 35–36, 71–73, 95, 116–17, 149, 165–207

Stratification of workers in health-care institutions, 41, 202
Stress, 28, 53, 147–49
Sweden, 53

Taxes, 104, 190–91, 194, 195, 203
Technologic progress and humanistic decline, 32–35
Technology, 4, 6–7, 21, 27–29, 32–35, 48–49, 77–96, 97–98, 110, 119, 123, 184, 204–5, 207
Torture, 205
Transition to socialism, 51–52, 166
Tuberculosis, 65–66

Underdevelopment, 5, 20–24, 50–52, 55, 65–73, 166, 169–71, 174, 178, 184–85, 195–96, 205–6
Undocumented clients, 113–15
Unemployment, 127–29, 147
Uneven development, 20–24, 27, 97–98, 113, 176, 194, 197, 203, 205
Unidad Popular government in Chile, 166–88
Unified health service *(Servicio Único),* Chile, 169
Unions, 10, 13–14, 19, 116–17, 179–81, 202, 205–6
United Farm Workers Union, 13–14, 19, 116–17
USSR, 9, 35, 49–51, 160, 195

Valenzuela Feijoo, J., 171
Vermont, 12
Vermont Asbestos Company, 12
Virchow, Rudolph, 37–39, 53, 55–73

Warner-Lambert Pharmaceutical Company, 83–93
White, Paul Dudley, 90
Women's movement, 110–13, 204–6
Work, health defined by, 123–24, 128–29
Worker-community control and coalitions, 115–17, 176–79, 187–88, 200, 202, 207
Working class, 5, 41–42, 56–60, 62–63, 64–69, 100–101
Workmen's compensation, 10

Yong Lords Party, 110

Ziem, Grace, 41–42
Zola, I. K., 123

About the Author

Howard Waitzkin is professor and director at the Division of Community Medicine, Department of Family and Community Medicine, University of New Mexico. Since receiving his doctorate in sociology and a degree in medicine from Harvard University, he has worked with several community-based health projects and has written numerous articles and books on health policy, community medicine, and patient-doctor communication, including *The Politics of Medical Encounters: How Patients and Doctors Deal with Social Problems* and *The Exploitation of Illness in Capitalist Society.*

8 29 2